HUMAN PARTURITION

BOERHAAVE SERIES FOR POSTGRADUATE MEDICAL EDUCATION
Vol. 15

PROCEEDINGS OF BOERHAAVE COURSES
ORGANIZED BY
THE FACULTY OF MEDICINE, UNIVERSITY OF LEIDEN,
THE NETHERLANDS

HUMAN PARTURITION

New concepts and developments

edited by

MARC J.N.C. KEIRSE M.D., D.Phil.
Leiden University Medical Centre

ANNE B.M. ANDERSON M.D., Ph.D.
University of Oxford

JACK BENNEBROEK GRAVENHORST M.D.
Leiden University Medical Centre

1979
LEIDEN UNIVERSITY PRESS

The distribution of this book is handled by the following team of publishers:

for the United States and Canada

Kluwer Boston, Inc.
160 Old Derby Street
Hingham, MA 02043
USA

for all other countries

Kluwer Academic Publishers Group
Distribution Center
P.O. Box 322
3300 AH Dordrecht
The Netherlands

Library of Congress Cataloging in Publication Data CIP

Main entry under title:

Human parturition.

(Boerhaave series for postgraduate medical education; v. 15)
Includes index.
1. Labor (Obstetrics) – Regulation. 2. Labor, Induced (Obstetrics) 3. Labor, Premature–Prevention. I. Keirse, Marc J.N.C. II. Anderson, Anne B.M. III. Bennebroek Gravenhorst, Jacob, 1931- IV. Series.
RG655.H85 618.4 79-17279

ISBN-13: 978-94-009-9588-8 e-ISBN-13: 978-94-009-9586-4
DOI: 10.1007/978-94-009-9586-4

Cover design: Paul Burg

PREFACE

In recent years there has been an impressive surge of interest in the mechanisms which control the onset and the maintenance of labour. Much of it stems from a constant awareness that gestational age at birth is still an important factor in neonatal mortality and morbidity. Advances in the sensitivity and specificity of immunoassay, the discovery of the prostaglandins, new skills in fetal surgery and chronic catheterisation in experimental animals have greatly stimulated further research in this area. In the meantime clinicians became continuously more aware that, despite considerable advances in perinatal medicine, gestational age at birth remains the major determinant of neonatal mortality and morbidity. It led them to seek new and better ways of controlling uterine function whether by influencing cervical ripeness, by stimulating or by inhibiting myometrial contractility.

This volume uniquely combines knowledge which has been gained from both experimental and clinical research on parturition. A brief outline of current evidence on the control of parturition in experimental animals may be fruitful in delineating problems and hypotheses for further study in human pregnancy. Much of our present day knowledge of human parturition has been gained by checking such data against experimental findings, careful measurements and clinical observations in human pregnancy.

It is hoped that the interdisciplinary nature of this volume will enhance the understanding of human parturition and stimulate further research in this area.

Thanks are due to Miss H. Wittenberg and Mrs M. Hogeweg for their assistance in the editing of this book.

February 1979

M.J.N.C. KEIRSE
A.B.M. ANDERSON
J. BENNEBROEK GRAVENHORST

CONTENTS

CONTRIBUTORS

Anne B.M. Anderson, M.D., Ph.D., Nuffield Department of Obstetrics and Gynaecology, University of Oxford, John Radcliffe Hospital, Oxford, OX3 9DU, England.

Jack Bennebroek Gravenhorst, M.D., Department of Obstetrics and Gynaecology, University of Leiden Medical Centre, Rijnsburgerweg 10, Leiden, The Netherlands.

Jaap Th.F. Boeles, M.D., Department of Physiology, University of Amsterdam, Jan Swammerdam Institute, Eerste Constantijn Huygensstraat 20, Amsterdam, The Netherlands.

Kees Boer, M.D., Netherlands Institute for Brain Research, IJdijk 28, Amsterdam, The Netherlands.

Andrew A. Calder, M.D., M.R.C.O.G., University Department of Obstetrics and Gynaecology, Royal Maternity Hospital, Rottenrow, Glasgow G4 ONA, Scotland.

John R.G. Challis, Ph.D., Departments of Obstetrics and Gynecology and Physiology, University of Western Ontario, University Hospital, London, Ontario, Canada.

Tom K.A.B. Eskes, M.D., Department of Obstetrics and Gynaecology, University of Nijmegen, St. Radboudziekenhuis, Geert Grooteplein Zuid 14, Nijmegen, The Netherlands.

Gerard G.M. Essed, M.D., Department of Obstetrics and Gynaecology, University of Nijmegen, St. Radboudziekenhuis, Geert Grooteplein Zuid 14, Nijmegen, The Netherlands.

Anthony P.F. 'Flint, Ph.D., Agricultural Research Council, Institute of Animal Physiology, Babraham Cambridge CB2 4AT, England.

Marc J.N.C. Keirse, M.D., D.Phil., Department of Obstetrics and Gynaecology, University of Leiden Medical Centre, Rijnsburgerweg 10, Leiden, The Netherlands.

Gerrit Jan Kloosterman, M.D., F.R.C.O.G., F.A.C.O.G., Department of Obstetrics and Gynaecology, University of Amsterdam, Wilhelmina Gasthuis, Eerste Helmersstraat 104, Amsterdam, The Netherlands.

Menno van Leeuwen, M.D., Department of Physiology, University of

Amsterdam, Jan Swammerdam Institute, Eerste Constantijn Huygensstraat 20, Amsterdam, The Netherlands.

Murray D. Mitchell, M.A., D.Phil., Nuffield Department of Obstetrics and Gynaecology, University of Oxford, John Radcliffe Hospital, Oxford, OX3 9DU, England.

Peter W. Nathanielsz, Ph.D., M.B., B.Chir., Department of Obstetrics, LA County Harbor – UCLA Medical Center, 1000 West Carson Street, Torrance, California 90509, U.S.A.

Robert E. Oakey, D.Sc., Ph.D., F.R.I.C., M.R.C. Path., Division of Steroid Endocrinology Department of Chemical Pathology, School of Medicine, University of Leeds, Leeds LS2 9LN, England.

Jeffrey S. Robinson, B.Sc., M.B., M.R.C.O.G., Nuffield Department of Obstetrics and Gynaecology, University of Oxford, John Radcliffe Hospital, Oxford OX3 9DU, England.

Dick F. Swaab, M.D., Netherlands Institute for Brain Research, IJdijk 28, Amsterdam, The Netherlands.

Michel Thiery, M.D., Ph.D., Department of Obstetrics, University of Gent, De Pintelaan 135, B-9000 Gent, Belgium.

Alexander C. Turnbull, M.A., M.D., F.R.C.O.G., Nuffield Department of Obstetrics and Gynaecology, University of Oxford, John Radcliffe Hospital, Oxford OX3 9DU, England.

Nils Wiqvist, M.D., Department of Obstetrics and Gynaecology, University of Göteborg, Sahlgrenska Sjukhuset, S-41345 Göteborg, Sweden.

George M.J.A. Wolfs, M.D., Department of Obstetrics and Gynaecology, Zeeweg Ziekenhuis, Velsen, The Netherlands.

PARTURITION IN SMALL MAMMALS

JOHN R.G. CHALLIS AND PETER W. NATHANIELSZ

Prior to 1965 the small laboratory rodent was the experimental model most commonly used in the investigation of the mechanisms of parturition. Sensitive assay methodology and techniques to monitor biophysical variables in the absence of the effects of anesthesia have to a large extent overcome the problems of size. From the outset it should be appreciated that rodent species demonstrate a wide variety of reproductive patterns and extrapolation of data to humans must be undertaken with caution. Of particular importance is the duration of the dependence of pregnancy on the corpus luteum, the wide variation in the number of fetuses in the litter, and the differences in the maturity of the fetuses at term.

Several recent reviews (1-5) have discussed the control of parturition in small mammals in great detail. The object of the present article is to outline the general principles of parturition as they relate to these species, and to examine the applicability, where appropriate, of these observations to man.

ROLE OF THE FETUS

In the rabbit, ovarian progesterone production is essential for the maintenance of pregnancy, and the factors which lead to the onset of labor are those which participate in regression of the corpus luteum. In contrast, with progressively greater dependence on progesterone production by the placenta as in the rat and guinea-pig, the possibility of local control mechanisms becomes more important. In polytocous animals any local mechanism must provide inherent synchrony between fetuses in order that non-viable littermates are not expelled as a result of premature myometrial activity elsewhere in the uterus. Thus, it seems unlikely that parturition could be triggered by a single fetus, but more likely by at least a "majority decision". In general, we have only scanty information pertaining to the size of the majority.

Fetal decapitation in the rabbit resulted in substantial variation in the date of delivery, although the mean length of pregnancy was unaltered (6). Progressive maturation of fetal pituitary-adrenal function is demonstrable

M.J.N.C. Keirse et al. (eds.), Human Parturition, 1-10.

after day 23-24 (7), although present information links these events more closely with the stimulus to organ maturation in the fetus than with the trigger to birth. In the guinea-pig fetal hypophysectomy led to fetal adrenal atrophy whilst injection of ACTH into the fetus led to fetal adrenal hypertrophy and a shortening of gestation length if all the fetuses were treated (8). Premature parturition did not ensue if a proportion of the fetuses was left uninjected.

The role of the fetal rat in the initiation of parturition is less clear. Fetectomy (9), or fetal brain aspiration (10) was without effect on gestation length, although the course of labor was protracted. The latter effect was attributed to the absence of arginine vasotocin-like material, normally present in the fetal pituitary at a higher concentration that either oxytocin or vasopressin (11). Maturation of fetal pituitary-adrenal function occurs during late pregnancy and is associated with a rise in fetal pituitary ACTH, and in fetal adrenal and plasma corticosterone concentrations (4). However, there is little evidence to suggest that maturation of this axis is critical as a trigger to the onset of parturition. While the fetus may still have a role in the timing of the onset of labor, that role is a relatively minor one, and of greater significance in relation to the duration of labor itself. In this respect the similarities between the rat and human are striking (11; Swaab and Boer, this volume).

PROGESTERONE

The regulation of plasma progesterone levels in these small mammals has been elegantly reviewed elsewhere (5). In the rabbit, ovarian progesterone production continues throughout gestation and is necessary for pregnancy maintenance. The function of the corpus luteum depends to a considerable extent on the luteotrophic action of estrogen which is primarily of ovarian origin. Thus, the corpus luteum regresses after estrogen withdrawal either in an animal which has become dependent on exogenous estrogen for maintenance of the corpus luteum, or after follicle irradiation, or after administration of an anti-estrogen (4, 5). Exogenous prostaglandin also causes regression of the corpus luteum. In late pregnancy there is an increase in prostaglandin production which probably alters the regulatory balance between luteotrophic and luteolytic control of the corpus luteum and leads to its demise.

Progesterone production in the rat is also predominantly ovarian in origin but is supplemented by a placental contribution in late gestation, such that by day 18 of pregnancy ovariectomy can be performed with less than 10 per cent abortions (12). In early pregnancy the corpus luteum depends upon pituitary luteotrophic support; in the second half of gestation trophic support is provided from the trophoblastic tissue (5). Plasma progesterone levels decrease before parturition, in large part due to a decline in ovarian progesterone secretion. Regression of the corpus luteum occurs simultaneously with an increase in the activity of the ovarian enzyme 20α-hydroxysteroid dehydrogenase, and leads to the formation of a biological inactive metabolite of progesterone, 20α-dihydroprogesterone (5, 13). It has been suggested that the rise in enzyme activity occurs in response to $PGF_{2\alpha}$(13), the production of which increases in late pregnancy.

The placenta of the guinea-pig actively synthesizes progesterone, and ovariectomy during the second half of pregnancy does not lead to abortion (14). In this species the plasma progesterone concentration rises to values in excess of 200-300 ng/ml after day 18-20 of pregnancy (0.3 gestation length). This is due to a fall in the progesterone metabolic clearance rate resulting from the appearance of a specific high affinity binding protein for progesterone in plasma (15). The animal has therefore developed a mechanism for maintaining a "reservoir" of progesterone in its plasma. However, the inability of exogenous progesterone to prolong pregnancy, the failure of exogenous progesterone, administered by every conceivable route, to suppress myometrial contractility in non-pregnant guinea-pigs (16), and the lack of decline in peripheral progesterone levels pre-partum (15) makes the purpose of this reservoir unclear.

A voluminous debate has arisen in the literature regarding the significance of changes in plasma progesterone concentration in the control of late pregnancy and the initiation of parturition. The importance of withdrawal of the progesterone block (17) which has often been interpreted as a decline in plasma progesterone levels is of varying significance in different species. Recent advances in steroid receptor technology have indicated that for some species such debate may be of little more than academic interest. In the rat, Davies and Ryan (18) showed that the fall in concentration of progesterone in uterine tissue during late pregnancy (19) was preceded by a decrease in the progesterone receptor capacity of myometrial cytosol. They pointed out that a decline in the ability of the target tissue to bind a steroid is an effective way of modulating the activity of that steroid. If such a change in progesterone binding occurs in human myometrium it would help resolve the apparent anomaly that most workers have failed to demonstrate significant changes in plasma progesterone concentrations pre-partum. Nuclear and cytosol receptor measurements on myometrium obtained at elective cesarean section from patients not in labor and compared with determinations on patients in active labor would be of great interest in this respect.

ESTROGENS

In the rabbit and guinea-pig the major circulating estrogen of pregnancy is not known, although neither estradiol nor "total unconjugated estrogens" respectively appear to change significantly in peripheral blood before parturition (1). Exogenous estradiol or diethylstilbestrol prolonged pregnancy in the guinea-pig (21), possibly through an effect on relaxin or relaxin receptors, and in apparent contradistinction to the effect of estrogen in most other animal species.

In the rat, parturition is preceded by an increase in ovarian estrone and estradiol secretion (22). Ovariectomy in late pregnancy does not result in parturition or abortion, unless exogenous estradiol is given (23). The effect of estrogen appears to be mediated by prostaglandins because the frequency of estrogen-induced deliveries in ovariectomized animals can be reduced by the simultaneous administration of naproxen, a prostaglandin synthetase inhibitor (24).

The potential importance of uterine estrogen receptors and enzyme activities, and the paucity of relevant information must again be stressed. In the rabbit, for example, the lack of change in plasma estradiol concentrations (perhaps related to the luteotrophic action of the steroid) is associated with a significant rise in the concentration of estradiol and in the ratio of estradiol: estrone in the myometrium (20). It is known (25) that the activity of 17 β hydroxysteroid oxidoreductase increases in late pregnancy, favoring estradiol-17 β formation from estrone. It seems likely that the rise in tissue estrogen levels involves changes in receptor capacity. Recently an increase in both cytosol and nuclear estradiol receptor capacity was demonstrated in rat myometrium (26).

PROSTAGLANDINS

An increase in prostaglandin production appears to be a common event in the final pathway of the parturient mechanism in most species. The prostaglandin effect may be two-fold; a luteolytic action on the corpus luteum of pregnancy and a myometrial stimulatory action on the uterus. In both the rat and rabbit, exogenous $PGF_{2\alpha}$ stimulates myometrial contractility, but the oxytocic effect is preceded by luteal regression, and a fall in circulating progesterone levels (27, 28). Pregnancy can be prolonged in both these species by administration of prostaglandin synthetase inhibitors, or by antibodies to $PGF_{2\alpha}$ (29, 30, 31), providing evidence for a role of endogenous prostaglandins. It is of note that following administration of indomethacin, plasma progesterone levels decreased at the expected time, although parturition was delayed. This suggests that the major site of the inhibitor's action was on myometrial prostaglandin synthesis, and that withdrawal of luteotrophic support, either alone or in conjunction with low prostaglandin levels, is sufficient to induce demise of the corpus luteum. In both the rabbit and rat there is an increase in uterine prostaglandin production in late pregnancy, coincident with the fall in plasma progesterone levels, and the increase in myometrial contractility (1, 2). In all the above respects; viz, increase in endogenous prostaglandin production, prolongation of pregnancy by prostaglandin synthetase inhibitors, and the oxytocic action of exogenous prostaglandins, similar information is available for human beings as for the rat and rabbit.

The control of prostaglandin production is multifactorial, and may depend on estrogen, progesterone, oxytocin and uterine stretch. The interaction of these factors is best demonstrated in the rat. Csapo (23, 24) showed that ovariectomy on day 17 did not induce abortion in that proportion of animals which had accomplished an adequate luteo-placental shift in progesterone production. Administration of naproxen further reduced the incidence of abortion, indicating that progesterone withdrawal *per se* allowed an increase in prostaglandin biosynthesis and was a major regulatory influence. In addition, Csapo showed that whilst exogenous estradiol increased the incidence of premature delivery, this effect was also blocked by naproxen, showing the stimulatory effect of estrogen on prostaglandin biosynthesis. The action of the steroids could be exerted either directly on prostaglandin synthetase, or on the metabolic pathways. Flower (32) has shown that the activity of 15-hydroxy-prostaglandin dehydrogenase (PGDH) in uterus and lung is high during pregnancy, but decreased dramatically between days 21-23. Thus, low levels of PGF can be maintained for most of pregnancy as a result of a high rate of metabolism; the fall in PGDH activity near term allows higher tissue and plasma levels of PGF to be achieved. PGDH activity appears to be influenced by steroid hormones. Exogenous progesterone increased, while exogenous estradiol decreased PGDH (32), allowing one to speculate that a further function of progesterone in pregnancy is to maintain high levels of the enzyme and thereby ensure low tissue PGF concentrations. Similar findings have recently been made in the rabbit by Powell (33).

Williams et al. (34) demonstrated that rat uterine homogenates, incubated with an excess of arachidonic acid progressively synthesized more PGF with advancing pregnancy. Thus, a rise in prostaglandin synthetase may also be important; maximum activity was measured on day 21-22, just prior to parturition.

PGF release by the uterus *in vitro* increases with tissue taken later in pregnancy, and correlates with the amount of spontaneous contractility that is developed (35). The endometrium appears to be a more important site of production than myometrium. *In vitro* both spontaneous and oxytocin-induced contractility of the uterus from non-pregnant animals can be blocked with indomethacin, although indomethacin treatment has no effect on prostaglandin-induced contractility. During indomethacin treatment, prostaglandin release was suppressed, and these experiments have been interpreted as indicating that oxytocin may act on the myometrium in part by increasing prostaglandin biosynthesis (35).

Previous studies have been interpreted in terms of the primary prostaglandins. The demonstration that the rat uterus contains high levels of 6-keto-$PGF_{1\alpha}$ during pregnancy (36) suggests the need to re-evaluate earlier experiments in relation to other pathways of arachidonic acid metabolism.

OXYTOCIN

During pregnancy in the rat and rabbit the spontaneous and oxytocin-induced contractility of the uterus increases (37). The change in oxytocin sensitivity has been attributed to progesterone withdrawal. A further influence on oxytocin sensitivity was suggested by the studies of Soloff (38). He showed that oxytocin binding sites were present in the uterus of the ovariectomized rat, and their capacity and affinity were increased within 12 h of estrogen administration. Thus, the enhanced sensitivity of the rat uterus to oxytocin following estrogen treatment, or at term when estrogen levels are elevated, may result from an increase in the affinity and number of oxytocin receptors in the uterus. Competition for oxytocin binding was exhibited by oxytocin and its analogues, but not by prostaglandins, confirming the separate nature of the prostaglandin and oxytocin receptor systems (39).

RELAXIN

In an elegant series of cross-circulation experiments, Porter (40, 41) has demonstrated the presence of a further myometrial inhibitory factor in the blood of pregnant guinea-pigs, rabbits and rats. It has been proposed that this substance may be relaxin. In the post-partum rat, progesterone administered in amounts which achieved concentrations in plasma and uterus similar to the maximum values previously found in pregnant animals, failed to suppress myometrial contractility (42). However, porcine relaxin inhibited uterine activity in the same preparation. Measurements of tissue and plasma relaxin concentrations in small mammals during late gestation are needed to substantiate the role of this/these compound(s).

MATERNAL INFLUENCES

Boer et al. (43) observed an abrupt increase in the incidence of labour in rats at about 12.00 h on day 22, with a second smaller peak on day 23. Lincoln and Porter (44) examined the effect of photoperiod on the timing of birth, and showed that despite shifting the light/dark interval by +8 or −8 h, 82 percent of births continued to occur during the 14 h of light. The relationship of this periodicity in delivery to maternal hormone levels and function of the autonomic nervous system will be of considerable interest.

MYOMETRIAL EFFECTS

The rat uterus has been used extensively in studies to examine the subcellular control of myometrial contractility. Korenman and Krall (45) have shown the central role of adenyl cyclase in this mechanism and have demonstrated changes in cAMP levels in the smooth muscle resultant upon binding to the cell surface by β-adrenergic agents. Treatment with β-agonists results in an increase in protein kinase activity and increased ATP-dependent Ca^{++} transport by cellular membrane preparations. A myometrial membrane fraction has been prepared from the rat uterus which has the ATP-dependent Ca^{++} transport properties consistent with an intracellular compartment able to bind or release Ca^{++} and respectively inhibit or activate contractility. Prostaglandins appear to interact with this system either by directly decreasing the ATP-dependent binding of Ca^{++} to cell membrane fractions, or by restricting the ability of β-agonists to elevate cAMP, and thus maintaining free Ca^{++} levels.

An exciting new development into our understanding of the control of myometrial contractility has recently been made by Garfield et al. (46). These workers have examined by electron microscopy both longitudinal and circular muscle of rat myometrium from pregnant animals before term, at delivery, and post-partum. They observed that gap junctions (low resistance pathways) were only present at the time of delivery or immediately post-partum, and were absent at other times in pregnancy. They suggest that the appearance of these junctions may be necessary for development of the synchronous myometrial activity which leads to delivery of the fetus.

ACKNOWLEDGEMENTS

J.R.G.C. is a Canada MRC Scholar, and gratefully acknowledges support of Canada MRC Grant No. Ma-6070. P.W.N. acknowledges the support of the Wellcome Trust for work referred to in this review.

REFERENCES

1. Thorburn GD, Challis JRG and Robinson JS: Endocrine control of parturition. In: *Biology of the Uterus*, Wynn RM (ed.), New York, Plenum Press, 1977, p. 653-732.
2. Nathanielsz PW: Parturition in rodents. *Seminars in Perinatology* 2, 223-234 (1978).
3. Nathanielsz PW: Endocrine mechanisms of parturition. *Ann Rev Physiol* 40, 411-445 (1978).
4. Thorburn GD and Challis JRG: Endocrine control of parturition. *Physiol Rev* in press (1979).
5. Anderson LL: Uterine control of ovarian function. In: *Biology of the Uterus*, Wynn RM (ed.), New York, Plenum Press, 1977, p. 587-651.
6. Jost A: Does the foetal hypophyseal-adrenal system participate in delivery in rats and in rabbits? In: *Foetal and Neonatal Physiology*, Comline RS, Cross KW, Dawes GS and Nathanielsz PW (eds.), Cambridge, Cambridge University Press, 1973, p. 589-593.
7. Albano JDM, Jack PM, Joseph T, Gould RP, Nathanielsz PW and Brown BL: The development of adrenocorticotrophin-sensitive adenylate cyclase activity in the foetal rabbit adrenal; a correlated biochemical and morphological study. *J Endocrinol* 271, 333-341 (1976).
8. Donovan BT and Peddie MJ: Foetal hypothalamic and pituitary lesions, the adrenal glands and abortion in the guinea pig. In: *Foetal and Neonatal Physiology*, Comline RS, Cross KW, Dawes GS and Nathanielsz PW (eds.), Cambridge, Cambridge University Press, 1973, p. 603-605.
9. Selye H, Collip JB and Thomson KL: Endocrine interrelations during pregnancy. *Endocrinology* 19, 151-159 (1973).
10. Swaab DF and Honnebier WJ: The influence of removal of the fetal rat brain upon intrauterine growth of the fetus and the placenta and on gestation length. *J Obstet Gynaecol Br Commonw* 80, 589-597 (1973).
11. Swaab DF, Boer K and Honnebier WJ: Influence of the fetal hypothalamus and pituitary on the onset and course of parturition. In: *The Fetus and Birth*, Ciba Foundation Symposium no. 47, Amsterdam, Elsevier/Excerpta Medica/North-Holland, 1977, p. 379-393.
12. Csapo A and Wiest W: An examination of the quantitative relationship between progesterone and the maintenance of pregnancy. *Endocrinology* 85, 735-746 (1969).
13. Strauss JF, Sokoloski J, Ocaplo EP, Duffy P, Mintz G and Stambough RC: On the role of prostaglandins in parturition in the rat. *Endocrinology* 96, 1040-1043 (1975).
14. Heap RB and Deanesly R: Progesterone in systemic blood and placentae of intact and ovariectomized pregnant guinea-pigs. *J Endocrinol* 34, 417-423 (1966).

15. Challis JRG, Heap RB and Illingworth DV: Concentrations of oestrogen and progesterone in the plasma of non-pregnant, pregnant and lactating guinea-pigs. *J. Endocrinol* 51, 333-345 (1971).
16. Porter DG: The failure of progesterone to affect myometrial activity in the guinea-pig. *J. Endocrinol* 46, 425-434 (1970).
17. Csapo A: Progesterone block. *Am J Anat* 98, 273-292 (1956).
18. Davies IJ and Ryan KJ: The modulation of progesterone concentration in the myometrium of the pregnant rat by changes in cytoplasmic "receptor" protein activity. *Endocrinology* 92, 394-401 (1973).
19. Wiest WG: Progesterone and 20α-hydroxypregn-4-en-3-one in plasma, ovaries and uteri during pregnancy in the rat. *Endocrinology* 87, 43-48 (1970).
20. Challis JRG, Davies IJ and Ryan KJ: The concentrations of progesterone, estrone and 17 β-estradiol in the myometrium of the pregnant rabbit, and their relationship to the peripheral plasma steroid concentrations. *Endocrinology* 95, 160-164 (1974).
21. Illingworth DV, Challis JRG, Ackland N, Burton AM, Heap RB and Perry JS: Parturition in the guinea-pig, plasma levels of steroid hormones, steroid-binding proteins, and oxytocin, and the effect of corticosteroids, prostaglandins and adenocorticotrophin. *J Endocrinol* 63, 557-570 (1974).
22. Yoshinaga K, Hawkins RA and Stocker JL: Estrogen secretion by the rat ovary *in vivo* during the estrous cycle and pregnancy. *Endocrinology* 85, 103-112 (1969).
23. Csapo AI: The four direct regulatory factors of myometrial function. In: *Progesterone: Its Regulatory Effect on the Myometrium*, Wolstenholme GEW and Knight J (eds.), London, 1969, p. 13-42.
24. Csapo AI, Csapo EF, Faye E, Henzl MR and Salau G: The role of estradiol-17β in the activation of the uterus during premature labor and the effect of Naproxen an inhibitor of prostaglandin synthesis. *Prostaglandins* 3, 839-846 (1973).
25. Jutting G: Action of oestrogen on 17β-OH-Steroid NAD oxido-reductase of rabbit myometrium.. *Geburtsh Frauenheilk* 26, 636-639 (1966).
26. Soloff MS: Does increased oxytocin binding in the rat uterus trigger parturition? Endocrinol Soc Miami Beach (Abstr No. 497), 1978.
27. Buckle JW and Nathanielsz PW: Effect of low doses of $PGF_{2\alpha}$ infused into the aorta of unrestrained pregnant rats: observations on induction of parturition and effect on plasma progesterone concentration. *Prostaglandins* 4, 443-458 (1973).
28. Challis JRG, Porter DG and Ryan KJ: The effects of prostaglandin $F_{2\alpha}$ and ovariectomy on the peripheral plasma steroid concentrations and the evolution of uterine activity in the pregnant rabbit. *Endocrinology* 95, 547-553 (1974).
29. Aiken JW: Aspirin and indomethacin prolong parturition in rats: evidence that prostaglandins contribute to expulsion of foetus. *Nature (Lond)* 240, 21-25 (1972).
30. Chester R, Dukes M, Slater SR and Walpole AL: Delay of parturition in the rat by anti-inflammatory agents which inhibit the biosynthesis of PG's. *Nature (Lond)* 240, 37-38 (1972).
31. Challis JRG, Davies IJ and Ryan KJ: The effects of dexamethasone and indomethacin on the outcome of pregnancy in the rabbit. *J. Endocrinol* 64, 363-370 (1975).
32. Flower RJ: The role of prostaglandins in parturition with special reference to the rat. In: *The Fetus and Birth*, Ciba Foundation Symposium no. 47, Amsterdam, Elsevier/Excerpta Medica/North-Holland, 1977, p. 297-321.
33. Powell WS: Changes in the ω-hydroxylation of prostaglandins induced by pregnancy, pseudopregnancy and progesterone treatment. Endocrinol Soc Miami Beach (Abstr No 378), 1978.
34. Williams KI, Sneddon JM and Harney PJ: Prostaglandin production by the pregnant rat uterus in vitro and its relevance to parturition. *Pol J Pharmacol Pharm* 26, 207-215 (1974).
35. Williams KI and Vane JR: Inhibition of uterine motility: the possible role of prostaglandins and aspirin-like drugs. *Pharmacol Therap Bull* 89-113 (1975).

36. Kennedy TG and Zemecnik J: The concentration of 6-keto-prostaglandin $F_{1\alpha}$ (6-keto-$PGF_{1\alpha}$) is markedly elevated at the site of blastocyst implantation in the rat. Can Invest Reprod Winnipeg (Abstr 25), 1978.
37. Fuchs AR: Parturition in rabbits and rats. *Mem Soc Endocrinol* 20, 163-186 (1973).
38. Soloff MS: Uterine receptor for oxytocin: effects of estrogen. *Biochem Biophys Res Commun* 65, 205-212 (1975).
39. Soloff MS, Swartz T, Morrison M and Saffran M: Oxytocin receptors: oxytocin analogs but not prostaglandins compete with ^{3}H-oxytocin for uptake by rat uterus. *Endocrinology* 92, 104-107 (1973).
40. Porter DG: Myometrium of the pregnant guinea-pig: the probable importance of relaxin. *Biol Reprod* 7, 458-464 (1972).
41. Porter DG: Myometrial regulation in the pregnant rabbit. Evidence for a "new" hormone. *Biol Reprod* 10, 54-61 (1974).
42. Porter DG and Challis JRG: Failure of high uterine concentrations of progesterone to inhibit myometrial activity in the *post partum* rat *in vivo*. *J Reprod Fertil* 39, 157-162 (1974).
43. Boer K, Lincoln DW and Swaab DF: Effects of electrical stimulation of the neurohypophysis on labour in the rat. *J Endocrinol* 65, 163-176 (1975).
44. Lincoln DW and Porter DG: Timing of the photoperiod and the hour of birth in rats. *Nature* 260, 780-781 (1976).
45. Korenman SG and Krall JF: The role of cyclic AMP in the regulation of smooth muscle cell contraction in the uterus. *Biol Reprod* 16, 1-17 (1977).
46. Buckle JW and Nathanielsz PW: Modification of myometrial activity in vivo by administration of cyclic nucleotides and theophylline to the pregnant rat. *J Endocrinol* 66, 339-347 (1975).
47. Garfield RE, Sims S and Daniel EF: Gap junctions: their presence and necessity in myometrium during parturition. *Science* 198, 958-960 (1977).

PARTURITION IN SHEEP

MURRAY D. MITCHELL

The mechanism of parturition in sheep is probably better documented than in most other animal species. An outline of the compounds involved and concepts on their interactions in ovine parturition may be useful to compare and contrast with data in other species. In this chapter attention will be devoted to three major aspects of ovine parturition: activation of the fetal pituitary-adrenal axis, steroid hormones and finally, oxytocin and prostaglandins.

ACTIVATION OF THE FETAL PITUITARY-ADRENAL AXIS

Presumptive evidence for activation of the fetal pituitary-adrenal axis as a major determinant in the onset of labour in sheep came from the field observations of Binns (1) and Basson (2). They observed a natural prolongation of pregnancy in ewes ingesting teratogens that led to abnormalities of the fetal pituitary and hypothalamus and were associated with adrenal regression. It should be noted that these fetuses continued to grow past term *in utero* implying that in sheep fetal stretching of the uterus *per se* does not precipitate labour.

Experimental evidence for the participation of the fetal pituitary in the onset of labour came from the classical experiments of Liggins and co-workers (3). By surgical ablation of the fetal pituitary they were able to prolong pregnancy by several weeks, finally delivering fetuses by Caesarean section. These findings have been confirmed by two further independent studies (4,5) although the results of fetal decapitation (6) are at some variance with those of fetal hypophysectomy. The role of the fetal hypothalamus remains uncertain. Section of the stalk of the fetal pituitary before 116 days of pregnancy resulted in prolongation of gestation whereas the same procedure performed on or after this day resulted in premature delivery (7). In lambs delivered prematurely, by this procedure, adrenal weights were similar to those of lambs born at term, suggesting stimulation of precocious maturation. Stalk section did not interrupt fetal growth, even past term, in contrast

M.J.N.C. Keirse et al. (eds.), Human Parturition, 11-23.

to the growth retardation which is associated with hypophysectomy (8).

Bilateral fetal adrenalectomy causes prolongation of pregnancy by at least ten days (9. 10). Thus the presence of the fetal adrenal glands must be regarded as a necessity for the onset of labour. Further studies (11) have shown that it is cortical rather than medullary tissue that is required for the spontaneous onset of parturition at term.

Having firmly established a role for the fetal pituitary-adrenal axis in the onset of labour, historically the next step was to attempt premature activation of this axis and hence provide evidence for possible endogenous mediators of the event. Intrafetal administration of synthetic adrenocorticotrophin ($ACTH_{1-24}$) or cortisol successfully induced premature delivery at all times studied after 88 days of gestation (12). In the same study administration of other pituitary hormones such as somatotropin, thyrotropin, prolactin, follitropin and lutropin did not induce labour. When birth is induced by ACTH fetal adrenal weights are comparable with those of lambs born at term. The use of synthetic analogues of both ACTH and cortisol to induce labour is now common amongst research workers in this area.

Further evidence of activation of the fetal pituitary-adrenal axis prior to parturition has come from hormone measurements in fetal plasma. In particular the sharp increase in the concentration of cortisol during the 7-10 days before delivery (13, 14; fig. 1) is regarded as the earliest well-defined event which may be called 'the trigger for parturition'. The increase in the plasma concentration is due primarily to an increase in the rate of production by the fetus (7, 15, 16) although levels of corticosteroid binding globulin are also raised (17). Levels of the pituitary hormone ACTH have recently been shown to rise close to parturition (18, 19) which is consistent with an activation of the fetal pituitary-adrenal axis. But it should be emphasized that the levels of ACTH in fetal plasma rise at the same time as but not before the levels of cortisol (fig. 1). Hence a simple explanation that rising levels of ACTH are responsible for the increased fetal secretion of cortisol is not tenable. The necessity of this increased secretion of cortisol for normal parturition to occur has been underlined by recent results demonstrating that there is no rise in fetal plasma concentrations of cortisol after fetal hypophysectomy which leads to prolonged pregnancy (20). These data also emphasize the need for trophic support from the pituitary as a prerequisite for enhanced cortisol secretion and parturition.

The question naturally arises; what is the mechanism controlling the fetal cortisol surge at term? The answer remains controversial. It is possible that the large increase in adrenal cortical mass (21) may account for this phenomenon, but it may also be effect rather than cause. Although changes in the

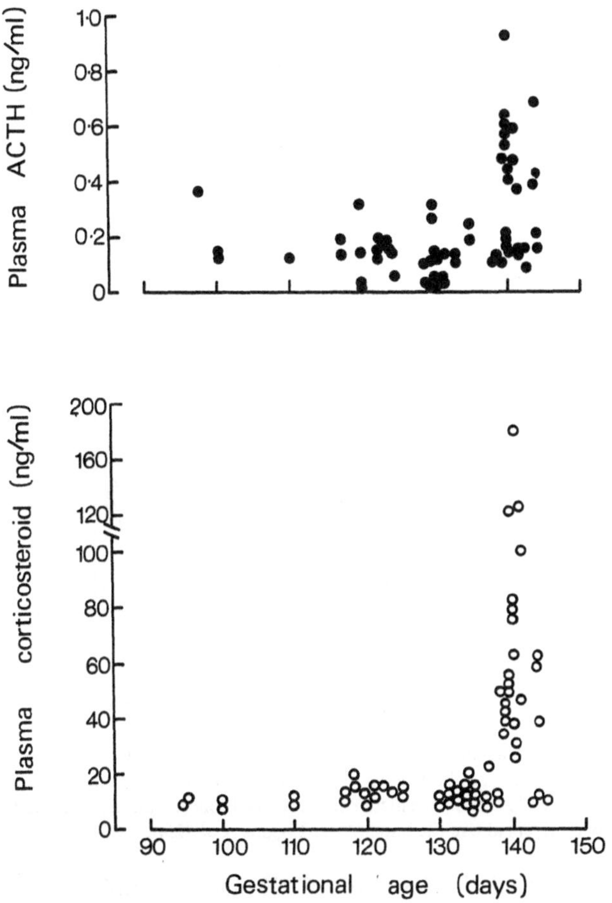

Fig. 1. Plasma corticosteroid (○) and ACTH (●) concentrations in 26 chronically catheterized fetal sheep during late pregnancy (After Jones *et al.* [19]).

activities of enzymes involved in the biosynthesis of cortisol e.g. steriod 11β and 17α hydroxylase, would seem an attractive mechanism, the available data do not support such an hypothesis. It has been shown that fetal adrenals obtained at mid-pregnancy respond well *in vitro* to ACTH (22). Further hypotheses have been put forward (23) suggesting tonic inhibition of fetal adrenal activity during pregnancy and its withdrawal before parturition or alterations in adrenal corticotropin receptor concentration. Both ideas remain to be tested experimentally. It is certain that the fetal adrenal becomes increasingly sensitive to ACTH stimulation near term (24, 25; fig. 2)

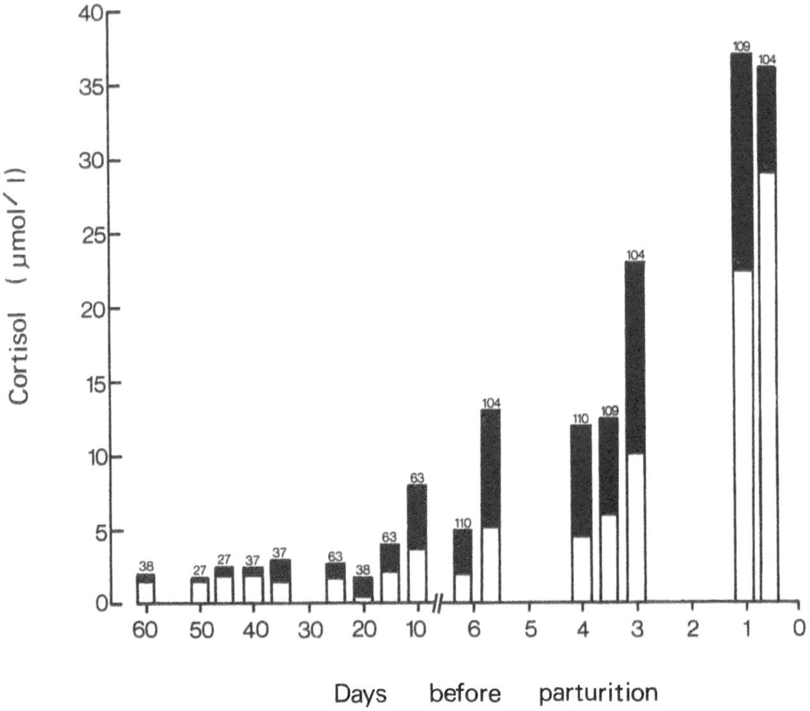

Fig. 2. Reponse to an intravenous fetal infusion of Synacthen ($ACTH_{1\text{-}24}$), 10 μg/min for 1 h at various stages of pregnancy. Solid bars show the fetal carotid plasma concentration of cortisol before Synacthen; open bars show the increment in cortisol concentration at 1 h. Individual sheep are identified by numbers above the bars. (After Liggins *et al.* [25]).

and hence basal circulating levels of ACTH may be a sufficient stimulus for the increase in cortisol secretion at that time. The factors involved in this heightened response to ACTH are at present unclear. As a note of caution, it should be remembered that ACTH is but one of a family of related peptides (Swaab and Boer, this volume) and that, in man, a switching between these related compounds may precede and influence the onset of labour (26). It is possible that another variation on this theme occurs in the sheep.

In summary, it may be concluded that there is an activation of the fetal pituitary-adrenal axis during late pregnancy which results in an enhanced rate of cortisol production and subsequently parturition. At present fetal cortisol may be considered as the trigger for parturition in sheep and its mechanism of action is discussed in the next section. The factors responsible for the increase in fetal cortisol production however, have yet to be fully elucidated and may still reveal an earlier trigger for parturition.

STEROID HORMONES

Progesterone derives almost totally from placenta during late gestation (27) and its rate of production is reflected well by the plasma concentration (28, 29). In general peripheral plasma levels are approximately one-fifth of uterine venous levels. Following the increase in fetal cortisol secretion, maternal plasma progesterone concentrations start to decline, somewhat variably, reaching low levels on the day of delivery (29, 30, 31). Similar qualitative changes occur if labour is induced by intrafetal glucocorticoid treatment (32, 33, 34; fig. 3). Delivery at term and following glucocorticoid administration is

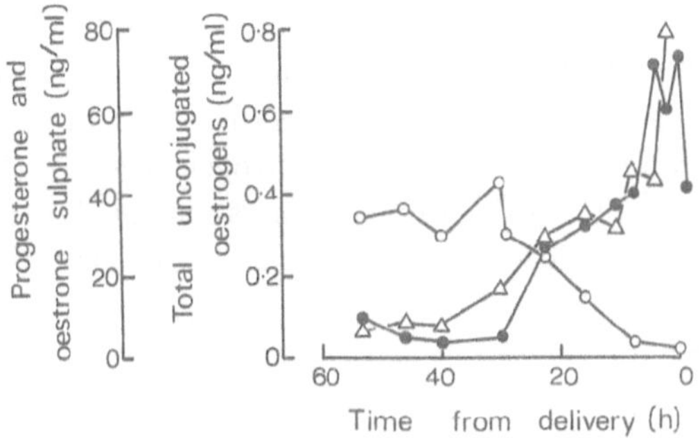

Fig. 3. Utero-ovarian venous plasma concentrations of progesterone (○), oestrone sulphate (●) and total unconjugated oestrogens (△) during delivery of an intact lamb (After Flint *et al.* [41]).

not delayed by treatment with progesterone in doses which are sufficient to maintain levels consistent with late pregnancy in plasma and myometrium (32, 35). If pharmacological doses of progesterone are administered, however, labour may be completely inhibited (32, 35).

The major oestrogens in maternal sheep plasma are oestrone, oestradiol-17α and oestradiol-17β in a ratio of 2:1:1 (36) with sulphoconjugated oestrogens being present in a two-fold excess (37). Plasma concentrations of unconjugated oestrogens are an accurate reflection of production (38) and remain low until the day of delivery when there is a rapid sustained rise in levels (36, 39). Oestrogen sulphate concentrations also rise at delivery (fig. 3) in both fetal (33) and maternal plasma (40, 41). The administration of oestrogen during late pregnancy usually, but not always, results in delivery (7, 33, 42).

The search for a mechanism to explain the increase in oestrogen production at term has, until recently, proved fruitless (43). Administration of DHEAS does not induce labour although androstenedione, in pharmacological doses, is effective (25, 33). The concept that increased adrenal precursor availability provided the key to the raised oestrogen levels found at term has now been revised. Two pieces of information were at variance with this concept. Firstly, although dexamethasone suppresses adrenal function (44) its use to induce labour is associated with oestrogen levels similar to (34) or higher (45) than those found during normal labour. Secondly, when parturition is induced by dexamethasone, after fetal adrenalectomy, oestrogen levels are again raised to levels comparable with normal delivery (41). The answer to these anomalies and an explanation for the trends in progesterone and oestrogen production during parturition have been provided recently in an elegant series of experiments (41, 46, 47, 48). Summarized simply, glucocorticoid acts on the fetal placenta to induce both increased 17α-hydroxylase and $C_{17\text{-}20}$-lyase activity which are the rate limiting steps in oestrogen biosynthesis during late pregnancy. The androgens thus formed from progesterone and pregnenolone are rapidly converted to oestrogens (fig. 4). Hence the fetal placenta may in one sense be autonomous in its control of oestrogen production. One question not answered is why there is a time-lag between the fall in

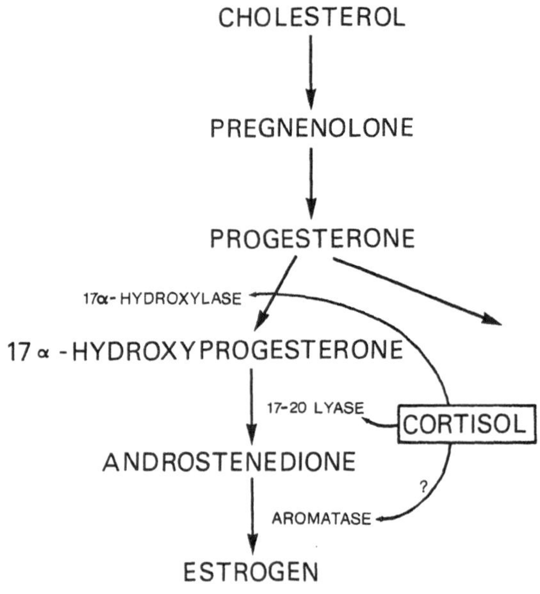

Fig. 4. Pathway of biosynthesis of progesterone and oestrogen in ovine placenta, indicating the possible sites of action of fetal cortisol on 17α-hydroxylase (46) $C_{17\text{-}20}$-lyase (47) and aromatase. The Δ^5 pathway which may contribute to oestrogen biosynthesis is omitted (After Liggins *et al.* [25]).

progesterone production and the increase in oestrogen production. Further investigations will be necessary before we have a full understanding of the control of oestrogen biosynthesis during parturition.

In summary, it may be concluded that progesterone and oestrogen production exhibit trends during parturition which are consistent with at least a permissive role for these steroids in the onset of labour. Increased fetal glucocorticoid secretion may directly produce the changes in placental enzyme activities resulting in the "withdrawal" of progesterone and the increase in oestrogens. How these changes finally promote uterine activity will now be discussed.

OXYTOCIN AND PROSTAGLANDINS

The earliest evidence (49) suggested that prostaglandin $F_{2\alpha}$ ($PGF_{2\alpha}$) was the only prostaglandin present in uterine tissues and uterine venous plasma and that its concentration in both tissue and plasma was elevated during labour (36, 49). Subsequently it has been shown that prostaglandin E_2 (PGE_2) is present in fetal and maternal plasma (50) and in intrauterine tissues (51) and that levels in fetal plasma are raised on the day of delivery (fig. 5). It is considered that the maternal cotyledon is the major source of $PGF_{2\alpha}$ during labour (49) with the myometrium a lesser source whereas the fetal cotyledon is almost certainly the major site of PGE_2 production (51, 52).

What controls the rise in prostaglandin levels during parturition? It is not due to a decreased rate of catabolism since the levels of the major circulating metabolite of $PGF_{2\alpha}$ (13,14-dihydro-15-keto $PGF_{2\alpha}$-PGFM) are also elevated in labour (53). Furthermore a recent study (54) showed that, with labour, the activity of 15-hydroxyprostaglandin dehydrogenase (a major catabolic enzyme) in maternal and fetal cotyledon is increased although in myometrium it falls. The concept of oestrogenic stimulation of PGF production has been well documented and has been demonstrated in the pregnant sheep (7, 34). Recently, however, it has been shown that a surge of oestrogen at parturition is not a prerequisite for a rise in plasma prostaglandin levels (45). The idea that progesterone withdrawal alone may be sufficient to release $PGF_{2\alpha}$ into uterine venous plasma had been suggested previously (33, 55) and has subsequently been confirmed experimentally by specific inhibition of progesterone synthesis (56).

The concentration of $PGF_{2\alpha}$ in uterine venous plasma shows a biphasic trend (33) and although steroid hormone changes may explain the first gradual increase in levels they do not explain the more sudden surge in levels

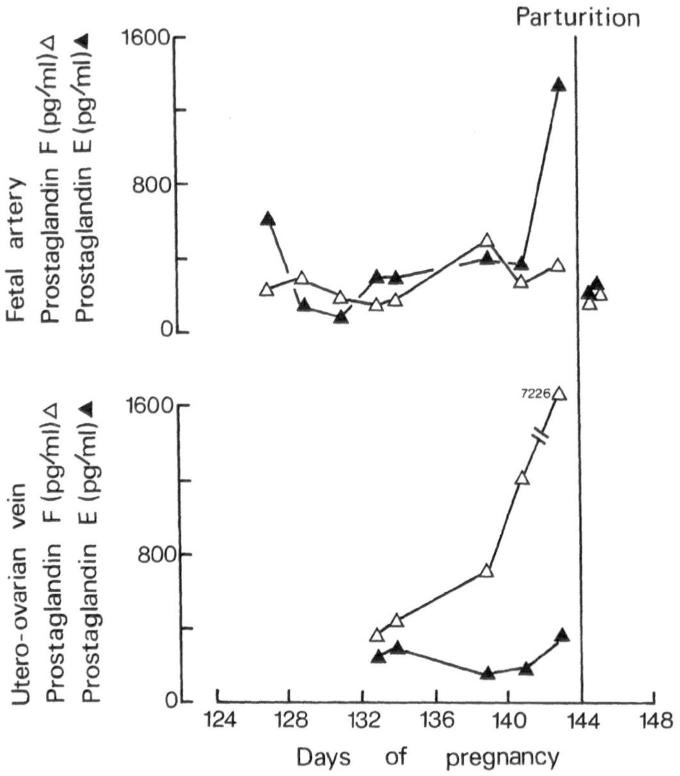

Fig. 5. Plasma concentrations of prostaglandins in a ewe and fetus during late pregnancy and parturition (After Challis *et al.* [50]).

during second stage labour. Although this surge was originally attributed to uterine contractions releasing $PGF_{2\alpha}$ (7, 33) it now seems likely that it is due to activation of the Ferguson reflex (57) by the presenting fetal parts. The Ferguson reflex is activated by cervical and vaginal stretching and results in the release of oxytocin from the posterior pituitary. Manual palpation of the vagina in late pregnant sheep results in a rise first of plasma oxytocin levels and then of prostaglandin levels (58; fig. 6). The magnitude of the effect on $PGF_{2\alpha}$ levels is increased close to delivery (59) and can be mimicked by the infusion of oxytocin (60). Hence the raised levels of oxytocin during late labour in sheep (61) are the likely stimulus for the rapid rise in prostaglandin levels at this time.

Having established that prostaglandin levels in plasma and tissues are raised during parturition, it is pertinent to question their function. Initially,

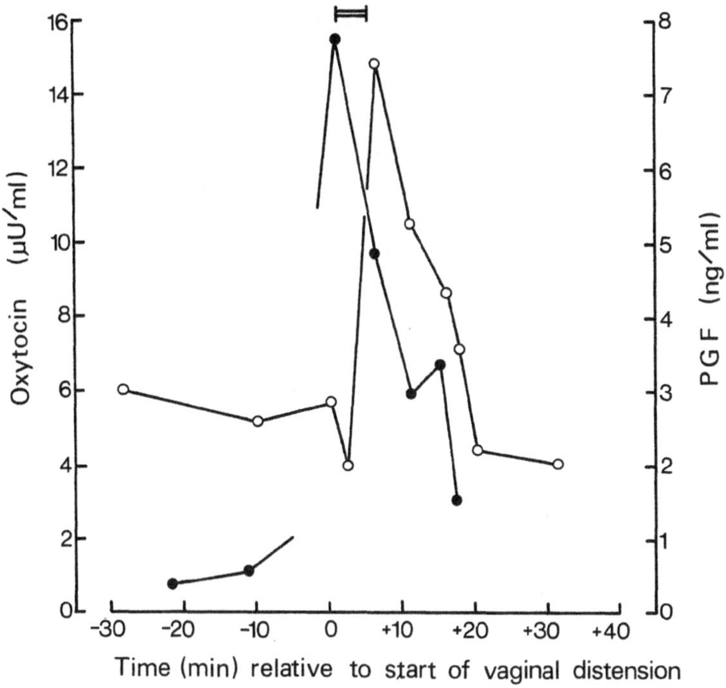

Fig. 6. Effect of vaginal distension (for 4 min as indicated by the horizontal bar) on jugular venous oxytocin (●) and utero-ovarian venous PGF (○) in one ewe 5 days before the birth of live twins at term (After Flint *et al.* [58]).

it seemed that the ovine uterus was insensitive to PGE and PGF and that infusion of $PGF_{2\alpha}$ would not have an oxytocic effect (32, 62, 63). Since then it has been shown that chronic (24 h) aortic infusion of $PGF_{2\alpha}$ (7) and acute administration of high doses of $PGF_{2\alpha}$ (64) will induce uterine contractions. The role of PGE in the fetus may well be to maintain the patency of the ductus arteriosus (65) although other functions have been suggested (66). It seems certain that prostaglandins play a crucial part in the mechanism of parturition in sheep and this has been highlighted in recent experiments where intrafetal dexamethasone infusion was accompanied by simultaneous maternal administration of a prostaglandin synthetase inhibitor (67). Despite the usual fall in progesterone levels and rise in oestrogen levels the animals did not go into labour until the inhibitor was withdrawn, when labour and delivery rapidly ensued. Hence the changes in steroid hormone concentrations during parturition probably play a permissive role while predisposing towards increased prostaglandin production.

An interesting finding in this study (67) was that the cervix did not soften and dilate during the administration of the prostaglandin synthetase inhibitor, despite the change in steroid hormone concentrations. Recent studies (25) have indicated that $PGF_{2\alpha}$, when infused into the lumen of the cervix, can cause local softening and dilation although this may be a pharmacological effect. In preliminary experiments it has now been established that cervical tissue *in vitro* can produce prostaglandins, predominantly PGE and that the rate of production of PGE is increased with labour (68). Nevertheless our knowledge of the mechanisms controlling cervical softening and dilation is very limited and presents considerable scope for future investigation.

In summary, it appears that the raised levels of prostaglandins found during parturition are controlled by the changing hormonal environment and that no one factor is primarily responsible. The increase in prostaglandin levels in tissues and plasma are the result of increased synthesis rather than decreased catabolism. Increased prostaglandin production is necessary both for the onset of labour and for cervical ripening.

CONCLUDING REMARKS

There are many aspects of parturition in sheep which have been omitted in this article. The exciting discoveries of thromboxane A_2 and prostacyclin will undoubtedly lead to an assessment of their functions in ovine parturition. The role of placental lactogen and a multiplicity of other hormones have not been discussed and neither has the influence of the adrenergic innervation of the uterus. These, and many other topics, may all have to be considered before the physiology of parturition will be fully understood. The basic outline of the hormonal events and interactions associated with parturition in sheep discussed in this article however is likely to be the framework for such studies.

REFERENCES

1. Binns W, Lynn JF, Shupe JL and Everett, GA: A congenital cylopian-type malformation in lambs induced by maternal ingestion of a range plant, *Veratrum californicum*. *Am J Vet Res* 24, 1164 (1963).
2. Basson PA, Morgenthal JC, Bilbrough RB, Marais JL, Kruger SP and van der Merwe JL de B: '*Grootlamsiekte*', a specific syndrome of prolonged gestation in sheep caused by a shrub, *Salsola tuberculata* (fenzl ex moq) schinz var. *tomentyosa*. CA Smith, ex gellen. *Onderstepoort J Vet Res* 36, 59-101 (1969).
3. Liggins GC, Kennedy PC and Holm LW: Failure of initiation of parturition after electrocoagulation of the pituitary of the fetal lamb. *Am J Obstet Gynecol* 98, 1080-1086 (1967):

4. Comline RS, Silver M and Silver IA: Effect of foetal hypophysectomy on catecholamine levels in the lamb adrenal during prolonged gestation. *Nature* 225, 739-740 (1970).
5. Bosc MJ: Conséquences sur la parturition, de l'hypophysectomie de la mère ou du foetus, chez la brebis traitée par la dexaméthasone. *CR Acad Sci* [D] (Paris) 274, 93-96 (1972).
6. Lanman JT and Schaffer A: Gestational effects of fetal decapitation in sheep. *Fertil Steril* 19, 598-605 (1968).
7. Liggins GC, Fairclough RJ, Grieves SA, Kendall JZ and Knox BS: The mechanism of initiation of parturition in the ewe. *Recent Prog Horm Res* 29, 111-150 (1973).
8. Liggins GC and Kennedy PC: Effects of electrocoagulation of the foetal lamb hypophysis on growth and development. *J Endocrinol* 40, 333-344 (1968).
9. Liggins GC, Holm LW and Kennedy PC: Prolonged pregnancy following surgical lesions of the foetal lamb pituitary. *J. Reprod Fertil* 12, 419 (1966).
10. Drost M and Holm LW: Prolonged gestation in ewes after foetal adrenalectomy. *J Endocrinol* 40, 293-296 (1968).
11. Liggins GC: Premature delivery of foetal lambs infused with glucocorticoids. *J Endocrinol* 45, 515-523 (1969).
12. Liggings GC: Premature parturition after infusion of corticotrophin or cortisol into foetal lambs. *J Endocrinol* 42, 323-329 (1968).
13. Bassett JM and Thorburn GD: Foetal plasma corticosteroids and the initiation of parturition in sheep. *J Endocrinol* 44, 285-286 (1969).
14. Comline RS, Nathanielsz PW, Paisey RB and Silver M: Cortisol turnover in the sheep foetus immediately prior to parturition. *J Physiol (Lond)* 210, 141P-142P (1970).
15. Beitins IZ, Kowarski A, Shermeta DW, De Lemos R and Migeon CJ: Fetal and maternal secretion rate of cortisol in sheep: diffusion resistance of placenta. *Pediatr Res* 4, 129-134 (1970).
16. Nathanielsz PW, Comline RS, Silver M and Paisey RB: Cortisol metabolism in the foetal and neonatal sheep. *J Reprod Fertil (Suppl)* 16, 39-59 (1972).
17. Fairclough RJ and Liggins GC: Protein binding of plasma cortisol in the foetal lamb near term. *J Endocrinol* 67, 333-341 (1975).
18. Rees LH, Jack PMB, Thomas AL and Nathanielsz, PW: Role of foetal adrenocorticotrophin during parturition in sheep. *Nature* 253, 274-275 (1975).
19. Jones CT, Boddy K and Robinson JS: Changes in the concentration of adrenocorticotrophin and corticosteroid in the plasma of foetal sheep in the latter half of pregnancy and during labour. *J Endocrinol* 72, 293-300 (1977).
20. Robinson JS, Challis JRG, Pooley G and Thorburn GD: Foetal and maternal cortisol and progesterone and maternal oestradiol in prolonged pregnancy after foetal hypophysectomy in sheep. *J Endocrinol* 72, 241-242 (1977).
21. Comline RS and Silver M: The release of adrenaline and noradrenaline from the adrenal glands of the foetal sheep. *J Physiol (Lond)* 156,424-444 (1961).
22. Wintour EM, Brown EH, Denton DA, Hardy KJ, McDougal JG, Oddie CJ and Whipp GT: The ontogeny and regulation of corticosteriod secretion by the ovine foetal adrenal *Acta Endocrinol* 79, 301-316 (1975).
23. Nathanielsz PW, Jack PMB, Krane EJ, Thomas AL, Ratter S and Rees LH: The role and regulation of corticotropin in the fetal sheep. In: *The Fetus and Birth*, Ciba Foundation Symposium no 47, Amsterdam, Excerpta Medica, 1977, p 73-91.
24. Madill D and Bassett JM: Corticosteroid release by adrenal tissue from foetal and newborn lambs in response to corticotrophin stimulation in a perifusion system *in vitro*. *J Endocrinol* 58, 75-87 (1973).
25. Liggins GC, Fairclough RJ, Grieves SA, Forster CS and Knox BS: Parturition in the sheep. In: *The Fetus and Birth*, Ciba Foundation Symposium no 47, Amsterdam, Excerpta Medica, 1977, p 5-25.
26. Chard T, Silman RE and Rees LH: The fetal hypothalamus and pituitary in the initiation of labour. In: *The Fetus and Birth*, Ciba Foundation Symposium no 47, Amsterdam, Excerpta Medica, 1977, p 359-370.

27. Linzell JL and Heap RB: A comparison of progesterone metabolism in the pregnant sheep and goat: sources of production and an estimation of uptake by some target organs. *J Endocrinol* 41, 433-438 (1968).
28. Short RV and Rowell JG: The half life of progesterone in the peripheral blood of a ewe at two stages of gestation. *J Endocrinol* 25, 369-374 (1962).
29. Bedford CA, Challis JRG, Harrison FA and Heap RB: The role of oestrogens and progesterone in the onset of parturition in various species. *J Reprod Fertil (Suppl)* 16, 1-23 (1972).
30. Bassett JM, Oxborrow TJ, Smith ID and Thorburn GD: The concentration of progesterone in the peripheral plasma of the pregnant ewe. *J Endocrinol* 45, 449-457 (1969).
31. Fylling P: The effect of pregnancy, ovariectomy and parturition on plasma progesterone level in sheep. *Acta Endocrinol* 65, 273-283 (1970).
32. Liggins GC, Grieves SA, Kendall JZ and Knox BS: The physiological roles of progesterone, oestradiol-17β and prostaglandin $F_{2\alpha}$ in the control of ovine parturition. *J Reprod Fertil (Suppl)* 16, 85-103 (1972).
33. Currie WB, Wong MSF, Cox RI and Thorburn GD: Spontaneous or dexamethasone-induced parturition in the sheep and goat: changes in plasma concentrations of maternal prostaglandin F and foetal oestrogen sulphate. *Mem Soc Endocrinol* 20, 95-118 (1973).
34. Flint APF, Anderson ABM, Patten PT and Turnbull AC: Control of utero-ovarian venous prostaglandin F during labour in the sheep: acute effects of vaginal and cervical stimulation. *J Endocrinol* 63, 67-87 (1974).
35. Bengtsson LP and Schofield BM: Progesterone and the accomplishment of parturition in axis in foetal sheep. *Acta Endocrinol (Suppl)* 199, 94 (1975).
36. Thorburn GD, Nicol DH, Bassett JM, Shutt DA and Cox RI: Parturition in the goat and sheep; changes in corticosteroids, progesterone, oestrogens and prostaglandin F. *J Reprod Fertil (Suppl)* 16, 61-84 (1972).
37. Wong MSF, Cox RI, Currie WB and Thorburn GD: Changes of oestrogen sulphoconjugates in the foetal plasma of sheep and goats during late gestation. *Proc Aust Soc Endocrinol* 15, 8 (1972).
38. Challis JRG, Harrison FA and Heap RB: The kinetics of oestrogen metabolism in the pregnant sheep. In: *Endocrinology of Pregnancy and Parturition: Experimental Studies in the Sheep*, Pierrepoint CG (ed), Cardiff, Alpha-Omega, 1973, p 73-82.
39. Challis JRG: Sharp increase in free circulating oestrogens immediately before parturition in sheep. *Nature* 229, 208 (1971).
40. Tsang CPW: Changes in plasma levels of estrone sulfate and estrone in the pregnant ewe around parturition. *Steroids* 23, 855-868 (1974).
41. Flint APF, Anderson ABM, Goodson JD, Steele PA and Turnbull AC: Bilateral adrenalectomy of lambs *in utero:* effects on maternal hormone levels at induced parturition. *J Endocrinol* 69, 433-444 (1976).
42. Hindson JC, Schofield BM and Turner CB: The effect of a single dose of stilboestrol on cervical dilatation in pregnant sheep. *Res Vet Sci* 8, 353-360 (1967).
43. Thorburn GD, Challis JRG and Robinson JS: Endocrine control of parturition. In: *Biology of the Uterus*, Wynn RM (ed), New York, Plenum Press, 1977, p 653-732.
44. Thomas SJ and Pierrepoint CG: Studies on the functional activity of the pituitary-adrenal axis in foetal sheep. *Acta Endocrinol (Suppl)* 199, 94 (1975).
45. Kendall JZ, Challis JRG, Hart IC, Jones CT, Mitchell MD, Ritchie JWK, Robinson JS and Thorburn GD: Steroid and prostaglandin concentrations in the plasma of pregnant ewes during infusion of adrenocorticotrophin or dexamethasone to intact or hypophysectomized foetuses. *J Endocrinol* 75, 59-71 (1977).
46. Anderson ABM, Flint APF and Turnbull AC: Mechanism of action of glucocorticoids in induction of ovine parturition: effect on placental steroid metabolism. *J Endocrinol* 66, 61-70 (1975).

47. Steele PA, Flint APF and Turnbull AC: Activity of steroid C-17, 20 lyase in the ovine placenta: effect of exposure to foetal glucocorticoid. *J Endocrinol* 69, 239-246 (1976).
48. Flint APF, Anderson ABM, Steele PA and Turnbull AC: The mechanism by which foetal cortisol controls the onset of parturition in the sheep. *Biochem Soc Trans* 3, 1189-1194 (1975).
49. Liggins GC and Grieves SA: Possible role for prostaglandin $F_{2\alpha}$ in parturition in sheep. *Nature* 232, 629-631 (1971).
50. Challis JRG, Dilley SR, Robinson JS and Thorburn GD: Prostaglandins in the circulation of the fetal lamb. *Prostaglandins* 11, 1041-1052 (1976).
51. Mitchell MD and Flint APF: Prostaglandin concentrations in intra-uterine tissues from late pregnant sheep before and after labour. *Prostaglandins* 14, 563-569 (1977).
52. Mitchell MD and Flint APF: Prostaglindin production by intra-uterine tissues from peri-parturient sheep: use of a superfusion technique. *J Endocrinol* 76, 111-121 (1978).
53. Mitchell MD, Flint APF and Turnbull AC: Plasma concentrations of 13, 14-dihydro-15-keto prostaglandin F during pregnancy in sheep. *Prostaglandins* 11, 319-329 (1976).
54. Keirse MJNC, Mitchell MD and Flint APF: Changes in myometrial and placental 15-hydroxyprostaglandin dehydrogenase with ovine parturition: production of prostaglandin metabolites *in vitro* and *in vivo*. *J Reprod Fertil* 51, 409-412 (1977).
55. Challis JRG, Forster CS, Furr BJA, Robinson JS and Thorburn GD: Production of prostaglandin $F_{2\alpha}$ in ewes following luteal regression induced with a prostaglandin analogue, Estrumate (cloprostenol ICI 80996) *Prostaglandins* 11, 537-543 (1976).
56. Mitchell MD and Flint APF: Progesterone withdrawal: effects on prostaglandins and parturition. *Prostaglandins* 14, 611-614 (1977).
57. Ferguson JKW: A study of the motility of the intact uterus at term. *Surg Gynecol Obstet* 73, 359-366 (1941).
58. Flint APF, Forsling ML, Mitchell MD and Turnbull AC: Temporal relationship between changes in oxytocin and prostaglandin F levels in response to vaginal distension in the pregnant and puerperal ewe. *J Reprod Fertil* 43, 551-554 (1975).
59. Mitchell MD, Flint APF and Turnbull AC: Increasing uterine response to vaginal distension during late pregnancy in sheep. *J Reprod Fertil* 49, 35-40 (1977).
60. Michell MD, Flint APF and Turnbull AC: Stimulation by oxytocin of prostaglandin F levels in uterine venous effluent in pregnant and puerperal sheep. *Prostaglandins* 9, 47-56 (1976).
61. Fitzpatrick RJ and Walmsley CF: The release of oxytocin during parturition. In: *Advances in Oxytocin Research*, Pinkerton JHM (ed), Oxford, Pergamon Press, 1965, p 51-71.
62. Keirse MJNC, Patten PT, Anderson ABM, Turnbull AC, Johns A, Wooster MJ and Pickles VR: Pregnant sheep myometrium responds to prostaglandins *in vitro* but not *in vivo*. *Int Res Commun Syst* 73-4, 8-5-1 (1973).
63. Oakes G, Mofid M, Brinkman CR and Assali NS: Insensitivity of the sheep to prostaglandins. *Proc Soc Exp Biol Med* 142, 194-197 (1973).
64. Mitchell MD, Flint APF and Turn bull AC: Stimulation of uterine activity by administration of prostaglandin $F_{2\alpha}$ during parturition in sheep. *J Reprod Fertil* 48, 189-190 (1977).
65. Coceani F, Olley PM and Bodach E: Prostaglandins: a possible regulator of muscle tone in the ductus arteriosus. In: *Advances in Prostaglandin and Thromboxane Research*, Vol. 1, Samuelsson B and Paolletti R (eds), New York, Raven Press, 1976, p 417-424.
66. Challis JRG, Hart I, Louis TM, Mitchell MD, Jenkins G, Robinson JS and Thorburn GD: Prostaglandins in the sheep fetus: implications for fetal function. In: *Advances in Prostaglandin and Thromboxane Research*, Vol. 4, Coceani F and Olley PM (eds), New York, Raven Press, 1978, p 115-132.
67. Mitchell MD and Flint APF: Use of meclofenamic acid to investigate the role of prostaglandin biosynthesis during induced parturition in sheep. *J Endocrinol* 76, 101-109 (1978).
68. Ellwood DA: Personal communication.

PARTURITION IN THE RHESUS MONKEY

J.S. ROBINSON, M.D. MITCHELL AND J.R.G. CHALLIS

There is now good evidence in the ruminant to believe that the fetus plays an important role in the initiation of its timely delivery (Mitchell, this volume). The initial observations on fetal malformations which resulted in prolonged pregnancy were followed by a combination of experimental techniques (e.g. ablative surgery and chronic fetal preparations with indwelling catheters) which are not possible in man. Therefore in order to see how far the results derived from sheep, for example, can be extrapolated to primates similar experiments need to be undertaken in a variety of different species. It is important to remember that man and the rhesus monkey differ greatly from the sheep and indeed there are well defined differences amongst the primates. The existence of a fetoplacental unit has been demonstrated in both man and the rhesus monkey but with difference in some placental enzymes. Also the placenta is relatively permeable to cortisol and the proportion of cortisol in the fetal circulation which is derived from the mother is much larger than that in sheep.

The purpose of this paper is to review briefly the control of parturition in the monkey. Since a number of reviews are available (1, 2, 3, 4) the reader will be referred to those for a more detailed description of certain aspects.

FETAL INFLUENCE ON GESTATIONAL LENGTH

The classic experiments in which the fetus was removed and the placenta left *in situ* were originally interpreted by van Wagenen and Newton (5) as evidence that the fetus has little influence on gestational length in the rhesus monkey. The placenta was delivered between 144 and 184 days of gestation at varying intervals after fetectomy. In similar experiments, Lanman *et al.* (6) noted that the placentae were frequently retained *in utero* well past normal term. Thus, a different conclusion that can be derived from these experiments is that there is a loss of the precise timing of delivery of the placenta in the absence of a fetus.

More recently, Kittinger (3) has described various neurosurgical ablative

M.J.N.C. Keirse et al. (eds.), Human Parturition, 25-39.

procedures which can be undertaken successfully in the rhesus monkey with fetal survival. These include fetal decapitation (experimental anencephaly, 4) in which the cerebral hemispheres and pituitary gland of the fetus were removed at 73-78 days of gestation. After making allowances for early post-operative abortions the length of gestation in the experiments in which the fetus was alive until shortly before delivery were described. Three animals delivered pre-term (<155 days), three at term (155-175 days) and in four pregnancy was prolonged (>175 days). There was no difference in amniotic fluid volume in experimental anencephaly compared to controls. These findings are similar to those in human pregnancy complicated by anencephaly in the absence of polyhydramnios (7) and both support a fetal role in the determination of the length of gestation.

The experiments of Liggins and his colleagues (8, Mitchell, this volume) clearly implicate the fetal pituitary and adrenal glands in the onset of parturition in the sheep. It is therefore pertinent to discuss the effects of ablation of these glands in the fetal primate. Chez *et al.* (9) destroyed either the maternal or fetal pituitary at 120-133 days by inserting yttrium-90 into the pituitary fossa. Maternal hypophysectomy did not affect gestational length in the animals in which the fetus continued to grow. Fetal hypophysectomy (and continued fetal growth) was associated with prolonged pregnancy in 4 out of 5 animals while sham operated fetuses delivered normally at term. Post-mortem examination of the hypophysectomized fetuses demonstrated a reduction in the size of the adrenal glands with a greater loss of the fetal than definitive zone of the cortex.

The role of the fetal pituitary-adrenal axis in the timely onset of parturition in the primate seemed to be an intriguing possibility. Unfortunately, the attempts to perform fetal adrenalectomy in the monkey gave inconclusive results. Mueller-Heubach *et al.* (10) removed the adrenals and reported that labour occurred about term. The result must be termed as inconclusive since in most fetuses fragments of the adrenal glands were found and only one pregnancy (associated with fetal death) went well past term. It would be interesting to repeat this difficult experiment but it should be noted that fetal adrenal aplasia in man is not always associated with prolonged pregnancy.

Fetal pituitary-adrenal axis

The prolongation of pregnancy after fetal hypophysectomy in the rhesus monkey naturally focuses attention on the pituitary-adrenal axis in view of its importance in the initiation of parturition in the ruminant. In the sheep ACTH concentration in fetal plasma does not increase before the rise of cortisol (11). This prompted Silman *et al.* (12) to examine the pituitary for the ACTH family of peptides. In pituitaries obtained from human fetuses melanocyte stimulating hormone (αMSH) and corticotrophin-like intermediate lobe peptide (CLIP) were present in large amounts. The ratio of these peptides to ACTH decreases at about the time of birth and it was speculated that this may provide a trigger for parturition. Further, experiments in rabbits suggested that αMSH is trophic for the fetal adrenal gland while ACTH is not and that the converse is true in the newborn rabbit (13). Silman *et al.* (14) have examined the pituitary content of ACTH family of peptides in the rhesus monkey. In this species, as in man, αMSH and CLIP are present in the fetal pituitary in large amounts but are only just detectable in the adult pituitary. The fetal monkey pituitary also contained βMSH and β-endorphin whereas the larger peptides ACTH, β-lipotrophin and α-lipotrophin were more characteristic of the pituitary after birth. While the importance of these observations remains to be established it is tempting to suggest that the switch from pattern in the fetus to another in which the larger molecules are present in the adult may play a role in the initiation of parturition in the monkey. Although these peptides are present in the pituitary the pattern of their release into the circulation in response to various stimuli is, as yet, unknown (as is their adrenocorticotrophic activity in this species).

The response of the fetal adrenal to ACTH has been tested by injections and by long term infusions in the rhesus monkey. In acute experiments the fetal adrenal gland appears to be insensitive to ACTH unless the pituitary-adrenal axis has been suppressed by prior administration of large amounts of dexamethasone (15). This has recently been confirmed in a small series of chronic experiments but it should be noted that increased adrenal sensitivity to ACTH was observed in two animals within 24 h of the onset of labour (16). Long term infusion of large amounts of ACTH into the chronically catheterised monkey fetus resulted in adrenal growth and an increase in cortisol concentration in the fetal circulation (4). This was associated with an increased concentration of oestrone in both the fetus and mother and a rise of plasma oestradiol concentration in the latter.

Since it is difficult to obtain serial blood samples from the rhesus monkey fetus under good physiological conditions an assessment of the change in fetal adrenocortical activity in late gestation has been made by measuring the concentrations of various steroid hormones in amniotic fluid (17). The concentration of cortisol in amniotic fluid increased gradually as gestation advanced with a more rapid rise in the last 10-20 days of pregnancy while cortisol concentration in maternal peripheral plasma remained unchanged. At the same time, increases in the concentrations of androstenedione, progesterone, oestrone and oestrone sulphate were observed in amniotic fluid but oestradiol concentration did not change significantly. Since the progesterone in amniotic fluid was suppressed by β-methasone it was reasoned that it was unlikely to be of placental origin and reflected fetal adrenal activity. Further, since oestradiol did not alter while the other steroids increased the changes observed were unlikely to be due to diminution of amniotic fluid volume. Measurement of amniotic fluid volume demonstrated that there was no significant decrease in late gestation (18, 4).

More recent observations on primate adrenal function have been made in the chronically catheterised fetus. Challis and Manning (19) have confirmed that the cortisol concentration in amniotic fluid correlates more closely with the concentration in fetal plasma than with that in maternal peripheral plasma. A further point which has to be taken into account in the assessment of fetal adrenal function is the time of day at which the samples were collected since a marked circadian variation of maternal cortisol concentration occurs and the placenta in this species is relatively permeable to cortisol (3). Taking these factors into account Jaffe and co-workers (16) have obtained blood samples from 20 fetuses with indwelling vascular catheters between 130 and 154 days of gestation. The fetuses were judged to be in good condition based on measurement of blood gases, pH and the fetal heart rate. A significant increase in cortisol concentration was observed after 150 days and a further rise occurred in labour. However, some reservation must be placed on these results since the age of the fetuses at delivery was not stated.

Maturation of the fetal pituitary-adrenal axis, as reflected by the cortisol and oestrogen concentrations, occurs in late pregnancy. Whether this is due to alteration of pituitary function or whether there are changes in the adrenal gland (e.g. receptor activity) has still to be determined. Another factor which has to be taken into account is the activity of enzymes required for production of cortisol by the adrenal cortex. Pepe *et al.* (20) examined the maturational changes occurring in the fetal adrenal gland in the baboon. They noted that activity of 3β-hydroxysteroid dehydrogenase increased with age whereas 17α and 21-hydroxylase were unchanged. This change may be more important for adrenocortical sufficiency after birth when placental progesterone is no longer available for adrenal cortisol production rather than for the increased cortisol concentrations observed prenatally.

MATERNAL PROGESTERONE AND OESTROGEN

Since detailed reviews (2, 1, 19) of the concentrations, sites of origin and regulation of these hormones are available only a brief outline will be given here. The concentration of progesterone in the maternal circulation varies greatly from species to species among the primates (21). In the rhesus monkey although three peaks of progesterone have been reported, the concentration in maternal peripheral plasma remains at levels similar to those in the luteal phase throughout most of pregnancy. The progesterone is derived from both the placenta and the ovary in late pregnancy (22, 23). Thau *et al.* (24) found decreasing concentrations of progesterone in the uterine venous plasma in the last third of gestation but the production rate and peripheral concentrations did not change greatly. Indeed, there is little to suggest that progesterone withdrawal is essential for the onset of parturition in the monkey. This is reinforced by the observation that daily injection of progesterone did not influence the length of gestation even though the plasma concentration was 10-20 times higher than normal (19). Similarly, Corner *et al.* (25) were unable to detect an alteration in spontaneous myometrial activity after progesterone treatment.

The rhesus monkey produces oestrone, oestradiol and oestriol but the proportion of oestriol is much less than that observed in women. The major metabolite in urine is oestrone (26,27). The concentration of oestradiol in plasma, however, is higher than that of oestrone (28, 29) and both increase during the last 5-10 days of pregnancy in most but not all animals. Plasma oestrogen concentrations in late pregnancy were unaltered by ovariectomy (23) but could be suppressed by dexamethasone (30, 31) or fetal death (22, 32) indicating that oestrogen production is largely of fetoplacental origin.

The importance of the increase of plasma oestrogen concentrations in relationship to the onset of parturition is still uncertain. Premature parturition has been observed in association with high oestradiol concentrations (33). In contrast, normal gestation length is observed in monkeys in which oestrogen concentrations have been suppressed by exogenous glucocorticoid (29) and exogenous oestradiol benzoate or valerate administration failed to induce parturition.

In view of difficulty of correlating maternal plasma oestrogens with the onset of parturition in the monkey we examined the changes of oestrone, oestrone sulphate and oestradiol in amniotic fluid (17). As mentioned previously oestrone and oestrone sulphate increased in the last 10-20 days of pregnancy. This rise of oestrogen correlated closely with the changes of prostaglandin F (PGF) and its principal metabolite 13, 14, dihydro-15-keto-prostaglandin $F_{2\alpha}$ (PGFM) in amniotic fluid (32). While a rise in oestrogens may not be obligatory for delivery under all circumstances it is likely that oestrogens may facilitate the onset of parturition by enhancing prostaglandin production.

PROSTAGLANDINS

It has been shown that administration of $PGF_{2\alpha}$, either intramuscularly or subcutaneously, results in abortion or pre-term delivery in the rhesus monkey (34, 35, 29). In these investigations relatively large doses of PGF were used but more recently it has been shown that smaller amounts of PGE_2 produce the same effect when injected extra-amniotically (36). These exogenous prostaglandins appear to act directly on the uterus in late pregnancy and to be independent of changes in hormone concentrations in maternal plasma. However, in early pregnancy the large amounts of PG used may have interfered with the trophic support provided by the conceptus to the corpus luteum.

In contrast to the effects of exogenous prostaglandins, inhibition of prostaglandin synthesis by indomethacin results in prolonged pregnancy (37). Indomethacin (10-28 mg/day) was given to the animals beginning between days 149 and 155 of pregnancy (normal term 167 $\pm$ 0.4 days, $n=310$) and continued until spontaneous vaginal delivery occurred or Caesarean section was performed. The mean age at delivery in the indomethacin-treated animals was 180 $\pm$ 2 days, five of the animals were delivered by Caesarean section between 180-187 days and the remainder vaginally at 171-176 days. Although 4 fetuses were dead at the time of delivery and others meconium-stained, fetal and placental weights were heavier than in control fetuses delivered at 161 days thus indicating that fetal growth continued when the mother was receiving indomethacin. A striking feature in these animals was the flaccid uterus at Caesarean section after the fetus and placenta had been removed and yet it responded normally to oxytocin (38). The extent of the inhibition of prostaglandin production was estimated by measurement of a metabolite of $PGF_{2\alpha}$ ($9\alpha,11\alpha$-dihydroxy-15-oxo-2,3,4,5-tetranorprosta-1, 20-dioic acid) in 24 hour urine collections obtained from one animal (4). The dose of indomethacin which successfully prolonged pregnancy led to a fall in the urinary excretion of the metabolite by 56 per cent.

Another interesting feature noted in these experiments was the reduction in amniotic fluid volume (mean 14 ml, range 4-44 ml) in the indomethacin-treated group compared to the normal range of 57 to 150 ml (mean 102 $\pm$ 12 ml) at 160 days. Novy (4) considered that this oligohydramnios may have resulted from disturbance of fetal renal function since it has been shown that PGE_2 enhances renal blood flow and urine production in the adult (39) whereas indomethacin causes renal vasoconstriction (40) and can result in oliguria in the human neonate (41, 42). This may not be the only explanation since the indomethacin may have altered pulmonary blood flow (43) and lung liquid production. Further, the amnion is a potent site of PG, particularly PGE production (44) and it may be speculated that reduction of this could alter permeability of the fetal membranes.

Prostaglandins in maternal plasma and amniotic fluid

The concentration of $PGF_{2\alpha}$ in maternal peripheral plasma does not change significantly with increasing gestational age in the macaque (45). However, in view of the efficiency of the metabolism of primary prostaglandins by the lung it was considered that measurement of the major circulating metabolite of PGF, 13,14-dihydro-15-keto-$PGF_{2\alpha}$ (PGFM), would more accurately relate to the production rate of $PGF_{2\alpha}$. In maternal plasma an increase in PGFM was observed post-partum when samples were collected within 12 h of delivery. Prepartum, PGFM levels were lower in the 5 days preceding delivery than earlier in pregnancy (32).

The mean concentrations of PGF and PGFM in amniotic fluid increased gradually during late pregnancy and rose significantly from 0.5 ng/ml up to 10 days prepartum to about 2 ng/ml during the last 5 days of pregnancy. A similar pattern but of lower magnitude, was seen in one animal with unexplained pre-term delivery at 124 days (32).

Except for the last few days before delivery, the concentration of PGFM in amniotic fluid was less than that in maternal peripheral plasma. The increase in amniotic PGFM and PGF appeared to follow closely the increase in the concentration of oestrone in amniotic fluid.

Prostaglandin production by uterine tissues in vitro

It has been shown that the highest concentrations of PGF in the human uterus are found in the decidua and fetal membranes (46, 59). However, these concentrations may be erroneously high due to trauma of the tissues during collection. In an attempt to overcome this difficulty a superfusion technique (47) has been used to estimate the production of prostaglandins and thromboxane by intrauterine tissues obtained at hysterotomy from rhesus monkeys during late pregnancy. This superfusion technique may avoid some of the problems with tissue collection as a 90 min wash-out period was allowed before fractions were collected for analysis. Tissues were obtained from 4 monkeys between 140-149 days (late pregnancy) and from 4 between 160-168 days (near term) (44). All tissues produced significantly more PGE than PGF and, excepting the decidua, more PGFM than PGF. During late pregnancy and near term the amnion and the decidua produced more prostaglandins (per unit weight) than the placenta, chorion or myometrium. Production of PGE by all tissues was significantly lower at term whereas production of PGF by the fetal membranes, myometrium and decidua parietalis was significantly greater (fig. 1).

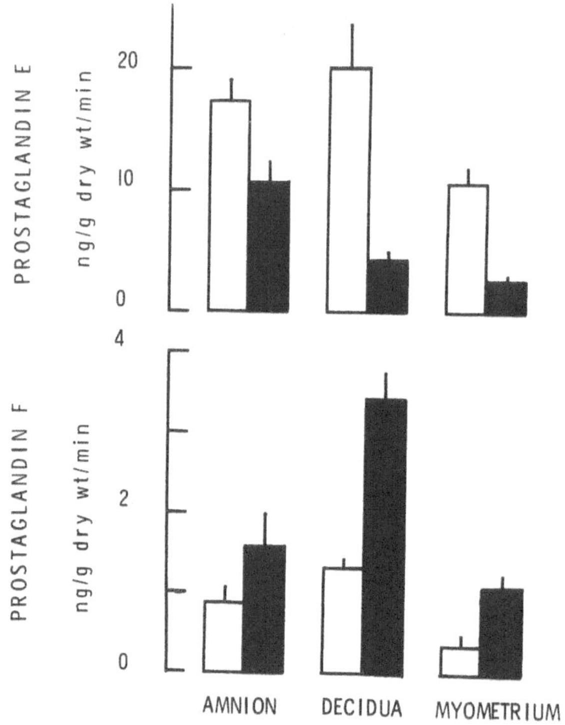

Fig. 1. Production of prostaglandin E and prostaglandin F in late pregnancy (140-149 days of gestation, open columns) and near term (160-168 days, closed columns) by intrauterine tissues from the rhesus monkey superfused *in vitro*. Prostaglandin E production decreases while prostaglandin F production increases with increasing gestational age.

In addition to the primary prostaglandins the prostaglandin endoperoxides can be converted to thromboxane A_2 (TXA_2) (48) or to prostacyclin (PGI_2) (49). These compounds are rapidly converted to their more stable metabolites thromboxane B_2 (TXB_2) and 6-keto-prostaglandin $F_{1\alpha}$. Since TXA_2 and PGI_2 act on smooth muscle their concentrations in uterine tissues pre-partum may be of considerable significance. Recently a sensitive radioimmunoassay has been developed for TXB_2 (50). Using this assay TXB_2 production by intrauterine tissues superfused *in vitro* has been reported (51). The greatest capacity for production of TXB_2 was found to be in the decidua but since no change with gestational age was observed it was considered unlikely that thromboxanes were important in the mechanisms responsible for the initiation of parturition in this species. The only tissue which showed a significant increase in TXB_2 production near term was the myometrium but the magnitude of this change was small and it was not considered to be important physiologically. It was speculated that since TXA_2 is a potent vasoconstrictor the high decidual and myometrial production of TXB_2 may reflect involvement of thromboxanes in the haemostatic mechanisms after delivery of the fetus and separation of the placenta.

These results of prostaglandin and thromboxane production *in vitro* lead to an interesting conclusion that a specific alteration in the direction of prostaglandin production occurs with increasing gestational age. This has been defined further by the significant fall in the PGE:PGF ratio near term (44) and these findings are similar to those in the sheep (47). The demonstration that oestrogen can direct prostaglandin synthesis from E to F in microsomal preparations of rat uteri (52) supports the suggestion that the increased PGF concentrations in amniotic fluid may be due to oestrogens acting on the fetal membranes and uterine tissues (1). This is an alternative hypothesis to that proposed by Challis *et al.* (1), to relate the importance of increasing concentrations of oestrogen in amniotic fluid to the increased PGF. At that time it was considered that the oestrogen acted on lysosomes in the decidual cell releasing phospholipase A_2 which in turn led to increased availability of arachidonic acid for prostaglandin synthesis. Implicit in that hypothesis and in Gustavii's hypothesis (53) was that the availability of arachidonic acid may be rate limiting in prostaglandin production and hence the onset of labour. Schultz *et al.* (54) reported that 1 g arachidonic acid injected into amniotic fluid could result in the successful termination of pregnancy in man. More recent experiments in the rhesus monkey failed to confirm these findings. The arachidonic acid was injected extra-amniotically so that it would be available to the decidua and fetal membranes (the most potent sites of prostaglandin production). The administration of 100 mg arachidonic acid extra-amniotically was not followed by any significant change in the concentrations of PGE, PGF or PGFM in amniotic fluid or maternal plasma (fig. 2). In contrast 2.5 mg PGE_2 given by the same route successfully induced delivery and resulted in increased prostaglandin concentrations. Since no change in prostaglandins occurred after arachidonic acid it may be suggested that prostaglandin synthesis is inhibited. The nature of the inhibitor remains to be established but recently an endogenous inhibitor of prostaglandin synthesis has been found in the α-globulin fraction of human plasma (55). Such a substance could be the pregnancy-associated α_2-globulin which has been localised immunocyto-

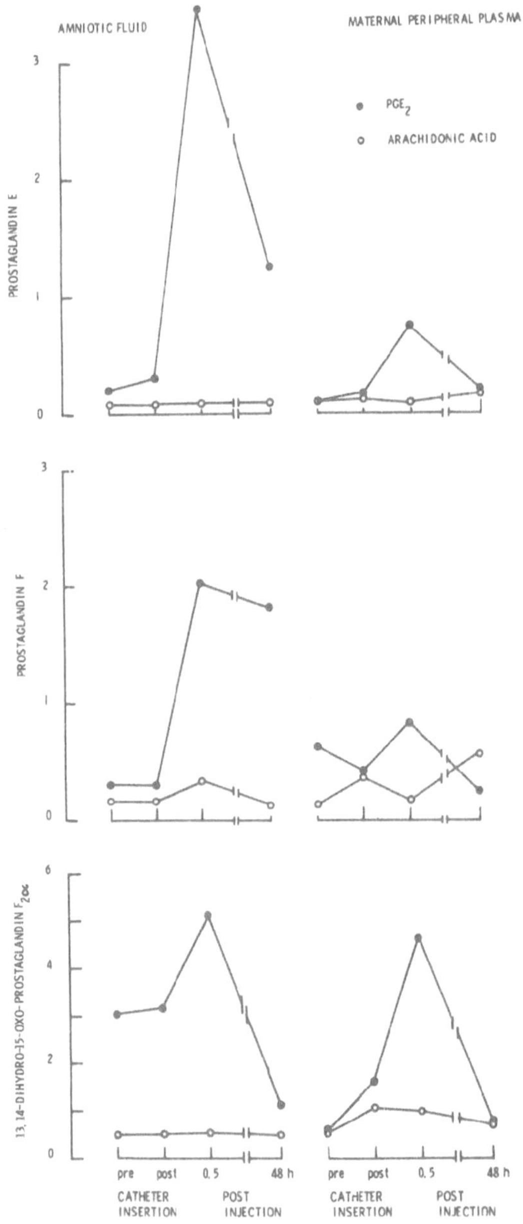

Fig. 2. The concentrations of prostaglandin E, prostaglandin F and 13, 14-dihydro-15-keto-prostaglandin $F_{2\alpha}$ in amniotic fluid and maternal peripheral plasma in monkeys treated with 100 mg arachidonic acid or 2.5 mg prostaglandin E_2 in 10 ml Hyskon extra-amniotically. The treatments were given via a catheter inserted into the extra-amniotic space. Each point is the mean of two values from different animals.

chemically in the decidual cell in human endometrium obtained at Caesarean section (56). However, it should be remembered that other substances present in amniotic fluid and maternal blood (e.g. oxytocin and progesterone) may influence the direction of prostaglandin production at term.

Any hypothesis which proposes that the fetus initiates its own timely delivery has to include mechanisms by which the dead fetus will be delivered. We have observed spontaneous delivery of a dead fetus in two animals after intrauterine death between 140-160 days, following attempted fetal hypophysectomy at 120-130 days (32). In both animals pregnancy was prolonged, and the fetus delivered on days 188 and 194. The concentrations of progesterone in maternal blood did not change significantly until after delivery but oestradiol concentration fell to 50-100 pg/ml. No obvious change in the concentration of PGFM occurred in maternal peripheral plasma after fetal death but it had increased two-fold in samples collected on the morning after delivery. Similar steroid hormone changes were reported by Bosu *et al* (22) after fetal death. Whether the time of delivery is related to progressive degenerative changes, vascular congestion and tissue necrosis (57) or to the gradual removal of a substance derived from the fetus which suppresses prostaglandin production remains to be established. However, the net effect is that prostaglandin production as shown by raised concentrations of PGFM increased at the time of delivery of the dead fetus.

CONCLUDING REMARKS

The involvement of the fetus in the onset of parturition in the primate remains somewhat uncertain at present. The surgical manipulations mentioned in this review allow speculation that the monkey fetus may control the precise timing of its own delivery. However, the nature of the trigger remains to be established. Since the fetal pituitary-adrenal axis appears to be essential in the sheep, the function of this axis in late gestation in the monkey has been described. In the pituitary there is a change in the content of the ACTH family of peptides but nothing is known, at present, about the signal (from the hypothalamus?) inducing this change.

At the adrenal level there is an increasing body of evidence to support increased activity of the adrenal cortex in late gestation. Examples of this are the increased cortisol concentrations in fetal plasma and amniotic fluid and also the rise in oestrogen concentrations. But neither of these seem to be essential to the normal onset of labour at term since dexamethasone fails to induce labour in this species. Daily administration of this glucocorticoid from 150 days onwards (46) suppressed oestrogen concentrations yet labour occurred normally at term. However, it is still likely that the oestrogen rise would facilitate the increased production of prostaglandins (1). Recently a dramatic fall in the sex steroid binding protein in the last few days of pregnancy in the rhesus monkey has been demonstrated (58). This may augment the effects of oestrogen in late pregnancy by altering the ratio of the free and physiologically active steroid to the bound hormone. To be effective at the tissue level this may have to be associated with an alteration in steroid hormone receptor population.

At present, the involvement of prostaglandins in the parturient processes is clearly recognised. Our experiments on the administration of arachidonic acid suggest that prostaglandin production is suppressed during pregnancy. It is likely that the conceptus is responsible for this suppression. A clear understanding of factors regulating prostaglandin production, both fetal and maternal, would provide further insight into the control of parturition in the monkey. Finally, the role of oxytocin from both the mother and fetus in these processes needs elucidation.

REFERENCES

1. Challis JRG, Robinson JS and Thorburn GD: Retal and maternal endocrine changes during pregnancy and parturition. In: *The Fetus and Birth*, Ciba foundation Symposium no 47, Amsterdam, Elsevier/Excerpta Medica/North-Holland, 1977, p 211-227.
2. Thorburn GD, Challis JRG and Robinson JS: Endocrine control of parturition. In: *Biology of the Uterus*, Wynn RM (ed), New York, 1977, p 653-732.
3. Kittinger, GW: Endocrine regulation of fetal development and its relation to parturition in the rhesus monkey. In: *The Fetus and Birth*, Amsterdam, Elsevier/Excerpta Medica/North-Holland, 1977, p 235-249.
4. Novy, MJ: Endocrine and pharmacological factors which influence the onset of labour in rhesus monkeys. In: *The Fetus and Birth*, Amsterdam, Elsevier/Excerpta Medica/North-Holland, 1977, p 259-288.
5. van Wagenen G and Newton WH: Pregnancy in the monkey after removal of the fetus. *Surg Gynecol Obstet* 77, 539-543 (1943).
6. Lanman JT, Thau R, Sundaram K, Brinson A and Bonk R: Ovarian and placental origins of plasma progesterone following fetectomy in monkeys *(Macaca mulatta)*. *Endocrinology* 96, 591-597 (1975).
7. Honnebier WJ and Swaab DF: The influence of anencephaly upon intrauterine growth of the fetus and placenta upon gestation length. *J Obstet Gynaecol Br Commonw* 80, 577-588 (1973).
8. Liggins GC, Fairclough RJ, Grieves SA, Kendall JZ and Knox BS: The mechanism of the initiation of parturition in the ewe. *Rec Prog Horm Res* 29, 111-150 (1973).
9. Chez RA, Hutchinson DL, Salazar H and Mintz DH: Some effects of fetal and maternal hypophysectomy in pregnancy. *Am J Obstet Gynecol* 108, 643-650 (1970).
10. Mueller-Heubach E, Myers RE and Adamson K: Effects of adrenalectomy on pregnancy length in the rhesus monkey. *Am J Obstet Gynecol* 112, 221-226 (1972).

11. Rees LH, Jack PMB, Thomas AL and Nathanielsz PW: Role of fetal adrenocorticotrophin during parturition in the sheep. *Nature (Lond)* 253, 274-275 (1975).
12. Silman RE, Chard T, Lowry PJ, Smith I and Young IM: Human foetal pituitary peptides and parturition. *Nature (Lond)* 260, 716-718 (1976).
13. Challis JRG and Torosis JD: Is αMSH trophic to adrenal function in the foetus? *Nature (Lond)* 269, 818-819 (1977).
14. Silman RE, Holland D, Chard T, Lowry PJ, Hope J, Robinson JS and Thorburn GD: The ACTH 'family tree' of the rhesus monkey changes with development. *Nature (Lond)* 276, 526-528 (1978).
15. Jaffe RB, Serrón-Ferré M, Huhtaniemi I and Korenbrot, C: Regulation of the primate fetal adrenal gland and testis *in vitro* and *in vivo*. *J Steroid Biochem* 8, 479-490 (1977).
16. Jaffe RB, Serón-Ferré M, Parer JT and Lawrence CC: The primate fetal pituitaryadrenal axis in the perinatal period. *Am J Obstet Gynecol* 131, 164-168 (1978).
17. Challis JRG, Hartley P, Johnson P, Patrick JE, Robinson JS and Thorburn GD: Steroids in the amniotic fluid of the rhesus monkey *(Macaca mulatta)*. *J Endocrinol* 73, 355-363 (1977).
18. Minei LJ and Suzuki K: Role of fetal deglutition and micturition in the production and turnover of amniotic fluid in the monkey. *Obstet Gynecol* 48, 177-181 (1976).
19. Challis JRG and Manning FA: Control of parturition in subhuman primates. *Seminars Perinatol* 2, 247-260 (1978).
20. Pepe GJ, Titus JA and Townsley JD: Increasing fetal adrenal formation of cortisol from pregnenolone during baboon *(Papio papio)* gestation. *Biol Reprod* 17, 701-705 (1977).
21. Lanman JT: Parturition in non human primates. *Biol Reprod* 16, 28-38 (1977).
22. Bosu WTK, Johansson EDB and Gemzell C: Influence of oophorectomy, luteectomy, foetal death and dexamethasone on the peripheral plasma levels of oestrogen and progesterone in the rhesus monkey (*Macaca mulatta)*. *Acta Endocrinol* 75, 601-616 (1974).
23. Hodgen GD and Tullner WW: Plasma estrogens, progesterone and chorionic gonadotrophin in pregnant rhesus monkeys *(Macaca mulatta)* after ovariectomy. *Steroids* 25, 275-282.
24. Thau R, Lanman JT and Brinson A: Declining plasma progesterone concentration with advancing gestation in blood from umbilical and uterine veins. *Biol Reprod* 14, 507-509 (1976).
25. Corner GW, Ramsey EM and Stran H: Patterns of myometrial activity in the rhesus monkey in pregnancy. *Am J Obstet Gynecol* 85, 179-185 (1963).
26. Hopper BR and Tullner WW: Urinary estrogens: excretion patterns in pregnant rhesus monkeys. *Steroids* 9, 517-527 (1967).
27. Liskowski L, Wolff RC, Chandler J and Myers RK: Urinary estrogen excretion in pregnant rhesus monkeys. *Biol Reprod* 3, 55-60 (1970).
28. Bosu WTK, Johansson EDB and Gemzell C: Peripheral plasma levels of oestrogens, progesterone and 17β – hydroxyprogesterone during gestation in the rhesus monkey. *Acta Endocrinol* 74, 348-360 (1973).
29. Challis JRG, Davies IJ, Benirschke K, Hendrickx AG and Ryan KJ: The concentrations of progesterone, estrone and estradiol-17β in the peripheral plasma of the rhesus monkey during the final third of gestation and after the induction of abortion with $PGF_{2}\alpha$. *Endocrinology* 95, 547-553 (1974).
30. Bosu WTK, Johansson EDB and Gemzell C: Peripheral plasma levels of oestrogen and progesterone in pregnant rhesus monkeys treated with dexamethasone. *Acta Endocrinol* 74, 338-347 (1973).
31. Challis JRG, Davies IJ, Benirschke K, Hendrickx AG and Ryan KJ: The effects of dexamethasone on plasma steroid levels and fetal adrenal histology in the pregnant rhesus monkey. *Endocrinology* 95, 1300-1305 (1974).
32. Mitchell MD, Patrick JE, Robinson JS, Thorburn GD and Challis JRG: Prostaglandins in the plasma and amniotic fluid of rhesus monkeys during pregnancy and after intrauterine fetal death. *J Endocrinol* 71, 67-76 (1976).

33. Atkinson LE, Hotchkiss J, Fritz GR, Surve AH, Neill JD and Knobil E: Circulating levels of steroids and chorionic gonadotrophin during pregnancy in the rhesus monkey, with special attention to rescue of the corpus luteum in early pregnancy. *Biol Reprod* 12, 335-345 (1975).
34. Kirton KT, Pharriss BB and Forbes AD: Some effects of prostaglandin E_2 and $F_{2\alpha}$ on the pregnant rhesus monkey. *Biol Reprod* 3, 163-168 (1970).
35. Kirton K, Duncan G, Oesterling T and Forbes A: Prostaglandins and reproduction in the rhesus monkey. *Ann NY Acad Sci* 180, 163-168 (1971).
36. Robinson JS, Chapman RLK, Challis JRG, Mitchell MD and Thorburn GD: Extra-amniotic arachidonic acid administration and the suppression of uterine prostaglandin synthesis during pregnancy in the rhesus monkey. *J Reprod Fertil*, 54, 369-373 (1978).
37. Novy MJ, Cook MJ and Manaugh L: Indomethacin block of normal onset of parturition in primates. *Am J Obstet Gynecol* 118, 412-416 (1974).
38. Manaugh L and Novy MJ: Effects of indomethacin on corpus luteum function and pregnancy in rhesus monkeys. *Fertil Steril* 27, 588-598 (1976).
39. Lonigro AJ, Itskowitz HD, Croshaw K and McGiff JC: Dependency of renal blood flow on prostaglandin synthesis in the dog. *Circ Res* 32, 712 (1973).
40. McGiff JC, Croshaw K and Itskowitz HD: Prostaglandins and renal function. *Fed Proc* 33, 39 (1974).
41. Friedman WF, Hirschklau MJ, Printz MP, Pitlick PT and Kirkpatrick SE: Pharamacologic closure of patent ductus arteriosus in the premature infant. *New Eng J Med* 295, 526-529 (1976).
42. Heyman MA, Rudolph AM and Silverman NH: Closure of the ductus arteriosus in premature infants by inhibition of prostaglandin synthesis. *New Eng J Med* 295, 530-533 (1976).
43. Cassin S, Tyler T and Leffler C: Pulmonary vascular responses to prostaglandins and prostaglandin synthetase inhibitors in perinatal goats. In: *Advances in Prostaglandin and Thromboxane Research*, vol. 4, Coceani F and Olley PM (eds), New York, Raven Press, 1978, p 249-256.
44. Mitchell MD, Clover L, Thorburn GD and Robinson JS: Specific change in the direction of prostaglandin synthesis by intra-uterine tissues of the rhesus monkey (Macaca mulatta) during late pregnancy. *J Endocrinol* 78, 343-350 (1978).
45. Challis JRG, Davies IJ, Hendrickx AG and Ryan KJ: Prostaglandin F in the peripheral plasma of the rhesus monkey in normal pregnancy and after the administration of dexamethasone and $PGF_{2\alpha}$. *Prostaglandins* 6, 389-396 (1974).
46. Karim SMM, Hillier K and Devlin J: Distribution of E_1, E_2, $F_{1\alpha}$ and $F_{2\alpha}$ in some animal tissues. *J Pharm Pharmacol* 20, 749-753 (1968).
47. Mitchell MD and Flint APF: Prostaglandin production by intrauterine tissues from periparturient sheep: use of a superfusion technique. *J Endocrinol* 76, 111-121 (1978).
48. Hamberg M, Svensson J and Samuelsson B: Thromboxanes: a new group of biologically active compounds derived from prostaglandin endoperoxides. *Proc Natl Acad Sci USA* 72, 2994-2998 (1975).
49. Moncada S, Gryglewski R, Bunting S and Vane JR: An enzyme isolated from arteries transforms prostaglandin endoperoxides to an unstable substance that inhibits platelet aggregation. *Nature (Lond)* 263, 663-665 (1976).
50. Mitchell MD, Bibby JG, Hicks BR, Redman CWG, Anderson ABM and Turnbull AC: Thromboxane B_2 and human parturition: concentrations in plasma and production in vitro. *J Endocrinol* 78, 435-441 (1978).
51. Mitchell MD, Hicks BR, Thorburn GD and Robinson JS: Production of thromboxane B_2 by intrauterine tissues from late pregnant rhesus monkeys *(Macaca mulatta)*. *J Endocrinol*, 79, 103-106 (1978).
52. Ham EA, Cirillo VJ, Zanetti ME and Kuehl FA: Estrogen-directed synthesis of specific prostaglandins in uterus. *Proc Natl Acad Sci USA* 72, 1420-1424 (1975).

53. Gustavii B: Human decidua and uterine contractility. In: *The Fetus and Birth*, Ciba Foundation Symposium no 47, Amsterdam, Elsevier/Excerpta Medica/North-Holland, 1977, p 343-353.
54. Schultz FM, Macdonald PC and Johnston JM: Arachidonic acid in human amniotic fluid and its relationship to labor. *Gynecol Invest* 5, 62 (1974).
55. Saed SA, McDonald-Gibson WJ, Cuthbert J, Copas JL, Schneider C, Gardiner PJ, Butt NM and Collier HOJ: Endogenous inhibitor of prostaglandin synthetase *Nature (Lond)* 270, 32-36 (1977).
56. Horne CHW, Bohn H and Towler CM: Pregnancy associated α_2 glycoprotein. In: *Plasma hormone assays in evaluation of fetal wellbeing*, Klopper A (ed.), Edinburgh, 1976, p 147-173.
57. Myers RE, Symchych P, Strauss L, Comas A, Figueroa-Longo J, Kerenyi T and Adamson K: Morphological changes of uterine wall following intra-amniotic injection of hypertonic saline in the rhesus monkey. *Am J Obstet Gynecol* 119, 877-888 (1974).
58. Schiller HS, Holm RA and Sackett GP: Alterations in steroid binding plasma proteins in *Macaca nemestrima* during pregnancy. *Am J Physiol* 234, E489-493 (1978).
59. Willman EA and Collins WP: Distribution of prostaglandins E_2 and $F_{2\alpha}$ within the foeto-placental unit throughout human pregnancy. *J Endocrinol* 69, 413-419 (1976).

SOME PHYSIOLOGICAL ASPECTS OF UTERINE CONTRACTILITY IN MAN

MENNO VAN LEEUWEN, JAAP TH.F. BOELES AND GEORGE M.J.A. WOLFS

Vertebrate smooth muscle has, for practical purposes, been categorized as belonging to either the single-unit or the multi-unit type (1). Single-unit or unitary muscles behave, as the word implies, as single units, presumably because electrical conduction takes place from cell to cell. The activity of such muscles is myogenic, in contrast to the multi-unit muscles, which are normally supplied with motor nerves. This latter type of smooth muscle consists of many independent units. If these do contract in an orderly manner, it is because of proper motor timing. The uterus is generally said to be a single-unit muscle. If one considers the well-coordinated contractions of labour or the contractions during menstruation, the uterus would certainly qualify for the single-unit category. At other times, however, the myometrium behaves as if it consisted of multiple, rather independent units, as will be shown in the next pages.

MEASURING UTERINE ACTIVITY

Mechanical activity

A well-known clinical method of measuring the mechanical activity of the human uterus *in vivo* is the recording of the intrauterine pressure. Usually this is not done for the purpose of studying the mechanism of labour, but it is used in conjunction with a continuous recording of the fetal cardiotachogram, as a means of monitoring the condition of the unborn child. Often it is not really the intrauterine pressure that is being recorded, but a so-called external tocodynamogram, i.e. a recording of local mechanical activity of the uterus by means of a displacement transducer. This method, of course, does not permit the measurement of the pressure acting on the child, particularly not a continuously elevated "resting" pressure. From a point of view of fetal monitoring this is a serious drawback.

Intrauterine pressure can be measured relatively easily. It has been shown that it is not necessary to puncture the amniotic sac. An open-tip catheter,

M.J.N.C. Keirse et al. (eds.), Human Parturition, 41-48.

inserted between the membranes and the uterine wall, yields a pressure curve which is practically indistinguishable from a pressure record simultaneously obtained via a catheter in the amniotic fluid (2).

Such a pressure curve, however, measures the net result of the activity or non-activity of all parts of the uterus. It fails to give a good impression, at least not in any straightforward manner, of the degree of organization in the uterus. For any attempt at understanding the mechanics of labour, insight into the temporo-spatial organization of uterine activity and its possible changes during the course of labour, is of considerable importance. It is, moreover, not inconceivable that a better understanding of this aspect of uterine activity could be meaningfully applied in clinical practice, e.g. to judge the progress of labour or the effects of attempts to either stimulate or inhibit uterine activity.

Cibils and Hendricks (3) clearly showed by means of pressure catheters implanted into the uterine wall of the (post-partum) human uterus, that the mechanical activity does not always occur synchronously throughout the uterus and that local contractions do not necessarily show on the record of intrauterine pressure. This is to be expected if relatively small parts of the myometrium shorten, simultaneously stretching passive parts.

The electrical activity

Implantation of multiple pressure catheters in the myometrium is not generally practicable. It is much simpler to measure the electrical activity. From a technical point of view this is, in principle, not complicated, and it offers the possibility of observing the activity of fairly small regions of the uterine muscle. Most recordings of electrohysterographic activity, however, have been made with electrodes affixed to the abdominal wall (4-6). A simpler technique is hardly thinkable, but it is fraught with problems. For the abovementioned purpose of obtaining a close-up view of detailed activity of the uterus, one would like to have one's electrodes as close to the myometrium as possible, if not in it. Any intervening tissue or organ will indeed reduce the signal-to-noise ratio. This is the most likely explanation for findings that electrograms obtained simultaneously from internal and external electrodes resembled each other only roughly and did not show the same relations in time with the intrauterine pressure (7). Statements to the effect that electrical activity similar to that recorded during labour, could be obtained from the abdomen of a male by stretching the skin (7), or during a Valsalva manoeuvre (8), certainly do not inspire much confidence in the method of external electrohysterography.

It is relatively easy, and certainly if intrauterine pressure is being measured by means of a catheter in the extraovular, intrauterine space, to also introduce a catheter carrying a number of small electrodes, whose connecting wires run through the lumen of the catheter to the outside world. For the non-pregnant uterus Van Geldorp et al. (9) have developed a technique for inserting a bipolar needle electrode in the fundus or even an intrauterine contraceptive device modified to contain the electrodes. This device can be left in situ more or less chronically and permits recordings to be made repeatedly, with very little discomfort to the wearer of the IUD (Dr. H.J. van Geldorp, personal communication). A technique using intrauterine needle electrodes has also been applied to the human parturient uterus, by Sakaguchi and Nakajima (10).

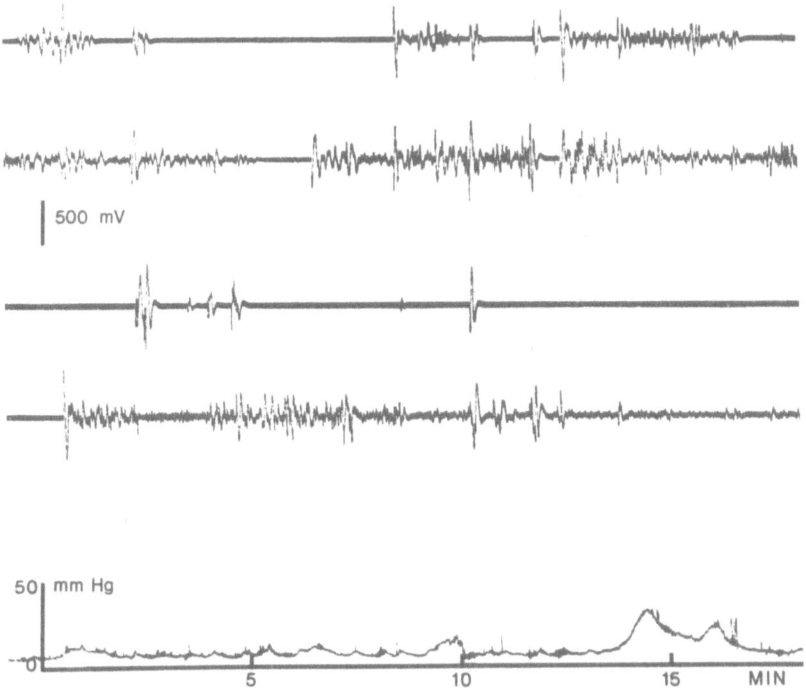

Fig. 1. Non-synchronous activity early during the first stage of labour. Electromyograms and intrauterine pressure.

ELECTRICAL AND MECHANICAL ACTIVITY OF THE HUMAN UTERUS *IN VIVO*

During labour

The general picture in spontaneous as well as in induced labour is as follows: if measurements are started during very early labour, little activity can be measured. The electrical activity is irregular and of low voltage; there is no rhythmic activity (fig. 1). The intrauterine pressure curve is in agreement with this: it shows small, irregular pressure elevations, without any obvious relationship with the electromyogram (EMG). Recordings from several electrodes simultaneously show little synchrony. Over a period of several hours this situation gradually develops into a pattern of regular, rhythmic activity. The electrical activity starts to be grouped into bursts, which increase in voltage. During the progress of labour many short bursts make way for fewer, longer bursts with longer intervals between them. At the same time the

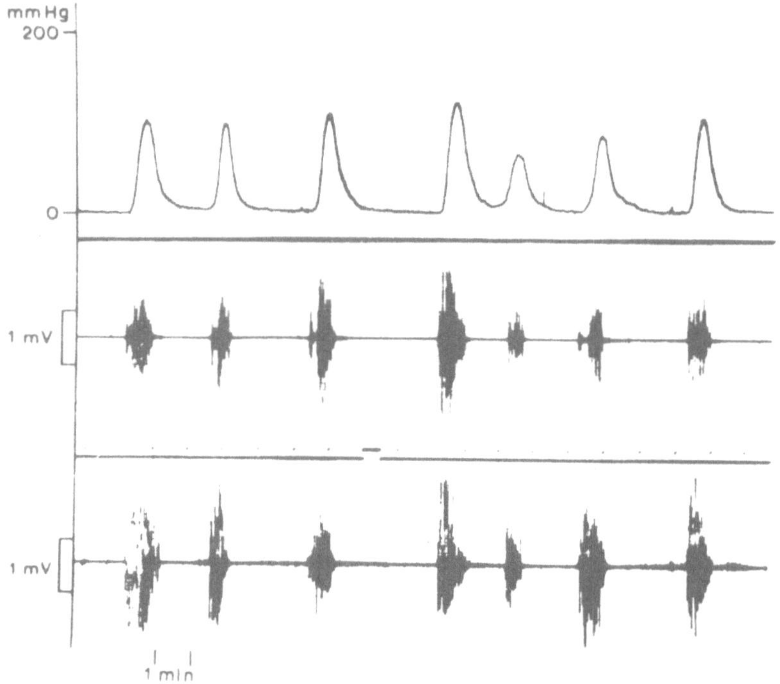

Fig. 2. A typical example of well-coordinated labour activity. Electrical activity only during the rising phase of intrauterine pressure. (From Wolfs and van Leeuwen [11].)

mechanical activity increases, the irregularities disappear and regular contractions result, which increase in amplitude and rate of rise (fig. 2). The EMG now has a clear-cut relationship to the pressure waveform; each increase in pressure is accompanied by an EMG-burst (10-12). In spontaneous, but often not in oxytocin-induced labour, the final stage of this process is characterized by EMG-bursts which start several seconds before any noticeable increase in intrauterine pressure and which stop when the pressure has reached its peak, or perhaps it is better to say that the intrauterine pressure starts to decline as soon as all electrical activity, i.e. active contraction, has ceased.

The non-pregnant uterus

The non-pregnant uterus seems to repeat the above picture during each menstrual cycle. During the first days of menstruation EMG-bursts, lasting about 30 s, are accompanied by intrauterine pressure waves of about 30 to 50 mm Hg (fig. 3). Between the bursts no significant electrical or mechanical activity can be measured. Electrical activity then decreases in the course of the menstrual cycle, and becomes more or less continuous, to increase again at the end of the luteal phase, when the burst activity of menstruation reappears. The more or less continuous, low-voltage electrical activity during the late follicular phase, is not in any obvious way correlated with the small changes in intrauterine pressure (9).

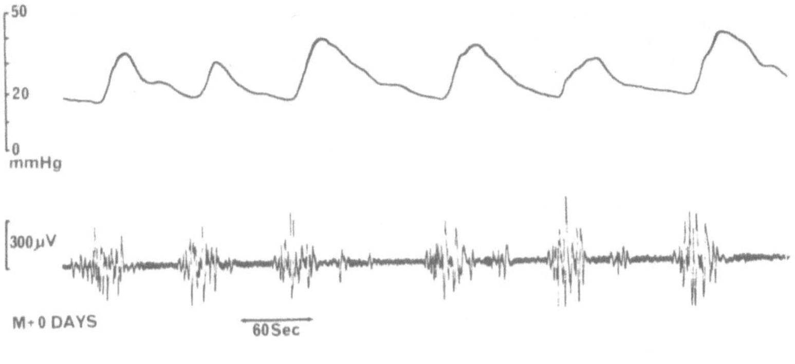

Fig. 3. Electromyogram and intrauterine pressure of the non-pregnant human uterus on day 1 of menstruation. (By courtesy of Dr H. J. van Geldorp.)

GENERAL DISCUSSION

The distinction between single-unit and multiple-unit smooth muscle appears to be of limited value as far as uterus is concerned. If one assumes that the only function of the uterus is to contract forcefully, the single-unit view seems very appropriate. It is, however, an equally important uterine function *not* to contract rhythmically and forcefully, e.g. during most of the 40 weeks of gestation. In the course of labour, and during the menstrual cycle, a change-over from a multi unit-like activity to a more unitary behaviour can be observed.

All of the electrical and mechanical phenomena described for the uterus during labour can adequately be explained by a process of gradually increasing synchronization of myometrial cells. The low-voltage, irregular to rather continuous electrical activity accompanied by irregular and small increases in intrauterine pressure are in this view caused by a very small degree of synchronization. In the final stage, the uterus is maximally synchronized and contracts in a coordinated way, as one muscle. The difference between these extremes is like that between a fibrillating heart and a normally beating one, with similar functional consequences. It is perhaps useful to mention that the drastic changes in the intrauterine pressure waveform that occur in the course of labour, might be ascribed to nothing but an increasing degree of synchronization of myometrial cells, as fig. 4 attempts to illustrate. This, of

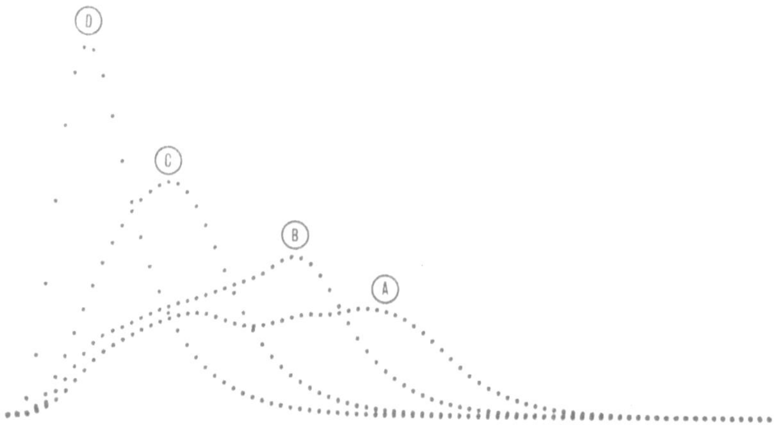

Fig. 4. Illustration of the fact that improved synchronization of uterine activity might account for the changes in the shape of the intrauterine pressure waveform during labour. In this computer simulation the uterus is assumed to consist of a large number of contractile units. All units are activated at random, within a given length of time, which is made shorter as one goes from curve A towards curve D.

course, is not intended to propose that the increase in contractile strength that occurs in the course of labour is to be attributed solely to changes in temporo-spatial organization of uterine activity. We do think, however, that such changes contribute significantly, and are in particular responsible for the changes in shape of the pressure waveform.

The mechanism responsible for the synchronization process is as yet unknown. Undoubtedly, humoral factors may play an important role. Our experience with oxytocin as an inducer of labour seems to indicate that this hormone is not by itself capable of eliciting or accelerating the process of synchronization.

Synchronized behaviour of the uterus presupposes a good intercellular communication. The factors responsible for it can be assumed to be of two types: either they prevent such communication when present and good intercellular communication then becomes possible upon their withdrawal, or they are necessary for intercellular communication and probably increase during labour. In any case, it is clear that uncoordinated contractions are not very efficient in expelling the fetus. In this respect we are apparently dealing with an elegant mechanism of protection against pre-term labour. The recent publication by Garfield et al. (13) is extremely important in this regard. They report that no gap junctions (nexuses) can be found in the pregnant (rat) uterus, except if the animal is in labour. Furthermore, they mention that this is also the case in rabbits in which abortion is caused by bilateral ovariectomy, unless the pregnancy is maintained by the administration of progesterone. It is immediately clear that these observations, for the first time, offer an anatomical explanation for the increasing synchronization of uterine activity that is perhaps *the* characteristic of labour. It is of considerable interest to see if nexus formation plays such a crucial role in human parturition, too, and to try and understand the endocrinology of this mechanism. Also, it would be interesting to see if gap junctions come and go cyclically during the menstrual cycle.

Finally, a few remarks should be made about the comparability of the human and the animal uterus. It is of course, true, that great differences exist within the human uterus and that of most animals, and even between the uteri of various species. This is not only so from an anatomical point of view, but certainly also applies to physiological aspects. It is therefore interesting to find that our observations on the electrical and mechanical behaviour of the human parturient uterus agree so well with the results obtained in some non-primates (14, 15). On second thoughts this need not surprise us too much. The answer to the question how such similarity is possible in the face of so many differences, undoubtedly lies in the fact that we are dealing with mechanisms with a common "goal", viz. the retention of the fetus during the larger part of gestation and the eventual expulsion at the moment of birth. Apparently we must conclude that the ultimate mechanism through which this is achieved is a completely asynchronous behaviour of the uterus during the greater part of pregnancy which, towards the end, changes into well-coordinated contractions, as intercellular communication becomes estabilished. When we observe the activity of the uterus by means of electrodes and pressure catheters we are, irrespective of the species, looking at a final common mechanism, possibly reached by different routes.

REFERENCES

1. Bozler E: Action potentials and conduction of excitation in muscle. *Biol Symp* 3, 95-109 (1941).
2. Csapo A: Extra ovular pressure – its diagnostic value. *Am J Obstet Gynecol* 90, 493-504 (1964).
3. Cibils L and Hendricks CH: Uterine contractility on the first day of the puerperium. *Am J Obstet Gynecol* 103, 238-243 (1969).
4. Sureau C: Étude de l'activité électrique de l'utérus au course de la gestation et du travail. *Gynécol Obstét* 55 (2), 153-175 (1956).
5. Dill LV and Maiden RM: The electrical potentials of the human uterus in labor. *Am J. Obstet Gynecol* 52, 735-745 (1946).
6. Veit J: Das Elektrometrogram. *Zbl Gynäkol* 36, 161-162 (1912).
7. Hon EHG and Davis CD: Cutaneous and uterine electrical potentials in labor; an experiment. *Obstet Gynecol* 12/1, 47-53 (1958).
8. Freundlich JJ and Wingate MB: An evaluation of an external electromyographic system for recording uterine contractions during labor. *Am J Obstet Gynecol* 116, 822-826 (1973).
9. Van Geldorp HJ, Wolfs GMJA, Van Leeuwen M and Wallenburg HCS: The electric and mechanical activity of the non-pregnant human uterus in vivo. Presented at the 16th meeting of the Dutch Federative Society, 1975.
10. Sakaguchi M and Nakajima A: Electrical activity of the human uterus in labor. *Am J Obstet Gynecol* 108, 992-993 (1970).
11. Wolfs G and Van Leeuwen M: Electromyography of the human parturient uterus. In: *Recent Progress in Obstetrics and Gynaecology*, Persianinov LS and Chervakova TV (eds), Amsterdam, Excerpta Medica, 1974, p. 431-442.
12. Wolfs G, Van Leeuwen M, Rottinghuis H and Boeles JThF: An electromyographic study of the human uterus during labor. *Obstet Gynecol* 37, 241-246 (1971).
13. Garfield RE, Sims S and Daniel EE: Gap junctions: Their presence and necessity in myometrium during parturition. *Science* 198, 958-959 (1977).
14. Csapo A and Takeda H: Effect of progesterone on the electric activity and intrauterine pressure of pregnant and parturient rabbits. *Am J Obstet Gynecol* 9, 221-231 (1965).
15. Ichijo M and Ujiie Y: Studies on electrohysterogram. *Tohoku J Exp Med* 90, 9-24 (1966).

FUNCTION OF PITUITARY HORMONES IN HUMAN PARTURITION – A COMPARISON WITH DATA IN THE RAT

DICK F. SWAAB AND KEES BOER

A role for pituitary hormones in parturition has been proposed ever since the orginal observation by Dale in 1906 (1). While studying the effect of tissue extracts on blood pressure, he observed that pituitary extracts caused uterine contractions in a pregnant cat. In the same year as Dale's full paper on the oxytocin effect of neurohypophysial extracts appeared (1909) (2), Blair-Bell (3) reported his observations on the clinical application of such extracts. Since in the early fifties the structures of the neurohypophysial hormones oxytocin and arginine-vasopressin (AVP) (fig. 1a) have been elucidated and the hormones synthesized (4), an avalanche of information has become available on the production sites of these hormones in the neurones of the hypothalamus, including data on the mechanism of their transport and release. In spite of these advances and of the extensive clinical use of oxytocin for the initiation and augmentation of slow and dysfunctional labour (Turnbull, this volume), the possible function of this hormone in the physiology of labour is still in dispute.

In 1938, Bell and Robson (5) showed that in addition to the mother, the fetus might be another source of neurohypophysial hormones. During the last decade, the foresight of these authors has become apparent: the data on fetal neuroendocrine mechanisms operating in the process of labour in various species are overwhelming (e.g., 6). These data involve not only neurohypophysial hormones but also the family of ACTH and related peptides. However, their role in physiology of labour in man is far from elucidated.

The observations on the possible involvement of the maternal or fetal pituitary in human labour are necessarily based mainly on pathological material and on fragmentary and indirect observations. For this reason, and because experimental data appear to provide similar and complementary data, the observations in the human will be compared with experimental data, in particular in the rat.

M.J.N.C. Keirse et al. (eds.), Human Parturition, 49-71.

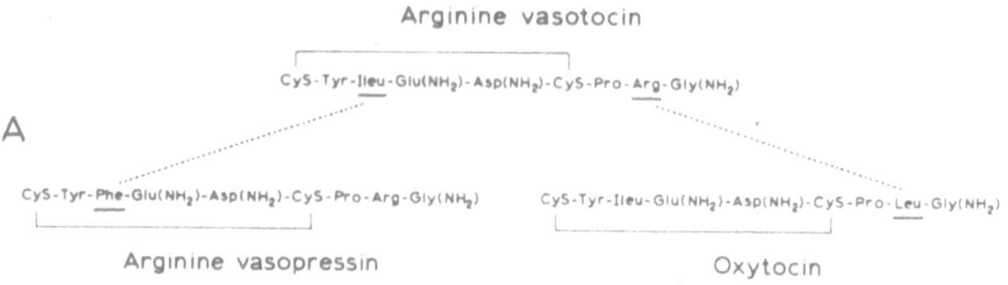

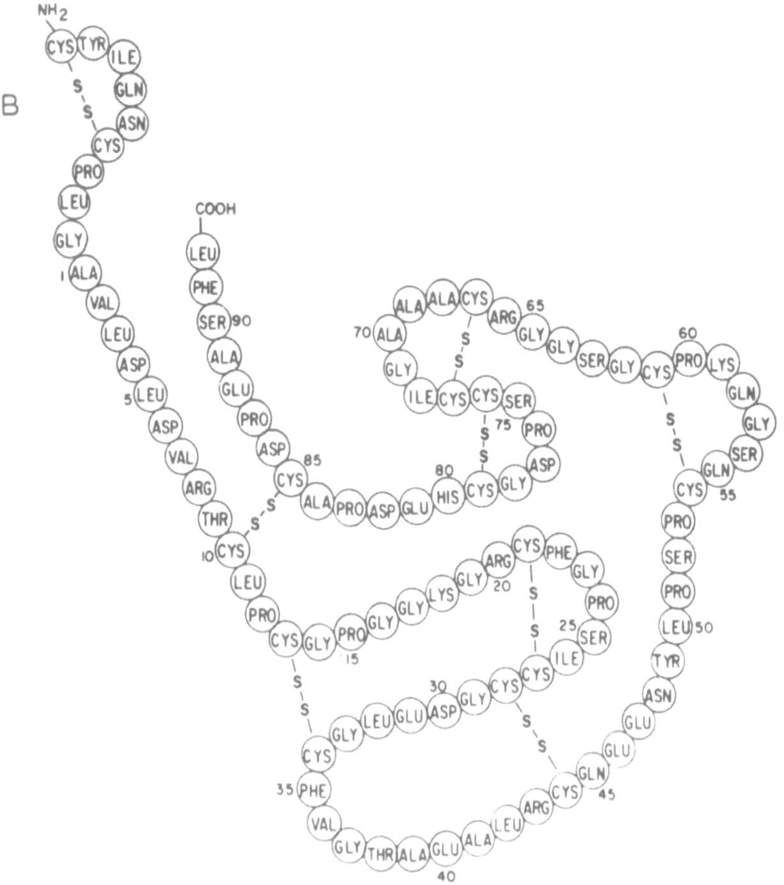

Fig. 1a. Hypothetical scheme for the molecular evolution of neurohypophysial peptides. It is assumed that arginine-vasotocin was the ancestral peptide and that principles changed during vertebrate phylogeny by steps involving one amino-acid substitution at a time. (Sawyer, 95.)
Fig. 1b. Suggested structure for the prohormone of oxytocin. The arrow shows where the transamidase would split the prohormone into oxytocin and neurophysin. (From B. T. Pickering, 100.)

NEUROHYPOPHYSIAL HORMONES

Oxytocin and vasopressin are synthesized as a hormone-neurophysin complex (fig. 1b) by the large hypothalamic neurons of the supraoptic (SON) and paraventricular (PVN) nuclei (fig. 2). During its transport along the nerve fibres to the neurohypophysis and to the external zone of the median eminence, this hormone complex (located in vesicles of about 140 nm diameter; cf. 7) is split into neurohypophysial hormones and their respective neurophysins (fig. 1b; 8). Release of neurohypophysial hormones from the nerve endings is regulated by action potentials, generated by nerve cell bodies in the hypothalamus, travelling along the nerve fibres to the pituitary (9, 10).

By means of immunohistochemistry it has been shown that individual neurones produce only one type of hormone, i.e., either oxytocin or vasopressin and its matching neurophysin (11, 12). Moreover, the earlier ideas on

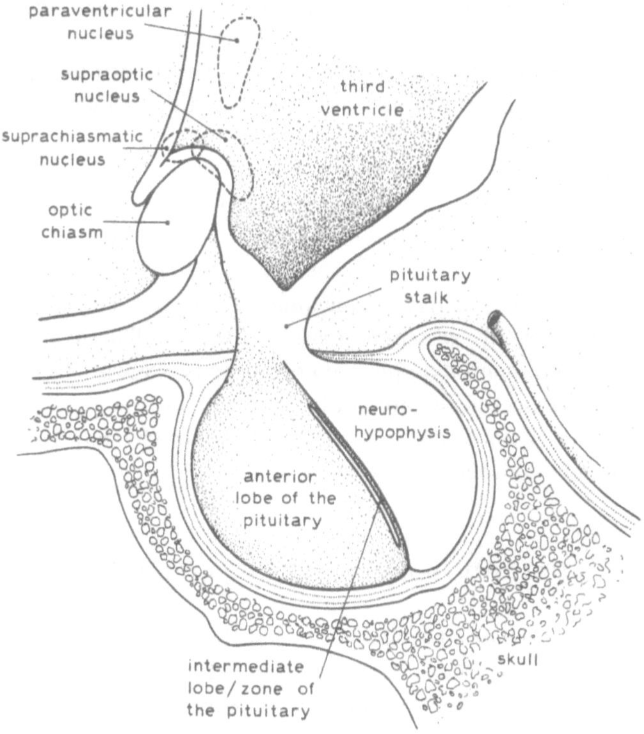

Fig. 2. Schematic reconstruction of the human hypothalamus and pituitary. (For explanation, see text.)

a designated function of the nuclei in the synthesis of one of the two hormones (i.e., that the PVN would synthesize mainly oxytocin, and the SON AVP) was contradicted by findings in the rat which showed the ratio of oxytocin- and vasopressin-producing cells to be about the same in both nuclei. However, since the SON is 2.5 times larger than the PVN, this nucleus is not only the main source of vasopressin, but also of oxytocin (11), as has been confirmed by direct measurements in these nuclei (13). Oxytocin and vasopressin are also produced in the human hypothalamus in separate neurones in the SON and PVN (14).

Neurohypophysial hormones are found in the fetus long before term. In the human they are present from 16 weeks of pregnancy, and in the rat from 17-18 days of pregnancy onwards (for review, see 15). It is not certain whether the neurohypophysial hormones in the fetus consist only of vasopressin and oxytocin; some authors assume the presence of a related "fetal" hormone for mammals (i.e., arginine-vasotocin, fig. 1a).

In addition to hypothalamo-neurohypophysial fibres, these neurosecretory cells have extrahypothalamic hormone-containing fibres that have been shown to be dispersed throughout the brain and even into the spinal cord (e.g., 16, 17). These fibres originate not only from the 'classical' neurosecretory nuclei, the SON and the PVN, the islands of the neurosecretory neurones and single neurones along their tracts, but also from the suprachiasmatic nucleus which contains only vasopressin (produced in vesicles that are smaller {about 90 nm} than those of the SON; 7). These vasopressin containing cells of the suprachiasmatic nucleus (fig. 2) also exist in man (14). The data on the extensive distribution of extrahypothalamic neurosecretory pathways, confirmed quantitatively by radioimmunoassay (13), fit well in the newly hypothesized function of neurohypophysial hormones in behaviour and memory (e.g., 18). With respect to the present topic of interest, the possibility exists that reproductive or allied behaviour may be influenced by the release of these hormones directly into the brain.

THE FAMILY OF ACTH/LPH AND RELATED COMPOUNDS

The intermediate lobe or intermediate zone of the pituitary (fig. 2) produces a number of peptides with melanocyte stimulating activity. Within these hormones a common sequence (adrenocorticotrophic hormone {ACTH} 4-10) of 7 amino acids occurs. These peptides are ACTH (1-39), α-MSH (α-melanocyte stimulating hormone = ACTH 1-13), β-MSH (=β/γ-lipotrophic hormone {LPH} 41-58 and which is probably an isolation artefact),

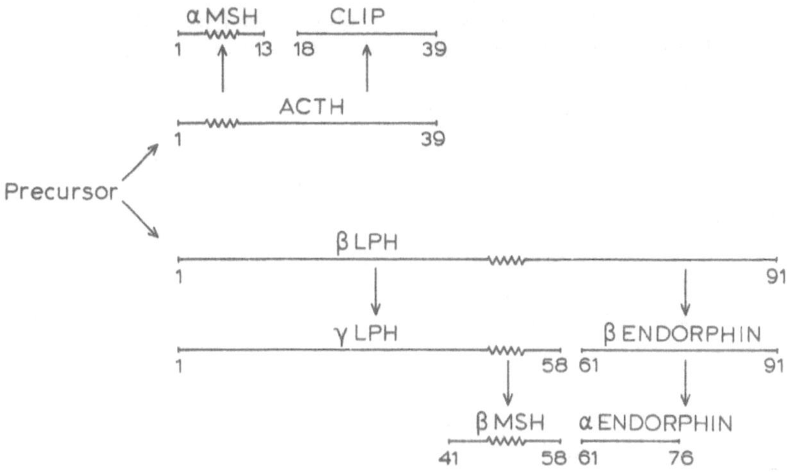

Fig. 3. The family of ACTH/LPH and related peptides. MSH: melanocyte stimulating hormone, CLIP: corticotropin-like intermediate lobe peptide, ACTH: adrenocorticotropic hormone, LPH: lipotropic hormone; ⁄\/\/ = common sequence of amino acids (ACTH 4-10).

γ-LPH (= β-LPH 1-58), and β-LPH (fig. 3). The fragment ACTH 18-39 is known as corticotrophin-like intermediate lobe peptide (CLIP). ACTH is supposed to be a precursor for both α-MSH and CLIP that would split within the pituitary cells by enzymatic action (19) . In a similar way the C-terminal fragments of β-LPH would split off β-endorphin (= β-LPH 61-91) and α-endorphin (= β-LPH 61-76) which have morphine-like effects. Studies on an ACTH producing tumor cell line make it conceivable that all these peptides arise from one common precursor, a glycoprotein of 31,000 D molecular weight (20,21; Tilders, personal communication). The manner in which this precursor would be cleaved enzymatically would thus determine which peptides are produced by a given cell, while the pattern of cleavage might vary during the course of fetal development (cf. 22, 23).

THE MATERNAL NEUROHYPOPHYSIS AND THE INITIATION OF PARTURITION

In the last decade, earlier ideas on the possible role of oxytocin as a major factor in the chain of events that result in labour have swung to the opposite view. Many authors deny a role of oxytocin in the initiation of parturition and doubt its functional significance in the course of labour except for the expulsion phase. This opinion is based mainly on the following findings:

(1) Labours at term have been described in hypophysectomized animals by some authors, although others observed a prolongation of pregnancy (for review, see 24).

(2) In women suffering from diabetes insipidus, either after a trauma, a tumor or due to a genetic cause, deliveries have been reported to occur at term (25, 26, 27, 28, 29, 30).

(3) The idea that oxytocin would only have a permissive function in the initiation of labour was sustained during the last few years by findings of Chard *et al.* (e.g. 31), who could not detect any oxytocin in maternal venous plasma.

Observations in man and rat, however, lead at present to the conviction that the above-mentioned findings can no longer be used as an argument against a role of oxytocin in the initiation of parturition.

Lesions of the hypothalamo-neurohypophysial system

The data on the initiation and course of labour after lesions of the HNS are quite confusing (see 24). Most of the confusion can probably be explained by misinterpretation of results due to a lack of knowledge of the exact consequences of the operations at the time the experiments were performed.

Hypophysectomy is presently known not to abolish completely neurohypophysial hormone release, while interruption or lesioning of the hypothalamo-neurohypophysial system at higher levels creates interpretation pitfalls since so many structures are lesioned, i.e., cell bodies, efferent fibres, blood vessels and nervous inputs.

Removal of the pituitary is followed by a rapid regeneration of the proximal part of the cut nerve fibres into a "miniature posterior lobe" (32, 33). Fisher *et al.* (34) noticed that if the median eminence was left intact after complete hypophysectomy, no permanent diabetes insipidus would result. However, even if severe diabetes develops and remains, the milk-ejection reflex is resumed within a short period of time: Benson and Cowie (32) reported an almost normal lactation performance in rats that became pregnant about 3 months after hypophysectomy, while Bintarningsih *et al.* (35) observed an intact milk-ejection reflex as early as 10 days following hypophysectomy. Radioimmunoassay of rat plasma neurohypophysial hormone levels 4 weeks after hypophysectomy revealed normal plasma oxytocin levels, in spite of low plasma vasopressin levels (36). The difference between the levels of the two hormones after hypophysectomy reflects either differences in the degree of damage inflicted on the system, or in the regeneration potency of the oxytocin and vasopressin nerve fibres. There is no reason to expect that in relation to oxytocin release pituitary stalk or median eminence lesions are better techniques than posterior lobectomy. On the contrary, the former techniques leave a large amount of neurohypophysial hormones *in situ* which will diffuse into the peripheral circulation and in case of vasopressin cause a temporary normal diuresis for 2-4 days (37) or 5-14 days (34).

Lesions of the magnocellular nuclei will usually be incomplete due to the number of nuclei and dispersed islands of neurosecretory cells, as well as the complex shape of the SON. The assessment of neurohypophysial hormone levels in the peripheral circulation is essential for the estimation of HNS lesions. In the case of oxytocin, no other criterium is available to ascertain it disappearance. Milk-ejection requires a pulse of oxytocin. An absence of the milk-ejection reflex might thus be due to the destruction of sensory afferents to the hypothalamus and the subsequent disappearance of oxytocin release pulses. However, this is no guarantee in itself that oxytocin is not released into the peripheral blood at a rate sufficient to induce uterine contractions (cf. 38).

In view of the data presented above, of the criticism by Fisher *et al.* (34) on previous hypophysectomy experiments, and the need for careful and continuous observation of the onset (and course) of parturition (cf. 39), very few useful studies are available and these may even lead to conclusions that differ from the original ones. Pencharz and Long (40), performing hypophysectomy in rats at the second half of pregnancy, clearly showed a prolongation of pregnancy and disturbances during delivery. The same was shown in cats by Fisher *et al.* (34) after median eminence lesions. Gale and McCann (41), partly repeating the latter experiments in rats, found a prolongation of pregnancy and a disturbance of labour in 22% of the rats that were lesioned between 7 and 9 days of gestation and that displayed severe diabetes insipidus. It is difficult to assess pregnancy length from their paper when lesions had been performed earlier than this period since implantation was also delayed. In lesions performed later than 9 days of gestation few birth impairments were seen, but parturition may well have been coincidental to the again normal interphase of neurohypophysial hormone release (cf. 34).

Diabetes insipidus

The relevance of diabetes insipidus for the knowledge of plasma oxytocin levels is little. Oxytocin and vasopressin are not both absent in hereditary hypothalamic diabetes insipidus. For instance, in the homozygous Brattleboro rat (a mutant species that is unable to produce vasopressin) high oxytocin levels are found (42), which could be explained by the chronic osmotic stimulation of the entire hypothalamo-neurohypophysial system. If oxytocin would play no role in the initiation of parturition, one would not expect a shorter length of gestation in these animals. However, their mean gestation is some 4 hours shorter than that of their homozygous normal controls (43). About the same advancement of labour can be induced by electrical stimulation of the pituitary stalk in the rat (39,60), by means of which neurohypophysial hormone release is increased (38). Thus maternal oxytocin appears to be able to induce labour. From these studies, however, it cannot be concluded that maternal vasopressin has no role to play in the initiation of parturition. Experiments by Fuchs (44) indicate that although vasopressin as such is not oxytocic during pregnancy, it potentiates the labour-inducing effect of oxytocin. The surplus of oxytocin may thus well have compensated for the lack of vasopressin in the Brattleboro rat.

Sende *et al.* (29) found measurable levels of oxytocin in a human pregnancy complicated by diabetes insipidus. We recently measured high (120 pg/ml) oxytocin blood levels in another woman at 36 weeks of pregnancy who suffered from diabetes insipidus due to a pituitary tumor, and who delivered in the Nijmegen University Clinic of Obstetrics and Gynaecology within 4 days after these values. Diabetes insipidus, either due to lesions or by a genetic cause, can thus be accompanied by normal or even increased oxytocin release.

Oxytocin in the maternal circulation

Oxytocin levels in peripheral blood are so low that the functional plasma oxytocin levels for the induction of labour in man would remain undetectable by bioassay (cf. 24). After the introduction of the much more sensitive radioimmunoassay method, Chard *et al.* (31) were still unable to detect plasma oxytocin before labour. The frequency of positive values was low during early labour, increased during the first stage of labour, and reached a maximum of 60% during expulsion (e.g., 45). Recently, however, more and more radioimmunoassay studies report increased oxytocin levels well before labour. This might have been expected in view of gradually increasing neurophysin levels found in the course of pregnancy (46). Kumaresan *et al.* (47) and Gazarek *et al.* (48) measured oxytocin in unextracted blood samples, and found oxytocin levels that were gradually increasing up to extremely high levels in the course of gestation (mean value about 330 pg/ml). Dawood *et al.* (49, 50) reported oxytocin levels during pregnancy between 1.9 and 69 pg/ml, while the levels were undetectable in 23% of the patients. We found levels around 20 pg/ml at term (15, table 1). In individual patients with hyponatremia which were followed for a different reason, we have observed definite increases in plasma oxytocin levels up to very high values one or two weeks before labour started (> 100 pg/ml, fig. 4).

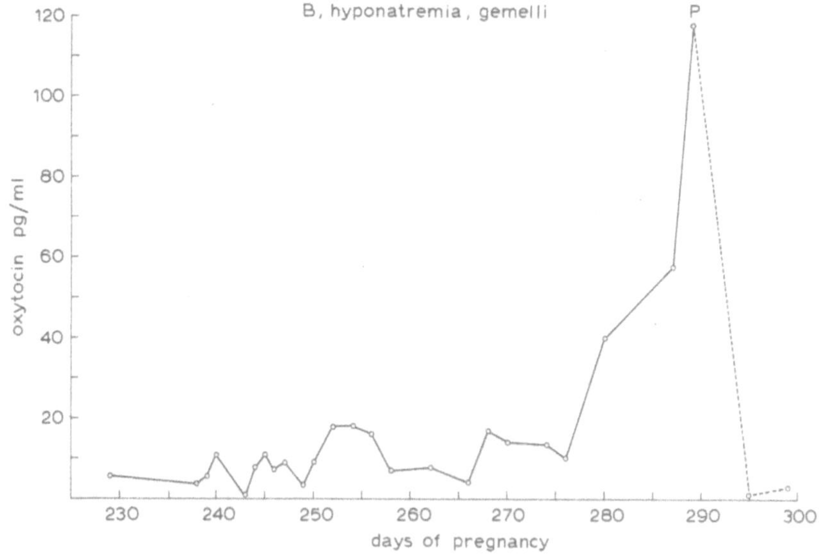

Fig. 4. Plasma oxytocin levels of a patient (B) during the course of a twin pregnancy. She had low plasma Na (around 120 mmol/l) and osmolality (around 250 mosm/kg), and a normal blood pressure and urine protein excretion. Note the rise of plasma oxytocin 9 days before parturition (P) and the fall of oxytocin levels after delivery (broken line). (Unpublished observations of Smorenberg-Schoorl and Swaab.)

In the rat we found that plasma oxytocin levels increase during gestation, and more rapidly after Day 15 (51). No further increase was observed during actual delivery (fig. 5). The increase in oxytocin levels before labour fully agrees with the observation that the electrical activity of identified PVN neurosecretory cells was elevated during the last days of pregnancy (10).

These data on the presence of oxytocin after hypophysectomy and in diabetes insipidus, the increased oxytocin levels well before labour, and the advancement of labour in rats with high oxytocin levels require a thorough reassessment of a role of this hormone in the initiation of parturition. The more so since a long term tonic release of oxytocin is effective in inducing uterine contractions (38), which means that additional increases of oxytocin levels at term may not be required for an initiating action of this hormone.

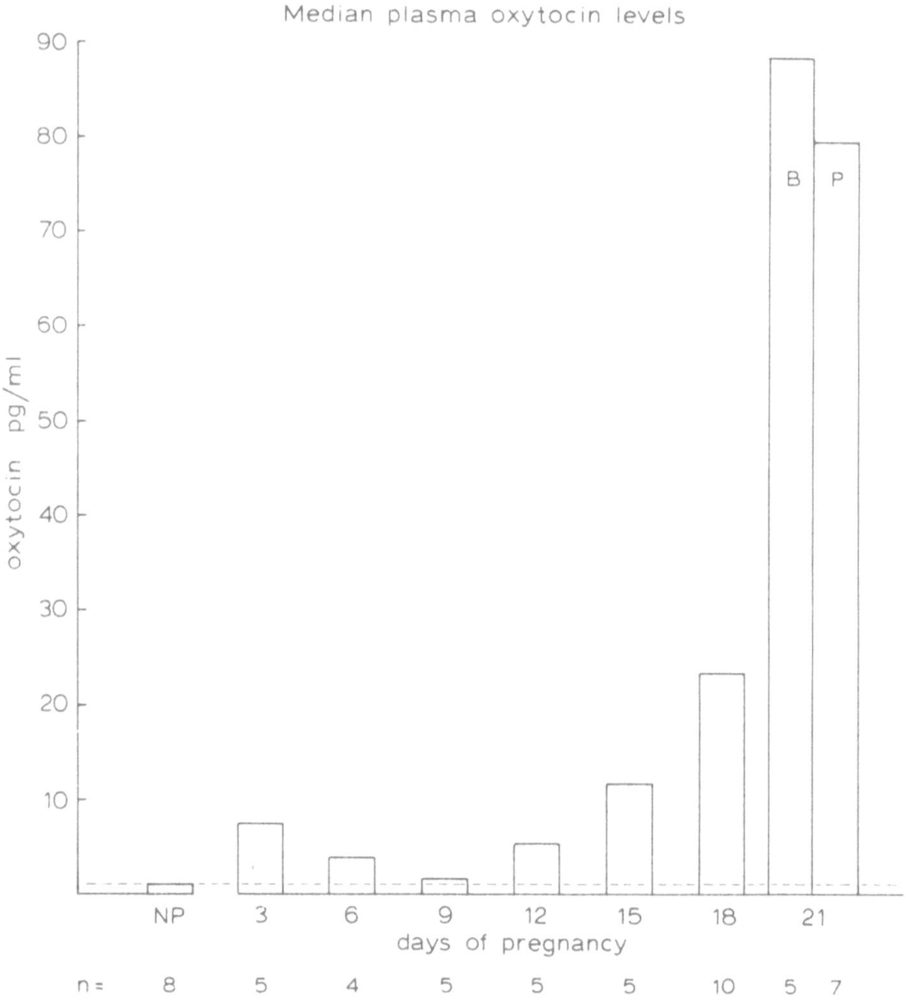

Fig. 5. The median plasma oxytocin levels in non-pregnant (NP) rats (stage of oestrous cycle not defined), in rats during the course of pregnancy and at day 21 before (B) and during (P) parturition. Blood was taken by decapitation between 2 and 3 in the afternoon (lights on from 07.00-19.00 h) except during parturition (between 09.00 and 17.00 h). Note the increase of oxytocin during the last days of pregnancy and the similar plasma oxytocin levels before and during parturition.

THE MATERNAL NEUROHYPOPHYSIS AND THE COURSE OF LABOUR

An accelerating or facilitating role of oxytocin in the course of labour has been less disputed than its possible inductive function (for clinical application of exogenous oxytocin see Turnbull, this volume). Increasing levels of oxytocin during the course of parturition have been found in jugular blood of man and domestic animals (for review, see 24). In human peripheral blood Chard *et al.* (31) found an increase in the percentage of positive samples during the course of stage I of labour that reached a maximum number during the expulsion phase. Dawood *et al.* (49, 50) found higher oxytocin levels during the first stage of labour than in pregnancy, while the highest levels were observed during stage II followed by a marked drop a few minutes later during the third stage. Vasicka *et al.* (52) found no significant difference between the oxytocin levels at term and in labour. During labour, however, they found moderate surges of oxytocin that could be related to specific events (see below).

In the rat the potency of the neurohypophysis to accelerate labour was apparent from the accelerated course of labour during electrical stimulation of the pituitary stalk (39). Since Brattleboro rats homozygous for diabetes insipidus delivered more rapidly than their controls (43), maternal oxytocin seems to be of importance for the course of labour in the rat as well. However, depending on the etiology and site of the lesion, diabetes insipidus can also be accompanied by a decreased oxytocin secretion. This is corroborated by the many animal experiments from which it appeared that the more central the lesion in the hypothalamo-neurohypophysial system, the more protracted was the course of labour (for review, see 24). Protracted labours have also been reported in human diabetes insipidus patients (e.g., 53, 29, 54), although the literature is certainly not unanimous on this point. The pluriformity in etiology and exact localization of the lesions that induce diabetes insipidus and the subsequent differences in oxytocin and vasopressin production and release during the course of pregnancy and labour make it necessary to perform systematically neurohypophysial hormone assays during pregnancy and labour in order to ascertain the effect of lesions and diabetes insipidus on the initiation and course of labour.

The Ferguson reflex

The increased oxytocin levels found during labour have been attributed to the stimulating effect of a neurohormonal reflex. Ferguson (55) showed in the post-partum rabbit and cat that stretch of the genital tract induced uterine contractions in two ways, one of which had to be dependent on the release of an oxytocic substance from the pituitary. The humoral component of this reflex was later elegantly demonstrated by Debackere *et al.* (56) in cross-transfused ewes. The Ferguson reflex can be evoked in many species. There exists a discrepancy, however, between the effect on the uterus and mammary gland. In man, Fisch *et al.* (57) and Sala *et al.* (58), among others, showed that dilation of the cervix caused coordinated uterine contractions but no milk-ejection. Cobo *et al.* (59) found no significant milk ejecting activity during labour in man. Similar observations were made in the rat by Boer (60): at term (under anaesthesia) spontaneous uterine contractions without pressure changes in the mammary gland were observed, although the latter was sensitive to bolus injections of normal doses of oxytocin. Only two papers have appeared on the occurrence of milk-ejection during labour in man (61, 62). The apparent rareness of milk-ejection during labour might be due to either a good sphincter function in the mammary gland (63) and /or a more tonic release of oxytocin during labour, that would not elicit milk-ejection. Uterine contractions can be raised by continuous low frequency stimulation of the neurohypophysis (38) or low dose infusions of oxytocin (44, see also the clinical use of oxytocin), while for recurrent milk-ejections high frequency pulses or bolus injections are required (38). From electrophysiological investigations in the suckling anaesthetized rat the PVN neurosecretory cells appeared to cause an intermittent release of oxytocin in pulses (64). Although, by analogy, a pulse-like release of oxytocin has been supposed during labour (65), various arguments plead against such a release pattern in labour. Using a similar electrophysiological set up as Lincoln *et al.* (64), Boer and Nolten (10) obtained evidence for an activated neurohypophysial hormone release already before the expulsion of rat pups that was tonic rather than pulsatile. There was no relationship between action potential pattern in the PVN and uterine contractions. Neither the "spurts of oxytocin" that were found by Vasicka *et al.* (52), nor the rather stable oxytocin levels determined by us in man (unpublished observations) before, during and after contractions revealed any correlation between oxytocin levels and uterine contractions. During labour the tonic elevation of oxytocin appears to dominate, while during milk ejection a more spurt-like release is required.

The importance of the Ferguson reflex in the physiology of labour is not yet clear. Most experiments that demonstrated clearly the presence of this reflex were performed in post-partum animals and under anaesthesia, while the stretch of the vagina has to be enormous in order to obtain a moderate effect on the paraventricular neurosecretory cells (66). Vasicka *et al.* (52) were the first to describe oxytocin surges during vaginal examination, after rupture of the membranes and after maximal cervical dilation and vaginal distention. These surges were not observed after local anaesthesia. This is consistent with the Ferguson reflex. However, the increase in oxytocin levels due to these events look relatively modest in relation to the high basic levels already present and are within the range of variation found in the course of pregnancy. The Ferguson reflex might thus exist also in physiological human deliveries but its efficacy in providing an important surplus stimulation of the uterus during labour can be doubted.

In view of the accelerated course of labour under conditions of increased oxytocin levels, the protracted course following some hypothalamo-neurohypophysial system lesions and the high oxytocin levels during labour, a facilitating function of maternal oxytocin in the course of labour is very likely.

THE FETAL BRAIN AND THE ONSET OF PARTURITION

A wealth of data show that, in sheep, the fetal hypothalamus is primarily responsible for the sequence of events that result in birth. Since this sequence involves fetal pituitary ACTH, an ACTH releasing factor (CRF) seems to be *the* hypothalamic stimulus initiating labour (for recent reviews, see 67, 68). The nature of CRF itself has been a topic of considerable discussion (e.g. 69). There is some evidence that AVP might be (one of) these hypothalamic factor(s) in the fetus (e.g. 70). Intravenous infusion of AVP into the sheep fetus results in increased ACTH release as mentioned by Jones and Rurak (71, discussion). A rise in fetal plasma AVP has been reported during the last few days before birth in the lamb (72) but has not been confirmed in later studies in which AVP was found to rise only during the last hours of pregnancy (73). It remains questionable, therefore, whether fetal AVP is indeed of any physiological importance for the initiation of labour in sheep. It is certainly not such a factor in rats since removal of the fetal brain does not prolong gestational length in this species (74), while homozygous Brattleboro rats with a homozygous litter even have a shorter gestation than their homozygous normal controls (43).

Data such as increased cortisol levels in the amniotic fluid and umbilical cord blood during pregnancy and labour indicate a role of the human fetus in the onset of parturition similar to that of the sheep (70), Yet, contrary to the general opinion expressed in the literature (e.g. 75) we found the mean gestational length in human anencephalics without hydramnios to be the same as that of the controls. However, a high percentage of both pre- and

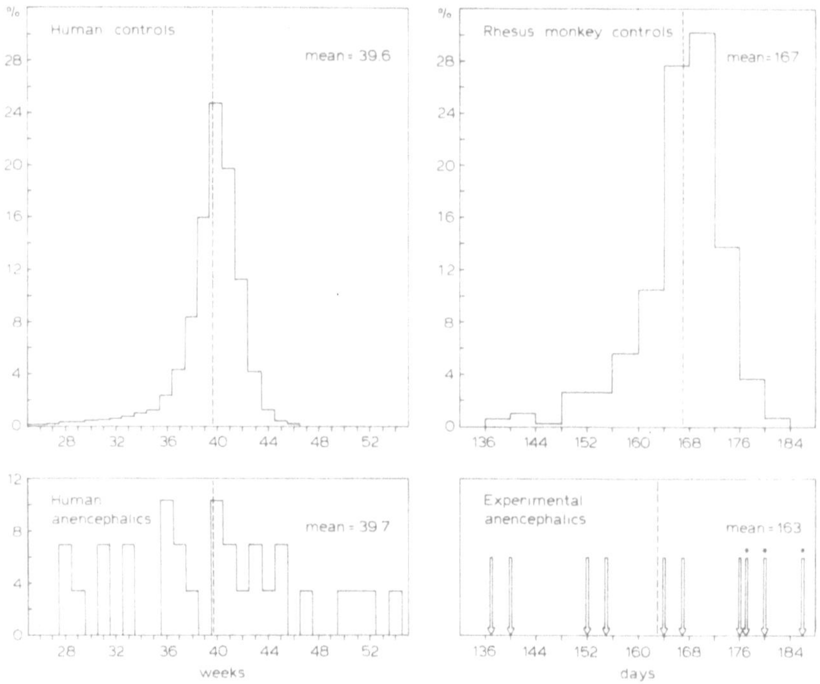

Fig. 6. The influence of anencephaly on the distribution of birth in man (left) and rhesus monkey (right). Left: frequency distribution of gestation length for a control group ($n = 49{,}996$) and for spontanous birth of anencephalic fetuses ($n = 29$) without hydramnios, omitting those who had stillborn fetuses with third degree maceration, fetuses which were given intrauterine injections, twins and those in which labour was induced (from Honnebier and Swaab, 76). Right: frequency distribution of gestation length in a group of 310 rhesus monkeys which produced live-born infants and after experimental anencephaly ((77) with permission of the Ciba Foundation). Each arrow indicates the birth of one anencephalic fetus. * = delivered by Caesarean section. Note the huge scatter of anencephalic births and the normal mean gestational length in both groups.

post-term labours were observed in human anencephalics (76) (fig. 6, left). A similar distribution of births was found in rhesus monkeys: the majority of the experimental anencephalics delivered either pre- or post-term (77) (fig. 6, right).

Additional data arguing against a crucial role of the human fetal brain in the determination of the mean pregnancy length are the few reported cases of acephaly (cf. 78), pituitary aplasia (cf. 79) and microcephaly accompanied by the absence of the hypothalamus (80) in which, on the average, delivery was not post-term. All these data show that in the primate the pituitary does not play the same triggering role in the initiation of labour as it does in sheep, but rather is involved in the precision of control of the initiation of labour within close limits around the species mean. It is not known whether the mechanisms by which the brain effects this 'timing' mechanism in man is also the fetal hypothalamo-hypophysial-adrenal system that initiates labour in sheep. Arguments in favour of this possibility are the findings that corticosteroid or ACTH administration in the human fetus initiated labour in postmature pregnancies (81, 82), but they did not induce labour at term (83, 84). Moreover, a tendency towards prolongation of the length of pregnancy was reported following β-methasone treatment in pre-term labour (85, 86).

One cannot be sure that ACTH is the most important adrenotropic factor in the fetus as it is in the adult. The development of the fetal zone of the adrenal and, via this development, also the timing mechanism of birth might be dependent on other adrenotropic factors. In anencephalics the fetal adrenal cortex is extremely hypoplastic. Since a high amount of ACTH 1-24 injected repeatedly into the shoulder of a human anencephalic resulted only in a moderately developed fetal zone, ACTH was thought not to account sufficiently by itself for the presence of a normal fetal adrenal zone. MSH was proposed as one of the possible additional adrenotropic factors (87). Challis and Torosis (88) have shown that the fetal rabbit adrenal does indeed secrete cortisol in response to α-MSH but not to ACTH, while the reverse was found in the newborn rabbit. The absence of α-MSH in anencephalics with adrenal hypoplasia, the simultaneous presence of an α-MSH containing intermediate lobe and a fetal adrenal cortex in normal fetuses, and the post-term switch in the α-MSH/ACTH ratio when the fetal zone involutes (22, 23) support the possible role of α-MSH as a fetal adrenotropic hormone. Moreover, recent findings show that α-MSH is steroidogenic for isolated human fetal adrenal cells in very small amounts (Challis, personal communication). The crucial demonstration that α-MSH is also circulating in the fetus is yet to be made, however.

THE FETAL BRAIN AND THE COURSE OF LABOUR

The integrity of the fetal brain appears to be necessary for a normal course of delivery in man and rat. In human anencephalics without hydramnios, expulsion of the fetus took twice as long as in controls, and the average time between birth of the fetus and birth of the placenta was nearly three times longer in the anencephalic group. In addition, in 10% of the anencephalics the placenta had to be removed manually while the overall mean in the University Clinic of Amsterdam was less than 2% (74). In this respect it is of interest that in the group of children who died during pregnancy (1968-1972: $n = 143$), a high number of placentas (8.4%) had to be removed manually (Huidekoper and Kloosterman, personal communication). All these data point to an active involvement of the fetus in the course of its own delivery and in the delivery of its placenta.

In the rat a protracted course of labour was found after removal of the fetal brain (74). That the fetal neurohypophysis may play a role in the acceleration of the course of labour was already proposed in 1938 by Bell and Robson (5), who found appreciable amounts of oxytocin in fetal pig and sheep pituitaries. This possibility is reinforced by the finding that uterine contractions could effectively be evoked in sheep (89) and in man (87) by injection of posterior lobe hormones into the fetal compartment, despite the conceptual difficulties in postulating the route which the fetal hormones should take to the myometrium (cf. 90). Furthermore, fetal rat pituitary extracts have the potency to induce uterine contractions (91). In addition, high levels of these hormones are present in human umbilical cord blood (cf. Table 1). These levels rise during the last hours of pregnancy in man (92) and sheep (73, 93). A fetal source of these neurohypophysial hormones is proven by the observation that the arterial umbilical cord hormone levels are higher than the venous ones (92, 49, 50). Although it is conceivable that the fetus contributes to the maternal neurohypophysial levels, it cannot totally account for the maternal plasma levels (49, 50).

Table 1. Neurohypophysial hormone levels in man: (pg/ml; mean ± SEM)*

	Oxytocin	Vasopressin	Vasotocin
midpregnancy amniotic fluid $n = 3$	< 4	< 1	<1
maternal plasma at term $n = 16$	20.6 ± 3.1	< 2	< 2
maternal plasma immediately after delivery $n = 5$	28.7 ± 6.2	< 2	< 2
umbilical cord plasma $n = 5$	68.1 ± 18.4	75.8 ± 50.6	< 2

* From Swaab *et al.* (15)

The fetus thus appears to have the means to stimulate the uterus and so to facilitate the course of labour by increasing its neurohypophysial hormone release. The high AVP levels in umbilical cord blood could, like from the maternal side, potentiate the oxytocin effects in these processes and might be of particular importance in the prevention of blood loss.

Characteristic for the fetal neurohypophysis in all species studied to date is the high vasopressor to oxytocic ratio. According to Perks and Vizsolyi (94) this might indicate that the supraoptic nucleus becomes active earlier in fetal development than does the paraventricular nucleus. This hypothesis, however, was based upon the assumption that the supraoptic nucleus would synthesize mainly vasopressin and the paraventricular nucleus mainly oxytocin; this has been proven not to be the case. In the adult rat, both nuclei show the same ratio of oxytocin- to vasopressin-containing cells (11). In their study on the nature of fetal seal neurohypophysial hormones, Perks and Vizsolyi (94) isolated a fraction with high activity on frog bladder permeability. Together with the amino acid analysis, this finding made it most probable that the fetal neurohypophysis contained, as a third hormone, arginine-vasotocin (AVT) (fig. 1a), a peptide hitherto thought to be confined to lower vertebrates (95, 96). AVT was also reported to be present in the pituitary of the ovine fetus (97, 98), the human fetus (98) and the rat fetus at term (99).

New observations make it questionable, however, that the compound measured in the fetal rat pituitary was indeed AVT. Recently, we have produced antibodies against AVT that permit a sensitive (up to 0.25 pg) and specific radioimmunoassay for this peptide, and are currently repeating the various observations on this peptide reported in the literature. Until now no AVT has been found with this assay method in either Wistar rat pituitaries, rat brains from day 17 of pregnancy throughout postnatal day 6, in 5 midpregnancy sheep pituitaries, or in human midpregnancy amniotic fluid and plasma (Table 1). These data argue against the importance, and even against the existence, of arginine-vasotocin in the fetus. However, the existence of other, e.g. AVT-like, fetal pituitary peptides remains possible.

SUMMARY AND CONCLUSIONS

Observations concerning the possible involvement of the maternal and fetal pituitary hormones in human and rat labour are presented. The clinical observations in man appear to correspond very well with the experimental data obtained in the rat.

The neurohypophysial hormones oxytocin and vasopressin are produced in the hypothalamic supraoptic and paraventricular nuclei, while the suprachiasmatic nucleus synthesizes only vasopressin. The adenohypophysis contains cells that synthesize a family of related hormones (ACTH, α-MSH, CLIP, β-LPH, γ-LPH and β-MSH) that probably arise by enzymatic cleavage out of one common glycoprotein precursor.

Recent observations show that maternal oxytocin is a putative factor of importance for both the initiation and the course of labour. In contrast to earlier suppositions in the literature, oxytocin is present in blood after hypophysectomy and in cases of diabetes insipidus. Since advanced labour was found under conditions of increased oxytocin levels and since increased oxytocin levels were recently found well before labour begins, a role of oxytocin in the initiation of labour has to be reconsidered.

The accelerated course of labour under conditions of increased oxytocin levels, the protracted course following some hypothalamo-neurohypophysial system lesions and the high oxytocin levels during labour make a facilitating function of maternal oxytocin in the course of labour most probable.

In sheep the fetal hypothalamus is primarily responsible for the determination of the mean gestation length, but in man the fetal brain seems to be rather involved in the precision of control of the initiation of labour within close limits around the species mean. Circumstantial evidence points to the possible role of the fetal hypophysial-adrenal system in this timing mechanism, and to the possibility that α-MSH rather than ACTH is the fetal adrenotropic hormone.

The fetal brain facilitates the course of labour of the fetus and of its placenta. For this action the neurohypophysial hormones are probably essential. They have the potency to evoke uterine contractions when injected at the fetal site. In addition, high levels of these hormones that are increasing during the course of labour are found in umbilical cord blood. The existence of arginine-vasotocin in the fetal mammalian neurohypophysis is doubted, but the existence of arginine vasotocin-like substances or even other exclusively fetal pituitary hormones that might be of importance in the process of labour are certainly possibilities.

Maternal and fetal neuroendocrine mechanisms are thus essential for the initiation and course of labour in both rat and man.

REFERENCES

1. Dale HH: On some physiological actions of ergot. *J Physiol* 34 (11), 163-206 (1906).
2. Dale HH: The action of extracts of the pituitary body. *Biochem J* 4, 427-447 (1909).
3. Blair-Bell W: The pituitary body and the therapeutic value of the infundibular extract in shock, uterine atony and intestinal paresis. *Br Med J* 2, 1609-1613 (1909).
4. Du Vignaud V: Hormones of the posterior pituitary gland: oxytocin and vasopressin. *Harvey Lectures*, ser. 50, 1-26 (1954-55).
5. Bell GH and Robson JM: The oxytocin content of the foetal pituitary. *Q J Exp Physiol* 27, 205-208 (1938).
6. Knight J and O'Connor M (eds), *The Fetus and Birth*. Ciba Foundation Symposium no 47, Amsterdam, Elsevier/Excerpta Medica/North-Holland, 1977.
7. Van Leeuwen FW, Swaab DF and De Raay C: Immunoelectron microscopic localization of vasopressin in the rat suprachiasmatic nucleus. *Cell Tissue Res* 193, 1-10 (1978).
8. Pickering BT: The molecules of neurosecretion: their formation, transport and release. In: *Perspectives in Brain Research*, Corner MA and Swaab DF (eds). Progress in Brain Research, vol. 45, Amsterdam, Elsevier, 1976, p 161-180.
9. Wakerley JB and Lincoln DW: The milk-ejection reflex of the rat: a 20- to 40-fold acceleration in the firing of paraventricular neurones during oxytocin release. *J Endocrinol* 57, 477-493 (1973).
10. Boer K and Nolten JWL: Hypothalamic paraventricular unit activity during labour in the rat. *J. Endocrinol* 76, 155-163 (1978).
11. Swaab DF, Nijveldt F and Pool CW: Distribution of oxytocin and vasopressin in the rat supraoptic and paraventricular nucleus. *J Endocrinol* 67, 461-462 (1975).
12. Vandesande F, Dierickx K and De Mey J: Identification of the vasopressin-neurophysin II and the oxytocin-neurophysin I producing neurons in the bovine hypothalamus. *Cell Tissue Res* 156, 189-200 (1975).
13. Dogterom J, Snijdewint FGM and Buijs RM: The distribution of vasopressin and oxytocin in the rat brain. *Neurosci Lett* 9, 341-346 (1978).
14. Dierickx K and Vandesande F: Immunocytochemical localization of the vasopressinergic and the oxytocinergic neurons in the human hypothalamus. *Cell Tissue Res* 184, 15-27 (1977).
15. Swaab DF, Boer GJ, Boer K, Dogterom J, Van Leeuwen FW and Visser M: Foetal neuroendocrine mechanisms in development and parturition. In: *Maturation of the Nervous System*, Corner MA *et al.* (eds.), Progress in Brain Research, vol. 48, Amsterdam, Elsevier, 1978, p 277-289.
16. Buijs RM, Swaab DF, Dogterom J and Van Leeuwen FW: Intra-and extrahypothalamic vasopressin and oxytocin pathways in the rat. *Cell Tissue Res* 186, 423-433 (1978).
17. Buijs RM: Intra- and extrahypothalamic vasopressin and oxytocin pathways in the rat. Pathways to the limbic system, medulla oblongata and spinal cord. *Cell Tissue Res* 192, 423-435 (1978).
18. De Wied D, Van Wimersma Greidanus TjB, Bohus B, Urban I and Gispen WH: Vasopressin and memory consolidation. In: *Perspectives in Brain Research*, Corner MA and Swaab DF (eds), Progress in Brain Research, vol. 45, Amsterdam, 1976, p 181-196.
19. Lowry PJ and Scott AP: Structural relationships and biosynthesis of corticotropin, lipotropin and melanotropin. In: *Melanocyte Stimulating Hormone: Control, Chemistry and Effects*, Tilders FJH Swaab DF and Van Wimersma Greidanus TjB (eds.), Basel, Karger, 1977, p 11-17.
20. Mains RE, Eipper BA and Ling N: Common precursor to corticotropins and endorphins. *Proc Natl Acad Sci USA* 74, 3014-3018 (1977).
21. Guillemin R, Vargo T, Rossier J, Minick S, Ling N, Rivier C, Vale W and Bloom F: β-Endorphin and adrenocorticotropin are secreted concomitantly by the pituitary gland. *Science* 197, 1367-1369 (1977).

22. Silman RE, Chard T, Landon J, Lowry PJ, Smith I and Young IM: ACTH and MSH peptides in the human adult and fetal pituitary gland. In: *Melanocyte Stimulating Hormone: Control, Chemistry and Effects*, Tilders FJH, Swaab DF and Van Wimersma Greidanus TjB (eds), Basel, Karger, 1977, p 179-187.
23. Visser M and Swaab DF: Life-span changes in α-melanocyte stimulating hormone (α-MSH) containing cells in the human pituitary *J Dev Physiol*, in press, 1979.
24. Fitzpatrick RJ: The posterior pituitary gland and the female reproductive tract. In: *The Pituitary Gland*, vol. III, Harris GW and Donovan BT (eds), London, Butterworths, 1966, p 453-504.
25. Chan SS, Fitzpatrick RJ and Jamieson B: Diabetes insipidus and parturition. *J Obstet Gynaecol Br Common W* 76, 444-450 (1969).
26. Cobo E, De Bernal M and Gaitan E: Low oxytocin secretion in diabetes insipidus associated with normal labour. *Am J Obstet Gynecol* 114, 861-866 (1972).
27. Moldavsky LF and Griffin ME: Diabetes insipidus in pregnancy. *Am J Obstet Gynecol* 100, 878-879 (1968).
28. Phelan JP, Guay AT and Newman C: Diabetes insipidus in pregnancy: a case review. *Am J Obstet Gynecol* 130, 365-366 (1978).
29. Sende P, Pantelakis N, Suzuki K and Bashore R: Plasma oxytocin determinations in pregnancy with diabetes insipidus. *Obstet Gynecol* (Suppl.) 48 (1), 38s-41s (1976).
30. Stephens CO and Hayes OJ: Diabetes insipidus associated with pregnancy. Report of a case. *Obstet Gynecol* 31, 79-82 (1968).
31. Chard T, Boyd NRH, Forsling ML, McNeilly AS and Landon J: The development of a radioimmunoassay for oxytocin: the extraction of oxytocin from plasma, and its measurement during parturition in human and goat blood. *J Endocrinol* 48, 223-234 (1970).
32. Benson GK and Cowie AT: Lactation in the rat after hypophysial posterior lobectomy. *J Endocrinol* 14, 54-65 (1956).
33. Moll J and De Wied D: Observations on the hypothalåmo-posthypophyseal system of the posterior lobectomized rat. *Gen Comp Endocrinol* 2, 215-228 (1962).
34. Fisher C, Magoun HW and Ranson SW: Dystocia in diabetes insipidus. *Am J Obstet Gynecol* 36 (1), 1-9 (1938).
35. Bintarningsih WR, Johnson RE and Li CH: Hormonally induced lactation in hypophysectomized rats. *Endocrinology 63, 540-548, (1958).*
36. Dogterom J, Snijdewint FGM, Peyet P and Swaab DF: Studies on the presence of vasopression, oxytocin and vasotocin in pineal gland, subcommisural organ and foetal pituitary glands. Failure to demonstrate vasotocin in mammals. *J Endocrinol*, in press, 1979.
37. Tilders FJH: Melanofoor stimulerend hormoon (MSH) bij zoogdieren. *Med Diss*, Amsterdam, Free university, 1975.
38. Boer K, Cransberg K Dogterom J and Pronker HF: The effect of low frequency *in vivo* pituitary stalk stimulation on neurohypophysial hormone release. In prep. (1979).
39. Boer K, Lincoln DW and Swaab DF: Effects of electrical stimulation of the neurohypophysis on labour in the rat. *J Endocrinol* 65, 163-176 (1975).
40. Pencharz RI and Long JA: Hypophysectomy in the pregnant rat *Am J Anat* 53, 117-139 (1933).
41. Gale CC and McCann SM: Hypothalamic control of pituitary gonadotrophins. Impairment in gestation, parturition and milk ejection following hypothalamic lesions. *J Endocrinol* 22, 107-117 (1961).
42. Dogterom J, Van Wimersma Greidanus TjB and Swaab DF: Evidence for the release of vasopressin and oxytocin into cerebrospinal fluid: measurements in plasma and CSF of intact and hypophysectomized rats. *Neuroendocrinology* 24, 108-118 (1977).
43. Boer K, Boer GJ and Swaab DF: Parturition in the Brattleboro rat. In prep. (1979). prep. (1979).

44. Fuchs AR: Parturition in rabbits and rats. In: *Endocrine Factors in Labour*, Klopper A and Gardner J (eds) . Cambridge, University Press, 1973, p 163-185.
45. Chard T: The role of oxytocin in the induction of labour. In: *Endocrinology*, Scow RO, Ebling FJG and Henderson JW (eds), Proc. 4th Int. Congress of Endocrinology, Washington D.C., 1972. Amsterdam, Excerpta Medica, 1973, p 1066-1070.
46. Legros JJ and Franchimont P: Human neurophysine blood levels under normal, experimental and pathological conditions. *Clin Endocrinol* 1, 99-113 (1972).
47. Kumaresan P, Anandarangam PB, Dianzon W and Vasincka A: Plasma oxytocin levels during human pregnancy and labor as determined by radioimmunoassay. *Am J Obstet Gynecol* 119, 215-223 (1974).
48. Gazárek F, Pohanka J, Talaŝ M, Fingerová H. Janousková M, Křikal Z and Hamal Z: Plasma oxytocin and oxytocinase levels in third trimester of pregnancy and at labour. *Endocrinol Exp* 10, 283-287 (1976).
49. Dawood MY, Raghavan KS and Pociask C: Radioimmunoassay of oxytocin. *J Endocrinol* 76, 261-270 (1978).
50. Dawood MY, Raghavan KS, Pociask C and Fuchs F: Oxytocin in human pregnancy and parturition. *Obstet Gynecol* 51, 138-143 (1978).
51. Boer K, Dogterom J and Snijdewint FGM: Neurohypophysial hormone release during the oestrous cycle, pregnancy and parturition in the rat. In prep., 1979.
52. Vasicka A, Kumaresan P, Han GS and Kumaresan M: Plasma oxytocin in initiation of labour. *Am J Obstet Gynecol* 130, 263-273 (1977).
53. Marañón G: Diabetes insipidus and uterine atony. A case observed over a period of 26 years. *Br Med J* 2, 769-771 (1947).
54. Jouppila P and Vuopala U: Diabetes insipidus and pregnancy. *Ann Chir Gynaecol Fenn* 60, 57-61 (1971).
55. Ferguson JKW: A study of the motility of the intact uterus at term. *Surg Gynecol Obstet* 73, 359-366 (1941).
56. Debackere M, Peeters G and Tuyttens N: Reflex release of an oxytocic hormone by stimulation of genital organs in male and female sheep studied by a cross-circulation technique. *J Endocrinol* 22, 321-334 (1961).
57. Fisch L, Sala NL and Schwarz RL: Effect of cervical dilatation upon uterine contractility in pregnant women and its relation to oxytocin secretion. *Am J Obstet Gynecol* 90, 108-114 (1964).
58. Sala NL, Fisch L and Schwarz RL: Effect of cervical dilatation upon milk-ejection and its relation to oxytocin secretion. *Am J Obstet Gynecol* 91, 1090-1094 (1965).
59. Cobo E, De Bernal MM, Quintero CA and Cuadrado E: Neurohypophyseal hormone release in the human. III. Experimental study during labor. *Am J Obstet Gynecol* 101 (4), 479-489 (1968).
60. Boer K: The rat hypothalamo-neurohypophyseal system: its involvement in the onset and course of labour. *Med Diss*, University of Amsterdam, 1976.
61. Gunther M: The posterior pituitary and labour. *Br Med J* 1, 567 (1948).
62. Sica-Blanco Y, Mendez-Bauer C, Sala N, Cabot HM and Caldeyrobarcia R: Neuvo metodo para el estudio de la functionalidad mamaria en la mujer. *Arch de Ginecol Obstet (Montevideo)* 17, 63-72 (1959).
63. Campbell B and Petersen WE: Milk 'let-down' and the orgasm in the human female. *Hum Biol* 25, 165-168 (1953).
64. Lincoln DW and Wakerley JB: Factors governing the periodic activation of supraoptic and paraventricular neurosecretory cells during suckling in the rat. *J Physiol* 250, 443-461 (1975).
65. Chard T: The posterior pituitary gland. *Clin Endocrinol* 4, 89-106 (1975).
66. Dreifuss JJ, Tribollet E and Beartschi AJ: Excitation of supraoptic neurones by vaginal distention in lactating rats; correlations with neurohypophysial hormone release. *Brain Res* 113, 600-605 (1976).

67 Liggins GC, Fairclough, RJ, Grieves SA, Forster CS and Knox BS: Parturition in the sheep. In: *The Fetus and Birth*, Ciba Foundation Symposium no 47, Amsterdam, Elsevier/ Excerpta Medica/North-Holland, 1977, p 5-30.
68. Nathanielsz PW, Jack PMB, Krane EJ, Thomas AL, Ratter S and Rees LH: The role and regulation of corticotropin in the fetal sheep. In: *The Fetus and Birth*, Ciba Foundation Symposium no 47, Amsterdam, Elsevier/Excerpta Medica/North-Holland, 1977, p 73-98.
69. Saffran M and Schally AV: The status of the corticotropin releasing factor (CRF). *Neuroendocrinology* 24, 359-375 (1977).
70. Challis JRG and Thorburn GD: The fetal pituitary-adrenal axis and its functional interaction with the neurohypophysis. In: *Fetal Physiology and Medicine*, Beard RW and Nathanielsz PW (eds.), London, WB Saunders Comp Ltd, 1976, p 233-250.
71. Challis JRG, Robinson JS, Rurak DW and Thorburn GD: The development of endocrine function in the human fetus. In: *The Biology of Human Fetal Growth*, Roberts DF and Thomson AM (eds.), London, Taylor and Francis Ltd, 1976, p 149-194.
72. Alexander DP, Bashore RA, Britton HG and Forsling ML: Maternal and fetal arginine vasopressin in the chronically catheterized sheep. *Biol Neonate* 25, 242-248 (1974).
73. Stark R: Discussion. In *The Fetus and Birth*, Ciba Foundation Symposium no 47, Amsterdam, Elsevier/Excerpta Medica/North-Holland, 1977, p 370.
74. Swaab DF, Boer K and Honnebier WJ: The influence of the fetal hypothalamus and pituitary on the onset and course of parturition. In: *The Fetus and Birth*, Ciba Foundation Symposium no 47, Amsterdam, Elsevier/Excerpta Medica/North-Holland, 1977, p 379-400.
75. Potter EL and Craig JM (eds): Central Nervous System. In: *Pathology of the Fetus and the Infant*. Yb. Med. Publishers, Chapter 24, Chicago, 1975, p 500-549.
76. Honnebier WJ and Swaab DF: The influence of anencephaly upon intrauterine growth of the fetus and placenta and upon gestation length. *J Obstet Gynaecol Br Commonw* 80, 577-588 (1973).
77. Novy MJ: Endocrine and pharmacological factors which modify the onset of labour in rhesus monkeys. In: *The Fetus and Birth*, Ciba Foundation Symposium no 47, Amsterdam, Elsevier/Excerpta Medica/North-Holland, 1977, p 259-295.
78. Liggins GC: The influence of the fetal hypothalamus and pituitary on growth. In: *Size at Birth*, Elliot K and Knight J (eds), Ciba Foundation Symposium no 27, Amsterdam, Elsevier, 1974, p 165-183.
79. Swaab DF and Honnebier WJ: The role of the fetal hypothalamus in development of the feto-placental unit and in parturition. In: *Integrative Hypothalamic Activity*, Swaab DF and Schadé JP (eds), Progress in Brain Research, vol. 41, Amsterdam, Elsevier, 1974, p 255-280.
80. Janigan DT, Smith OD and Nichols J: Observations on the central nervous system, pituitary and adrenal in two cases of microcephaly. *J Clin Endocrinol Metab* 22, 683-687 (1962).
81. Mati JKG, Horrobin DF and Bramley PS: Induction of labour in sheep and humans by single doses of corticosteroids. *Br Med J* 2, 149-151 (1973).
82. Nwosu UC, Wallach EE and Bolognese RJ: Initiation of labor by intra-amniotic cortisol instillation in prolonged pregnancy. *Obstet Gynecol* 47, 137-142 (1976).
83. Gamissans O, Pujol-Amat P, Davi E, Pérez- Picañol E, Pujol-Amat P and Wilson GR: Effect of ACTH administration into the fetus, on onset of labour and on maternal plasma steroid levels. In: *Research on steroids*, vol. 6, Vermeulen A (ed). Amsterdam, ASP Biol and med press, 1977, p 621-626.
85. Liggins GC and Howie RN: A controlled trial of antepartum glucocorticoid treatment for prevention of the respiratory distress syndrome in premature infants. *Pediatrics* 50, 515-525 (1972).
86. Schutte MF, Treffers PE, Koppe JG and Breur W: Klinische toepassing van corticosteroiden ter bevordering van de foetale longrijpheid. *Ned Tijdschr Geneeskd*, 123, 420-427 (1979).

87. Honnebier WJ, Jöbsis AC and Swaab DF: The effect of hypophysial hormones and human chorionic gonadotrophin (HCG) on the anencephalic fetal adrenal cortex and on parturition in the human. *J Obstet Gynaecol Br Commonw* 81, 423-438 (1974).
88. Challis JRG and Thorosis JD: Is α-MSH a trophic hormone to adrenal function in the fetus? *Nature* 269, 818-819 (1977).
89. Nathanielsz PW, Comline RS and Silver M: Uterine activity following intravenous administration of oxytocin to the foetal sheep. *Nature* 243, 471-472 (1973).
90. Liggins GC, Forster CS, Grieves SA and Schwartz AL: Control of parturition in man. *Biol Reprod* 16, 39-56 (1977).
91. Swaab DF and Boer K: Cerebro e hipofisis fetal en el cremento intrauterino y el parto. In: *Avances en Obstetrica y Ginecologia*, Conzales-Merlo J, Iglesias Guiu J and Burzaco YI (eds), Salvat Editores, Barcelona, 1978, p 149-158.
92. Chard T, Silman RE and Rees LH: The fetal hypothalamus and pituitary in the initiation of labour. In: *The Fetus and Birth*, Ciba Foundation Symposium no 47, Amsterdam, Elsevier/Excerpta Medica/North-Holland, 1977, p 359-378.
93. Forsling M, Jack PMB and Nathanielz PW: Plasma oxytocin concentrations in the foetal sheep. *Horm Metab Res* 7, 197-198 (1975).
94. Perks AM and Vizsolyi E: Studies of the neurohypophysis in foetal mammals. In: *Foetal and Neonatal Physiology*, Comline KS, Cross KW, Dawes GS and Nathanielsz PW (eds). Proc Sir Joseph Bancroft Centenary Symp., London, Cambridge Univ Press, 1973, p 430-438.
95. Heller H and Pickering BT: Identification of a new neurohypophysial hormone. *J Physiol* 152, 56P-57P (1960).
96. Sawyer WH: Biological assays for neurohypophysial principles in tissues and in blood. In: *The Pituitary Gland*, vol. 3, Harris GW and Donovan BT (eds). London, Butterworths, 1966, p 288-329.
97. Viszolyi E and Perks AM: Neurohypophysial hormones in fetal life and pregnancy. II. Chromatographic studies in the sheep *(Ovis Aries)*. *Gen comp Endocrinol* 29, 41-50 (1976).
98. Skowsky R and Fisher DA: Immunoreactive arginine vasopressin (AVP) and arginine vasotocin (AVT) in the fetal pituitary of man and sheep. *Clin Res* 21, 205 (1973).
99. Swaab DF, Van Leeuwen RW, Dogterom J and Honnebier WJ: The fetal hypothalamus and pituitary during growth and differentiation. *J Steroid Biochem* 8, 545-551 (1977).
100. Pickering BT and Jones CW: The neurophysins. In: *Hormonal Proteins and Peptides*, Li CH (ed), New York, Academic Press, 1978, p 103-158.

CORTICOSTEROIDS AND THE FETAL ADRENAL IN HUMAN PARTURITION

ROBERT E. OAKEY

The variety of means by which human parturition can be induced or delayed and the natural variability in the length of gestation in the human suggest that initiation of parturition is a complex process brought about by interaction of a number of systems. The purpose of this essay is to review the evidence for corticosteroid production by the adrenal of the mature human fetus since recent research has implicated fetal corticosteroids in the initiation of parturition in other species.

The recent growth of interest in the involvement of the human fetal adrenal has been stimulated by two separate lines of evidence. Since the turn of the century, numerous reports have drawn attention to an association between postmaturity and fetal anencephaly, a condition in which the fetal adrenal is unusually small (1-3). According to evidence reviewed by Anderson et al. (4), the degree of postmaturity in those pregnancies with an anencephalic fetus uncomplicated by hydramnios, is inversely proportional to the weight of fetal adrenal tissue. Conversely, it was noted (5) that infants born prematurely for no known cause and who came to post mortem had larger adrenal weights than expected. This finding implies a relationship between pre-term birth and advanced adrenal growth. More recent surveys, however have not always confirmed these views. For example, Honnebier and Swaab (6) found that anencephalic infants, born spontaneously, in pregnancies without hydramnios had a mean length of gestation which was not significantly different from that of normal infants. It was noted that there was a high proportion of both pre-term and post-term births among these pregnancies. Milic and Adamsons (7), however, described an increased duration of pregnancy in 22 patients with an anencephalic fetus, but whose pregnancies were otherwise uncomplicated. Postmaturity is also common in primary hypoplasia of the fetal adrenal (8). Although this evidence is by no means conclusive, sufficient observations have accumulated to enable acceptance of some role for the fetal adrenal in the initiation of parturition. This belief received support from the investigations of Liggins and others into the control of parturition in sheep (9). For example, destruction of the pituitary of the fetal lamb leads to prolonged gestation and diminished adrenal weight (10). On the other hand, stimulation

M.J.N.C. Keirse et al. (eds.), Human Parturition, 73-84.

of adrenal growth by infusions of adrenocorticotrophin into the fetus induces pre-term delivery once the adrenal glands have grown to a size comparable with those of a term fetus (11). Of particular interest is the demonstration by Bassett and Thorburn (12) of a marked increase in the concentration of corticosteroids in the fetal circulation a few days before delivery. This increased concentration of corticosteroid was not associated with any change in the corticoisteroid concentration in the maternal circulation and appears to be produced by the fetus. The blood samples for these measurements were obtained through indwelling catheters placed in fetal and maternal vessels some 10 days before collection of the samples on which measurements were made. Consequently, the changes observed reflect the activity of the undisturbed sheep and fetus.

Encouraged by the evidence from fetal pathology in the human and by the observations recorded in the sheep, many investigators have sought evidence of cortisol secretion by the human fetus near term and for a surge of cortisol in the fetal circulation before delivery. The results of such investigations have been equivocal and one purpose of this paper is to assess the current status of our information on the subject. There are two questions to consider. First, does the human fetus, alone or in association with the placenta, produce cortisol? Secondly, if so, is there a prepartum increase in the cortisol concentration of the fetal circulation as there is in the sheep?

In seeking evidence of cortisol secretion by the human fetus near term, it is not possible, for very good ethical reasons, to insert catheters into fetal and maternal vessels to obtain the necessary blood samples. Consequently, indirect approaches are required. It is possible to examine adrenal tissue, amniotic fluid, cord blood and maternal urine for evidence of cortisol secretion. Each of these sources will be considered in turn.

ADRENAL TISSUE

Near term, the human fetal adrenal gland is composed of two distinct zones of tissue. There is an inner zone, known as the fetal zone, in which the cells are relatively large and contain abundant cytoplasm. This zone occupies about 80 percent of the volume of the adrenal gland at term (13, 14) but after birth it degenerates and disappears during the first year of extrauterine life (15-17). An outer zone of tissue, the definitive zone, is also present. This zone is composed of small cells with prominent nuclei but sparse cytoplasm. Near term, this zone occupies about 20 percent of the volume of the gland and after birth it develops into the adrenal cortex of the adult.

At birth, the adrenal glands, weighing 2-9 g per pair, are much larger relative to body weight than are those of the adult (18). In the mature anencephalic fetus the adrenal glands weigh only 0.2-1.0 g per pair, because of the virtual absence of the fetal zone in this condition (18-20).

There have been many reports that the human fetal adrenal can secrete corticosteroids during incubations *in vitro* (e.g. 21-24) or can convert selected labelled precursors to corticosteroids *in vitro* (e.g. 25, 26). Much of this work was carried out with adrenal tissue obtained at mid gestation and therefore may not be strictly relevant to corticosteroid production at term. Adrenal tissue from a newborn infant, who died with severe hydrocephalus shortly after delivery at 42 weeks gestation, was studied by Villee and Loring (27). These authors reported the conversion of [^{3}H]-pregnenolone (3β-hydroxy-5-pregnen-20-one) to cortisol and corticosterone in yields of 7 percent and 10 percent respectively. At the same time [^{14}C]-progesterone was converted to cortisol and corticosterone in yields of 6 percent and 25 percent. Both the precursors (pregnenolone as sulphate and progesterone) are to be found in cord blood (28, 29). This report provides evidence of the potential of the adrenal of the mature fetus for synthesis of two important corticosteroids. Villee and Loring (27) did not separate the fetal and definitive zones so that the exact location within the tissue where the transformations took place is uncertain. However, Shahwan et al. (30) demonstrated that the definitive zone has the essential enzymes. These authors incubated the same precursors with adrenal tissue from newborn anencephalic infants. Labelled pregnenolone was converted to cortisol (2 percent) and corticosterone (8 percent), whilst the yields of cortisol and corticosterone from radioactive progesterone were 7 percent and 17 percent respectively. Whether the fetal zone contains the necessary enzymes to convert Δ^5-3β-hydroxysteroids (such as pregnenolone) to Δ^4-3-oxo steroids (such as cortisol) is unresolved. Histochemical evidence suggests that the 3β-hydroxysteroid dehydrogenase-isomerase complex, which plays a key role in this transformation, shows only weak activity in the fetal zone (31). However, these two reports demonstrate the potential of the mature fetal adrenal for cortisol biosynthesis from selected precursors.

AMNIOTIC FLUID

Amniotic fluid has been shown to contain androgens (32), oestrogens (33) and corticosteroid metabolites (34). Since this fluid is derived in part from fetal urine, it is reasonable to conclude that the steroids present are produced by the fetus, but their exact origin cannot be established unequivocably. Murphy et al. (35) measured the concentration of cortisol by competitive protein binding assay of defined specificity (36). The concentration of cortisol increased between 15th and 20th week of gestation and again between the 36th week and term. Similar information was collected by Turnbull et al. (37). When the increase in the volume of the amniotic fluid between the 20th week of gestation and term is also taken into account, these findings indicate an increased production of cortisol, presumably by the fetus, near term.

CORD BLOOD

Since fetal catheterisation is not practicable, analysis of cord blood has probably been the most popular experimental approach in attempts to solve the questions which are being considered. There are serious reservations about the value of measurements of corticosteroids in cord blood as indicators of the cortisol status of the fetus. Cord blood is necessarily obtained after delivery of the infant and usually after delivery of the placenta. Generally, it is obtained by cutting the umbilical cord and allowing blood to flow from the cut end nearer the placenta. In some instances, to avoid contamination with blood held in the placenta, the cord is clamped and only blood retained in the cord is collected. In many reports, the exact means by which the blood samples were obtained is not stated clearly.

Another complication in the use of cord blood to give evidence from the resting fetus, is the effect of the stress of delivery on steroid secretion by the fetal adrenal. No investigator wishing to study the adrenal physiology of the resting adult would expose his subject to several hours of severe pressure on head and trunk, to anaesthetic and analgesic agents and finally to an abrupt alteration from a fluid to gaseous environment. That an infant born after spontaneous vaginal delivery is exposed to all these factors, probably renders corticosteroid measurements on cord blood of little value. Ohrlander et al. (38) attempted to avoid this problem by measuring the cortisol concentration of fetal scalp blood obtained as soon as the cervix had dilated to 2 cm. Even at this stage, however, most fetuses had experienced uterine contractions of increasing severity for 4 h. These authors found that the mean concentration of cortisol in fetal scalp blood (25 nmol/l) was less than that of umbilical artery blood (400 nmol/l) whereas Sybulski et al. (39) recorded the reverse (scalp 700 nmol/l; umbilical cord 300 nmol/l).

Transfer of cortisol from the maternal circulation may also modify the concentration of cortisol in the cord. In late pregnancy, cortisol in maternal blood exists in three pools maintained in equilibrium (40). These pools comprise cortisol bound to albumin (13 percent), cortisol bound to cortisol binding globulin (80 percent) and non-protein-bound cortisol (7 percent). It is probable that the non-protein-bound fraction is the most readily transferred across the placenta. Any stress to the mother will increase the portion of cortisol in the plasma which is not bound to protein, thereby promoting transfer to the fetus at this time. Talbert et al. (41) found the concentration of non-protein-bound cortisol in maternal plasma, collected at the moment of delivery, to be 70 nmol/l for spontaneous vaginal deliveries and 10 nmol/l for caesarean section where the stress of delivery is considered to be less. Several authors have described changes in the concentration of cortisol in maternal plasma at the time of delivery. Buchan et al. (42) showed that women receiving pethidine for the relief of pain in labour had increasing concentrations of corticosteroids as delivery progressed. However, in patients having delivery under epidural anaesthesia, plasma cortisol concentration remained virtually unchanged through the first and second stages of labour. Even with epidural blockade, however, maternal plasma corticosteroids increased following forceps delivery of the baby. Changes in peripheral plasma cortisol concentrations during normal delivery were found to be much greater than those which occurred during abdominal surgery (43). Moreover, the increase could not be suppressed by treatment with dexamethasone. Isherwood (44) found a correlation between duration of labour and maternal peripheral corticosteroid concentrations. A substantial portion of the cortisol transferred across the placenta during labour is likely to be oxidised to cortisone by the activity of placental 11β-hydroxysteroid dehydrogenase. This enzyme reported by Osinski (45) has since been extensively studied (46, 47).

One result of all these factors is the general lack of agreement between different authors on the question of cortisol secretion by the fetus (as indicated by an umbilical artery-umbilical vein concentration gradient) or of a prepartum surge of cortisol (as indicated by higher concentrations of cortisol in cord blood after spontaneous delivery in comparison to values after induced delivery). Leong and Murphy (48) found that the concentration of cortisol in samples of umbilical artery serum was significantly greater than that in the paired sample of umbilical vein serum after 45 spontaneous vaginal deliveries and 14 induced vaginal deliveries. Similar analyses by Cawson et al. (49) showed no indication of an arterio-venous concentration gradient. Although Fencl et al. (50) do not show results from paired samples, the mean concentration of cortisol in the umbilical artery (160 nmol/l) was not significantly different from that in the umbilical vein (140 nmol/l). In an earlier report, Dormer and France (51) also failed to demonstrate an arteriovenous difference.

Murphy reported (52) that the concentration of cortisol in cord serum collected after vaginal delivery following induction of labour was significantly lower than that in cord serum after spontaneous delivery. This finding, confirmed for arterial serum (53) was interpreted as demonstrating increased secretion of cortisol by the fetus before spontaneous labour. Independent corroboration of these results was given by Cawson et al. (49). Other authors, for example Sybulski and Maughan (54) who studied 213 samples and Pokoly (55), were unable to confirm these findings.

There is therefore no clear consensus on the result of the analysis of cord blood samples. It seems unlikely that such analyses will provide the necessary evidence for the reasons presented above.

MATERNAL URINE

It is not at first apparent that analysis of maternal urine can provide evidence of corticosteroid production by the fetus. However, the careful observations by Frandsen and Stakemann (56) drew attention to the role of the fetal adrenal in the synthesis of oestrogens excreted in maternal urine. Comparison of the quantities of oestrone, oestradiol-17β and oestriol excreted near term by women with a normal pregnancy with those excreted by women with an anencephalic fetus indicated that 90 percent of oestriol and 75 percent of oestrone and oestradiol-17β arose from precursors by the fetal adrenal. In view of this observation, which has been confirmed many times (e.g. 57) there is no reason to suppose that a portion of any corticosteroids secreted by the fetal adrenal is not excreted eventually in maternal urine. The use of maternal urine in the search for evidence of fetal steroid production has two distinct advantages. First, collection of the specimen is not invasive and second, the sample can be collected without stress, so that the analytical results obtained should reflect steroid production in the resting, undisturbed state. With the experimental design utilised by Frandsen and Stakemann, comparison of the quantities of corticosteroids in maternal urine in normal pregnancies with those in pregnancies with an anencephalic fetus enables delineation of the contribution of the fetal zone, which is unusually small in the anencephalic fetus.

Evidence has been obtained by measurement of groups of corticosteroid metabolites and of individual metabolites isolated by sequential chromatography.

Appleby and Norymberski (58) demonstrated that the excretion of 17-oxogenic steroids in individuals increased in normal pregnancy. By term the mean excretion of this group of metabolites was 46.0 ± 11.0 μmol/24 h compared with 25.0 ± 3.9 μmol/24 h when the fetus was anencephalic (table 1; 59). It might be argued that the lower excretion in pregnancies with an

Table 1. Urinary excretion (μmol/24 h, mean ± S.D.) of corticosteroid metabolites near term by women with a normal fetus and women with an anencephalic fetus.

	Normal fetus	Anencephalic fetus	Reference
17-oxogenic steroids	46.0 ± 11.0 (n = 13)	25.0 ± 3.9 (n = 13)	(59)
17-deoxycorticosteroids	47.5 ± 12.5 (n = 12)	11.5 ± 0.4 (n = 10)	(63)
21-deoxyketols	4.0 ± 0.2 (n = 9)	1.5 ± 0.1 (n = 8)	(64)

anencephalic fetus is due to an altered corticosteroid metabolism in this condition, associated with a reduced oestrogen production. That this is unlikely is shown by two pieces of evidence. There is sufficient oestrogen produced in pregnancies with an anencephalic fetus to stimulate an induction of plasma protein synthesis similar to that found in normal pregnancy (60). Any alterations of corticosteroid metabolism are probably similar in normal pregnancy and when the fetus is anencephalic. Also the mean 17-oxogenic steroid excretion in 7 proven cases of placental sulphatase deficiency is normal although oestrogen production is even lower than in pregnancy with an anencephalic fetus (61). The reduced excretion of 17-oxogenic steroids in pregnancies with an anencephalic fetus is therefore probably related to the absence of most of the fetal zone of the fetal adrenal. The fetal zone in normal pregnancy appears to contribute to the 17-oxogenic steroids in maternal urine.

Another group of urinary corticosteroids which may be measured are the 17-deoxycorticosteroids (62) which include metabolites of corticosterone and 11-deoxycorticosterone. Daily excretion in the non-pregnant woman is 10.0 ± 4.8 μmol/24 h. By term of normal pregnancy, excretion has increased to 47.5 ± 12.5 μmol/24 h. If the fetus is anencephalic, excretion is only 11.5 ± 0.4 μmol/24 h (table 1, 63). The measurements implicate the fetal zone of the fetal adrenal in the production of these urinary metabolites.

A third group of metabolites which have been measured are the steroid 21-deoxyketols (58). These include metabolites of 17α-hydroxyprogesterone such as pregnanetriol and 17α-hydroxypregnanolone. In normal pregnancy, there is a 4-fold increase in the excretion of these compounds but this does not occur if the fetus is anencephalic (table 1; 64).

These reports provide evidence for the participation of the fetal zone in the production of each group of steroid metabolites – 17-oxogenic steroids, 17-deoxycorticosteroids and steroid 21-deoxyketols.

Extension of this work to the determination of individual corticosteroid metabolites reinforces these conclusions (65). It was found that there was no significant difference in the mean excretion of cortol, cortolone, tetrahydrocortisol, tetrahydrocortisone and tetrahydro-11-deoxycorticosterone by 9 women with a normal pregnancy when compared with the excretion of these compounds by 9 women with an anencephalic fetus. Since the first four of these compounds are metabolites of cortisol, it appears that the fetal zone takes little, if any, part near term in the production of cortisol. In pregnancies with an anencephalic fetus, any cortisol production must occur in the maternal adrenal and in the definitive zone of the fetal adrenal. Similarly, it may be argued that the fetal zone plays no part in the production of 11-deoxycorticosterone. In contrast, the mean excretion of tetrahydrocorticosterone, tetrahydro-11-deoxycortisol, pregnanetriol and 17α-hydroxypregnanolone was significantly lower when the fetus was anencephalic than when the fetus was normal. The fetal zone therefore appears to contribute to the production of corticosterone, the precursor of urinary tetrahydrocorticosterone. In this context, it is of interest to note that the production rate of corticosterone by the newborn infant may exceed that of cortisol (66). Pregnanetriol and 17α-hydroxypregnanolone are urinary metabolites of 17α-hydroxyprogesterone, which Tulchinsky and Simmer (67) identified as originating (as 17α-hydroxypregnenolone sulphate) in the fetal zone. Our evidence from analysis of maternal urine therefore supports their conclusions.

CONCLUSIONS

From this review of the literature, it is not possible to conclude that the human fetus secretes cortisol. The inability to demonstrate this in an unequivocal manner is due largely to the necessity to use indirect evidence. Incubation of adrenal tissue enables a potential for the synthesis of cortisol and corticosterone to be demonstrated. The definitive zone has the necessary enzymes. Analysis of amniotic fluid provides evidence of increasing cortisol production during gestation, but the source of this cortisol is uncertain. Although cord blood has been used by many investigators, the influences of the stress of delivery, of contributions from the mother and of the effects of placental enzymes complicate the interpretation of the results obtained as indicative of cortisol production before delivery. Analysis of maternal urine provides evidence from the resting subject but interpretation is complicated because metabolites, rather than the active hormones, are measured. This approach however, provides evidence to suggest that the fetal zone is involved in the production of corticosterone and 17α-hydroxyprogesterone, but not of cortisol.

Evidence that a prepartum surge of cortisol in fetal blood occurs in human pregnancy, as it does in the sheep, rests on analysis of cord blood. Confirmation of these reports in a manner which avoids interference by the stress of delivery is awaited.

ACKNOWLEDGEMENTS

I should like to thank Mrs. M. Cawood, Mr. M. J. Diver, Dr. C. A. Adejuwon and Mr. R. F. Heys for their collaboration and the Medical Research Council and the Wellcome Trust for financial support.

REFERENCES

1. Ballantyne JW: The problem of the postmature infant. *J Obstet Gynaecol Br Emp* 2, 521-554 (1902).
2. Malpas P: The incidence of human malformations and the significance of changes in the maternal environment in their causation. *J Obstet Gynaecol Br Emp* 44, 434-454 (1937).
3. Comerford JB: Pregnancy with anencephaly. *Lancet* i, 679-680 (1965).
4. Anderson ABM, Laurence KM and Turnbull AC: The relationship in anencephaly between the size of the adrenal cortex and the length of gestation. *J Obstet Gynaecol Br Commonw* 76, 196-199 (1969).
5. Anderson ABM, Laurence KM, Davies K, Campbell H and Turnbull AC: Fetal adrenal weight and the cause of premature delivery in human pregnancy. *J Obstet Gynaecol Br Commonw* 78, 481-488 (1971).
6. Honnebier WJ and Swaab DF: The influence of anencephaly upon intrauterine growth of the fetus and placenta and upon gestation length. *J Obstet Gynaecol Br Commonw* 80, 577-588 (1973.
7. Milic AB and Adamsons K: The relationship between anencephaly and prolonged pregnancy. *J Obstet Gynaecol Br Commonw* 76, 102-111 (1969).
8. O'Donohoe NV and Holland PDJ: Familial congenital adrenal hypoplasia. *Arch Dis Child* 43, 717-723 (1968).
9. Liggins GC, Fairclough RJ, Grieves SA, Kendall JZ and Knox BS: The mechanism of initiation of parturition in the ewe. *Recent Prog Horm Res* 29, 111-150 (1973).
10. Liggins GC, Kennedy PC and Holm LW: Failure of initiation of parturition after electrocoagulation of the pituitary of the fetal lamb. *Am J Obstet Gynecol* 98, 1080-1086 (1967).
11. Liggings GC: Premature parturition after infusion of corticotrophin or cortisol into foetal lambs. *J Endocrinol* 42, 323-329 (1968).

12. Bassett JM and Thorburn GD: Foetal plasma corticosteroids and the initiation of parturition in sheep. *J Endocrinol* 44, 285-286 (1969).
13. Elliott T and Armour RG: The development of the cortex in the human superenal gland and its condition in hemicephaly. *J Pathol Bact* 15, 481-488 (1911).
14. Swinyard CA: Growth of the human superenal glands *Anat Rec* 87, 141-150 (1943).
15. Brenner MC: Studies on the involution of the fetal cortex of the adrenal glands. *Am J Pathol* 16, 787-798 (1940).
16. Blackman SS: Concerning the function and origin of the reticular zone of the adrenal cortex. *Bull Johns Hopkins Hosp* 78, 180-208 (1946).
17. Lanman JT: The fetal zone of the adrenal gland. *Medicine* 32, 389-430 (1953).
18. Keene MFL and Hewer EE: Observations on the development of the human superenal gland. *J Anat Physiol* 61, 302-324 (1927).
19. Angevine DM: Pathologic anatomy of hypophysis and adrenals in anencephaly. *Arch Pathol* 26, 507-518 (1938).
20. Benirschke K: Adrenals in anencephaly and hydrocephaly. *Obstet Gynecol* 8, 412-415 (1956).
21. Goodyer CG, Torday JS, Hall CStG, Smith BT and Giroud CJP: Biogenesis of corticosteroids in monolayer cultures of human foetal adrenal cells. *Acta Endocrinol (Kbh)* 81, 774-786 (1976).
22. Roos BA: Effect of ACTH and CAMP on human adrenocortical growth and function *in vitro*. *Endocrinology* 94, 685-690 (1974).
23. Stark E, Gyevai A, Szalay K and Acs Z: Hypophysialadrenal activity in combined human foetal tissue cultures. *Can J Physiol Pharmacol* 43, 1-7 (1965).
24. Kahri, AI, Huhtaniemi I and Salmenpera M: Steroid formation and differentiation of cortical cells in tissue culture of human fetal adrenals in the presence and absence of ACTH. *Endocrinology* 98, 33-41 (1976).
25. Whitehouse BJ and Vinson GP: Pathway for cortisol biosynthesis in the fetal adrenal cortex. *Nature* 221, 1051-1052 (1969).
26. Villee DB and Driscoll SG: Pregnenolone and progesterone metabolism in human adrenals from twin female fetuses. *Endocrinology* 77, 602-608 (1965).
27. Villee CA and Loring JM: Synthesis of steroids in newborn human adrenal *in vitro*. *J Clin Endocrinol Metab* 25, 307-314 (1965).
28. Conrad SH, Pion RJ and Kitchin JD: Pregnenolone sulfate in human pregnancy plasma. *J Clin Endocrinol Metab* 27, 114-119 (1967).
29. Harbert GM, McGaughey HS, Scoggin WA and Thornton WN: Concentration of progesterone in newborn and maternal circulation at delivery. *Obstet Gynecol* 23, 413-426 (1964).
30. Shahwan MM, Oakey RE and Stitch SR: Corticosteroid synthesis *in vitro* by adrenal tissue from newborn anencephalic infants. *J Endocrinol* 44, 559-566 (1968).
31. Goldman AS, Yakovac WC and Bongiovanni AM: Development of activity of 3β-hydroxysteroid dehydrogenase in human fetal tissues and in two anencephalic newborns. *J Clin Endocrinol Metab* 26, 14-22 (1966).
32. Schindler AE and Siiteri PK: Isolation and quantitation of steroids from normal human amniotic fluid. *J Clin Endocrinol Metab* 28, 1189-1198 (1968).
33. Klopper AI: Estriol in liquor amnii. *Am J Obstet Gynecol* 112, 459-471 (1972).
34. Wade AP and Abramovich DR: The distribution of 17-oxosteroids and 17-hydroxycorticosteroids in amniotic fluid. *Steroids* 10, 669-686 (1967).
35. Murphy BEP, Patrick J and Denton RL: Cortisol in amniotic fluid during human gestation. *J Clin Endocrinol Metab* 40, 164-167 (1975).
36. Murphy BEP: Non-chromatographic radiotransinassay for cortisol: application to human adult serum, umbilical cord serum and amniotic fluid. *J Clin Endocrinol Metab* 41, 1050-1057 (1975).

37. Turnbull AC, Anderson ABM, Flint APF, Jeremy JY, Keirse MJNC and Mitchell MD: Human parturition. In: *The Fetus and Birth*, Amsterdam, Elsevier, 1977, p. 427-452.
38. Ohrlander S, Gennser G and Eneroth PD: Plasma cortisol levels in human fetus during parturition. *Obstet Gynecol* 48, 381-387 (1976).
39. Sybulski S, Goldsmith WJ and Maughan GB: Cortisol levels in fetal scalp, maternal and umbilical cord plasma. *Obstet Gynecol* 46, 268-271 (1975).
40. Rosenthal HE, Slaunwhite WE and Sandberg AA: Transcortin: a corticosteroid binding protein of plasma. X. Cortisol and progesterone interplay and unbound levels of these steroids in pregnancy. *J Clin Endocrinol Metab* 29, 352-367 (1969).
41. Talbert LM, Pearlman WH and Potter HD: Maternal and fetal serum levels of total cortisol and cortisone unbound cortisol and corticosteroid binding globulin in vaginal delivery and cesarean section *Am J Obstet Gynecol* 129, 781-786 (1977).
42. Buchan PC, Milne MK and Browning MCK: The effect of continuous epidural blockade on plasma 11-hydroxycorticosteroid concentrations in labour. *J Obstet Gynaecol Br Commonw* 80, 974-977 (1973).
43. Jolivet A, Blanchier H, Gautray JP and Dhem N: Blood cortisol variations during late pregnancy and labour. *Am J Obstet Gynecol* 119, 775-783 (1974).
44. Isherwood DM: Relation between corticosteroid and albumin concentrations in umbilical vein plasma and the duration of labour. *J Obstet Gynaecol Br Commonw* 84, 186-190 (1977).
45. Osinski PA: Steroid 11β-dehydrogenase in human placenta. *Nature* 187, 777 (1960).
46. Murphy BEP: Chorionic membrane as an extra-adrenal source of foetal cortisol in human amniotic fluid. *Nature* 266, 179-181 (1977).
47. Murphy BEP, Clark SJ, Donald IR, Pinsky M and Vedady D: Conversion of maternal cortisol to cortisone during placental transfer to the human fetus. *Am J Obstet Gynecol* 118, 538-541 (1974).
48. Leong MKH and Murphy BEP: Cortisol levels in maternal venous and umbilical cord arterial and venous serum at vaginal delivery. *Am J Obstet Gynecol* 124, 471-473 (1976).
49. Cawson MJ, Anderson ABM, Turnbull AC and Lampe L: Cortisol, cortisone and 11-deoxycortisol in human umbilical and maternal plasma in relation to the onset of labour. *J Obstet Gynaecol Br Commonw* 81, 737-745 (1974).
50. Fencl M deM, Osathanondh R and Tulchinsky D: Plasma cortisol and cortisone in pregnancies with normal and anencephalic fetuses. *J Clin Endocrinol Metab* 43, 80-85 (1976).
51. Dormer RA and France JT: Cortisol and cortisone levels in umbilical cord plasma and maternal plasma in normal pregnancies. *Steroids* 21, 497-510 (1973).
52. Murphy BEP: Does the human fetal adrenal play a role in parturition? *Am J Obstet Gynecol* 115, 521-525 (1973).
53. Campbell AL and Murphy BEP: The maternal-fetal cortisol gradient during pregnancy. *J Clin Endocrinol Metab* 45, 435-440 (1972).
54. Sybulski S and Maughan GB: Cortisol levels in umbilical cord plasma in relation to labor and delivery. *Am J Obstet Gynecol* 125, 236-238 (1976).
55. Pokoly TB: The role of cortisol in human parturition. *Am J Obstet Gynecol* 117, 549-553 (1973).
56. Frandsen VA and Stakemann G: The site of production of oestrogenic hormones in human pregnancy. Hormone excretion in pregnancy with an anencephalic foetus. *Acta Endocrinol (Kbh)* 38, 383-391 (1961).
57. Michie EA: Oestrogen levels in urine and amniotic fluid in pregnancy with live anencephalic foetus and the effect of intraamniotic injections of sodium dehydroepiandrosterone sulphate on these levels. *Acta Endocrinol (Kbh)* 51, 535-542 (1966).
58. Appleby JI and Norymberski JK: The urinary excretion of 17-hydroxycorticosteroids in human pregnancy. *J Endocrinol* 15, 310-319 (1957).
59. Heys RF and Oakey RE: Differences in 17-oxogenic steroid excretion in pregnancies with normal or an anencephalic foetus. *Acta Endocrinol (Kbh)* 72, 156-160 (1973).

60. Cawood ML, Heys RF and Oakey RE: Cortisol binding capacity and oestrogen concentrations in maternal and cord plasma in pregnancies with normal and anencephalic foetuses. *Clin Endocrinol (Oxf)* 5, 341-347 (1976).
61. Oakey RE: Placental sulphatase deficiency: antepartum differential diagnosis from foetal adrenal hypoplasia. *Clin Endocrinol (Oxf)* 9, 81-88 (1979).
62. Exley D and Norymberski JK: Urinary excretion of 17-deoxycorticosteroids in man. *J Endocrinol* 29, 292-302 (1964).
63. Diver MJ, Cawood ML, Heys RF and Oakey RE: The excretion of 17-deoxycorticosteroids by women pregnant with a normal or an anencephalic foetus. *Clin Endocrinol (Oxf)* 2, 227-232 (1973).
64. Adejuwon CA, Heys RF and Oakey RE: Differences in urinary excretion of steroid 21-deoxyketols by women pregnant with a normal or an anencephalic foetus. *Acta Endocrinol (Kbh)* 81, 598-604 (1976).
65. Cawood ML, Heys RF and Oakey RE: Corticosteroid production by the human foetus: evidence from analysis of urine from women pregnant with a normal or an anencephalic foetus. *J Endocrinol* 70, 117-126 (1976).
66. Hall CStG, Branchaud C, Klein GP, Loras B, Rothman S, Stern L and Giroud CJP: Secretion rate and metabolism of the sulphates of cortisol and corticosterone in newborn infants. *J Clin Endocrinol Metab* 33, 98-104 (1971).
67. Tulchinsky D and Simmer HH: Sources of plasma 17-hydroxyprogesterone in human pregnancy. *J Clin Endocrinol Metab* 35, 799-808 (1972).

ROLE OF PROGESTERONE AND OESTROGENS IN THE CONTROL OF THE ONSET OF LABOUR IN MAN: A CONTINUING CONTROVERSY

A.P.F. FLINT

The physiology and endocrinology of parturition are difficult to study in man. Ethical considerations and the inaccessibility of the human fetus preclude the use of the techniques that have been exploited so successfully in studies in animals (surgical ablation of fetal organs and the sampling of blood by means of indwelling catheters); for this reason much of the evidence on factors controlling the onset of labour in man is circumstantial, and emphasis has been placed on investigations carried out in "animal models". The hope has been that mechanisms discovered in animals may be applicable to man, and with respect to the role of changes in maternal circulating progesterone and oestrogens we are now in a position to investigate to what extent the control of parturition by these steroids, which is known to occur in the rabbit (1), the sheep (2) and the goat (3) exists in man.

PRODUCTION OF PROGESTERONE AND OESTROGENS IN PREGNANCY

The part played by the fetal adrenal in the onset of labour in the sheep and the goat is well established. At term in the sheep, rising fetal cortisol concentrations increase C_{21}-steroid 17α-hydroxylase, C-17,20 lyase and aromatase activities in the placenta (4-7). The placenta produces large amounts of progesterone in late pregnancy and these enzymatic changes are believed to cause the decrease in maternal circulating progesterone concentration, and the increase in oestrogen concentration, which always precede parturition in the sheep (Mitchell, this volume). Similar enzymatic changes occur in the placenta of the goat in response to increased fetal cortisol concentrations at term (8) but in this species the corpus luteum is responsible for the bulk of maternal progesterone production, and luteal regression is a necessary prelude to parturition; this is probably brought about by increasing placental oestrogen secretion coupled with decreased production of placental lactogen (3). In both these species, therefore, fetal circulating cortisol controls the maternal circulating concentrations of progesterone and oestrogen through its effects on the activities of key placental steroidogenic enzymes (9, 8).

M.J.N.C. Keirse et al. (eds.), Human Parturition, 85-100.

Synthesis of progesterone and oestrogens is controlled in an entirely different way in man during pregnancy. The fetal zone (also called the "definitive" or "provisional" zone) of the fetal adrenal, being deficient in 3β-hydroxysteroid dehydrogenase but containing sulphokinase, secretes dehydroepiandrosterone sulphate (DHEAS); the placenta, which contains sulphatase and aromatase, but only low activities of 17α-hydroxylase and C-17,20 lyase, uses this DHEAS as a substrate for oestrogen synthesis. The maternal circulating concentration of DHEAS, which is high before pregnancy, decreases during gestation as this also is converted to oestrogens by the placenta (10). Administration of large doses of DHEAS in pregnancy raises maternal circulating oestrogen concentrations (11, 12) so it seems unlikely that the placental enzymes are rate limiting in oestrogen synthesis. Thus as in the sheep and the goat, maternal circulating oestrogen concentrations are controlled to some extent by fetal adrenal activity; in man, however, this control is exercised through the secretion of DHEAS, rather than cortisol. This difference between man and the ungulates referred to above is reflected in the different responses of these species to intrafetal administration of glucocorticoid; in man, this causes a drop in maternal oestrogen and little change in progesterone concentrations, but does not cause labour. In the sheep and goat it causes the drop in maternal progesterone and the rise in oestrogen that normally precede labour, and the animals deliver.

EVIDENCE FOR A ROLE OF PROGESTERONE AND OESTROGEN IN THE ONSET OF LABOUR

Circumstantial evidence

A number of investigations have, over the past two or three decades, provided circumstantial evidence for the involvement of progesterone and oestrogens in the onset of labour in man. Urinary oestrogen production is high in women delivering early in gestation (13, 14, 15); and plasma oestradiol is higher at term in women in labour than in those not in labour (16). Progesterone levels are low in women in whom the duration of labour is short, and also in many patients who miscarry at the end of the first trimester (17, 18). Placental progesterone levels are low in women in labour (19) and uterine venous progesterone levels decrease towards term (18).

Effects of administration of progesterone or oestrogen

Many groups have tested the effects of administration of oestrogens and progesterone on uterine activity. Although the doses given were sometimes high, stimulatory effects have been claimed for oestradiol (20, 21, 22, 23). Other oestrogens (oestriol and stilboestrol, or equine oestrogens) have no effect (24, 25). Progesterone treatment, on the other hand, is generally ineffective in blocking labour (26, 27) or in prolonging gestation (28), although synthetic progestins have been claimed to be useful in treating patients with threatened abortion due to progesterone deficiency (29).

Peripheral plasma progesterone and oestrogen concentrations and the onset of labour

Measurement of progesterone and oestradiol in plasma from selected patients has revealed that in some cases there is a decrease in the systemic progesterone concentration before labour. Csapo et al. (17) sampling from 12 primigravid women, and Turnbull et al. (30) sampling from 33 very carefully selected primigravidae, found that mean progesterone levels dropped between 36 weeks gestation and term. The latter study showed that mean oestradiol levels rose rapidly at this time; levels of oestrone also increased, but less dramatically (fig. 1). The study of Csapo has recently been confirmed in a larger population of unstated parity (18).

Although these steroids had been measured in many previous studies, such dramatic changes at term had not been found (31, 32, 33, 34, 35, 36). It appears that they are not observed in every patient and are only reflected in mean concentrations when great care is exercised in standardizing the selected population and eliminating sources of variation. In the study of Turnbull et al. (30) a fall in progesterone concentration occurred in only two-thirds of the subjects examined; a rise in oestradiol occurred to varying degrees in all the women investigated between 36 weeks gestation and term, but very large changes were only found in about 40 percent of cases. A further study (37) in which patients were not so rigorously selected showed no such dramatic changes in progesterone and oestrogen, and confirmed that labour can be initiated without a fall in progesterone level or a rise in oestrogen. On the other hand, Dawood and Ratnam (38) taking single samples from patients of varying parity demonstrated a dramatic rise in peripheral plasma oestradiol concentrations during the last month of gestation.

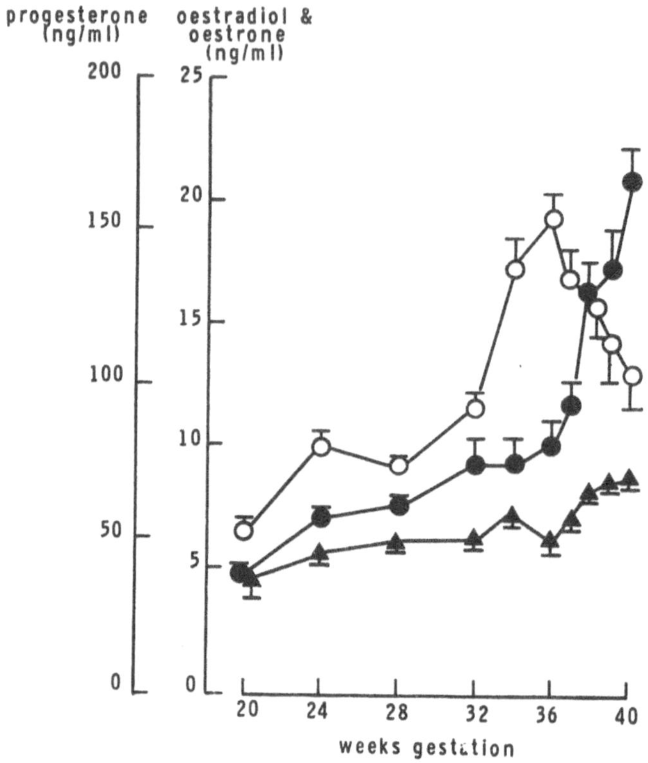

Fig. 1. Concentration of plasma progesterone (○), oestradiol-17β (●) and oestrone (▲) (means ± S.E.M.) measured serially in 33 primigravidae between the 20th week of pregnancy and the spontaneous onset of labour at term. (Data of Turnbull et al., 1974 [30]). These patients were selected on the basis of parity, age, stature and a history of normal menstrual cycles; all were certain of the date of their last menstrual period. Of 65 patients recruited into the study on these grounds, 33 spontaneously delivered single, normal infants vaginally within 12 days of expected term and the data shown are from these 33 subjects only.

Alternative modes of action of progesterone and oestrogen

The lack of any consistent changes in maternal peripheral circulating level of progesterone and oestradiol before labour is diffcult to reconcile with the control of the onset of labour by systemic effects of these steroids. However there are at least three ways, other than by changing peripheral concentrations, in which these steroids might exert their effects: (a) changes in steroid concentration could be local, occurring in intrauterine tissues but not being reflected in the peripheral circulation; (b) changes may occur in the production of steroid conjugates, but not in the unconjugated hormones, and (c) changes may occur in intra- or extra-cellular binding of the hormones to transport proteins or receptors.

The local action of progesterone and oestrogens: concentrations in amniotic fluid

The lack of a consistent fall in peripheral plasma progesterone concentration before labour and the inability to block labour by systemic administration of progesterone led Csapo (39, 40) to postulate that progesterone diffusing from the placenta exerts its effect locally on the myometrium underlying it (the local block theory). Support for this hypothesis comes from the observed distribution of progesterone between the placenta and the myometrium; progesterone concentrations are higher in myometrium underlying the placenta than in sites remote from it in uteri obtained before 38 weeks gestation (fig. 2). After 38 weeks the differences disappear (41, 42). However in the relatively small number of cases examined, Runnebaum and Zander (42) were unable to show any decrease in the myometrial progesterone concentration before labour.

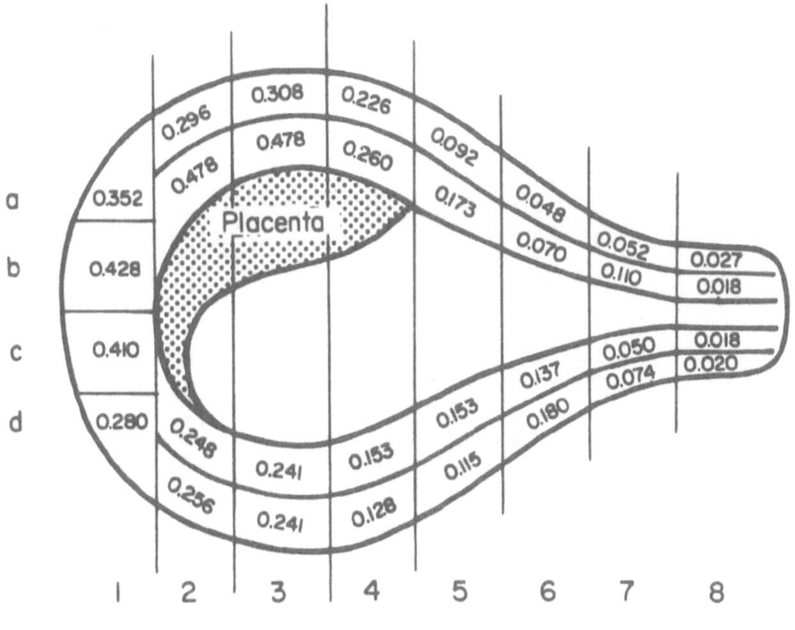

Fig. 2. Diagram illustrating concentrations of progesterone (μg/g wet tissue) measured in segments of a uterus at 14 weeks gestation, relative to the position of the placenta. (From Runnebaum and Zander, 1971 [42].)

This important hypothesis has been criticized on several grounds: (a) the myometrium underlying the placenta is permeated by venous sinuses draining the retroplacental space, which are filled with blood containing very high concentrations of progesterone: values for myometrial progesterone concen-

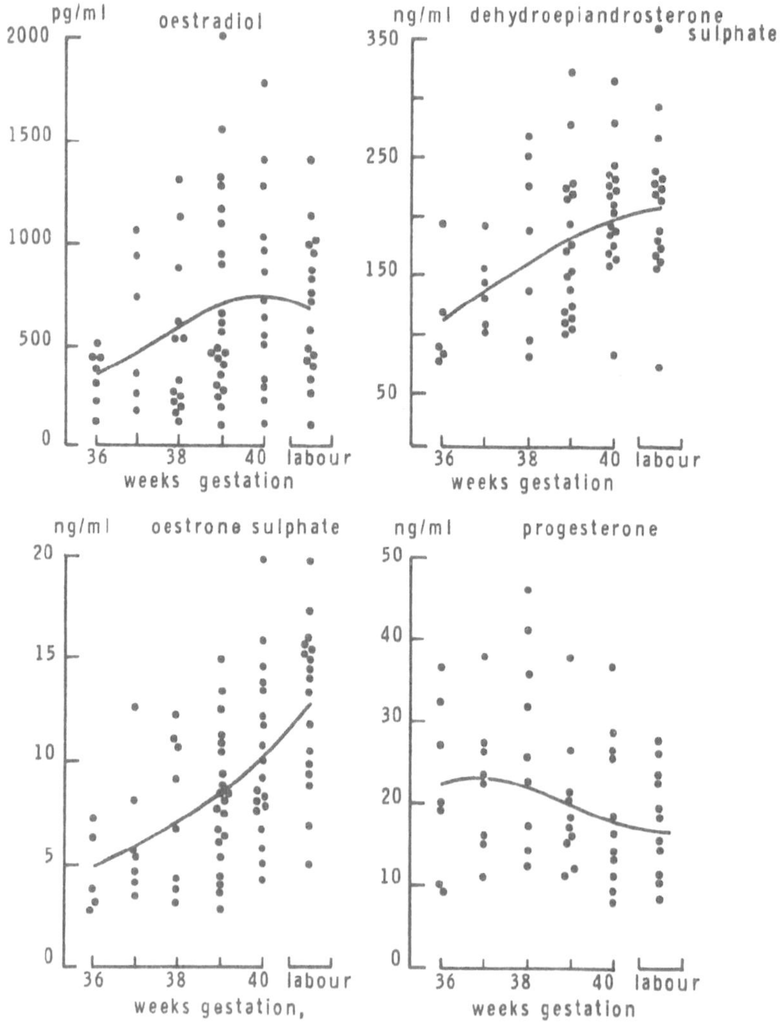

Fig. 3. Concentrations of oestradiol-17β, DHEAS, oestrone sulphate and progesterone in amniotic fluid obtained before the onset of labour and during spontaneous labour. Samples were obtained by both amniocentesis and at amniotomy: the way in which liquor was obtained had no effect on the levels of the steroids measured in it. (Data of Turnbull et al., 1977 [37].)

tration were not corrected for the steroid in this blood; (b) it is not certain how the progesterone diffuses away from the retroplacental space; the hypothesis would be more easily acceptable if a route were established; (c) the uterus is able to concentrate progesterone out of plasma, on account of the presence of specific receptors, so some gradient from plasma to myometrium might be expected (43), and (d) if the inhibitory effect of progesterone on the myometrium depends on its interaction with a cytoplasmic receptor protein, then it is not the concentrations of the steroid in the muscle which are important, but the degree to which the receptors are occupied. It seems possible that saturation may occur at relatively low progesterone concentrations.

The local block theory is supported by results of studies with animals. In non-pregnant rabbits treated unilaterally with intrauterine progesterone, differences can be seen between the contractility of the two horns (44) and similar claims have been made in rats in which the placentae have been unilaterally dislocated (40). It may also occur in sheep and goats: the fact that when one fetus of twins is infused with dexamethasone or corticotrophin in late pregnancy, it almost always delivers first (2, 3) can best be explained on this basis.

In an attempt to gain further support for a local action of these steroids, progesterone, oestradiol and oestrone sulphate, as well as DHEAS, have been measured in amniotic fluid (fig. 3). The amniotic fluid progesterone concentration is low in late pregnancy and tends to decrease towards term (45, 46); levels of oestradiol are variable but total unconjugated oestrogens (oestradiol + oestrone) tend to increase (46). Levels of oestrone sulphate and DHEAS rise more rapidly during this period (fig. 3). This rise in DHEAS is consistent with changes in the levels of amniotic fluid cortisol, which is also a product of the fetal adrenal, and which also rises before term (46, 48, 49, 37). However, in these studies on amniotic fluid steroid levels it should be noted that variations between individuals are usually large.

Changes in levels of steroid conjugates

Conjugates of progesterone metabolites (e.g. pregnanediol sulphates) circulate during pregnancy in very high concentrations (50, 51) but these compounds have not been measured in relation to the onset of labour, and they are not known to be biologically active.

By virtue of the presence of arylsulphatase (E.C. 3.1.6.1) and 17β-oxidoreductase in a number of intrauterine tissues (fig. 4; 52), some oestrogen conjugates may be converted to active oestrogens in their target organs, and in contrast to the progesterone metabolites, may indirectly be biologically

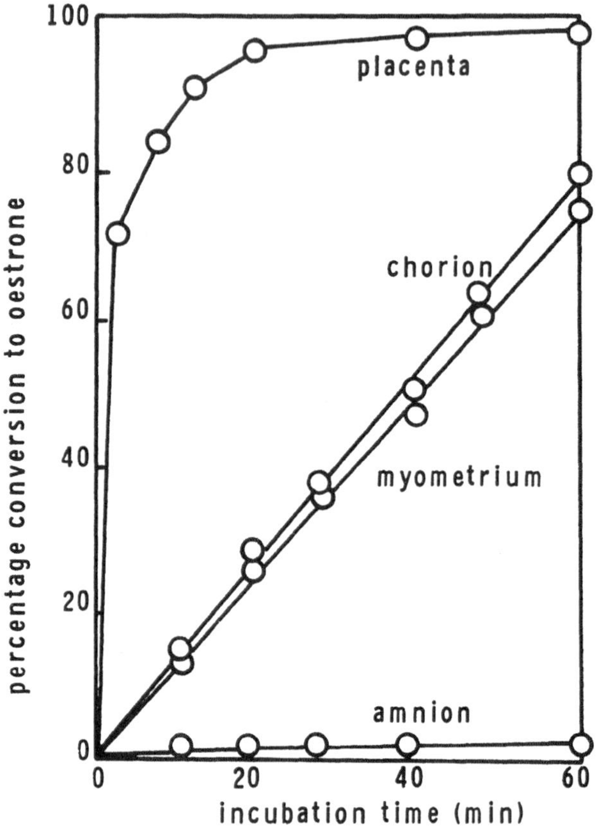

Fig. 4. Aryl sulphatase activity measured in homogenates of tissues obtained at Caesarean section from a patient at term. Labelled oestrone sulphate was used as substrate; incubation at 37 °C, in Tris buffer. (Data of Turnbull et al., 1977 [37].)

active. Of the oestrogen conjugates which have been measured in maternal peripheral plasma during pregnancy, oestrone 3-sulphate, oestradiol 17-sulphate, oestradiol 3,17-disulphate, the oestradiol diglucuronides and oestrone 3-glucuronide have also been measured in a limited number of cases in relation to the onset of labour, but the levels of these compounds are relatively low, and do not change any more dramatically before term. Mean concentrations of oestrone sulphate, however, rise rapidly during the last trimester, even in patients of varying parity in whom there is no dramatic increase in mean oestradiol levels (fig. 5). This increase in maternal systemic oestrone sulphate level parallels that in amniotic fluid (fig. 3).

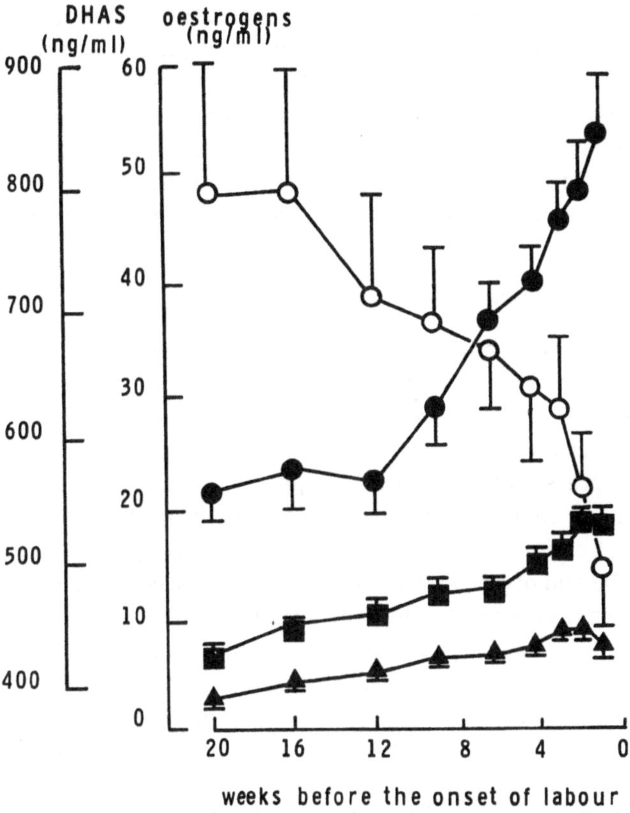

Fig. 5. Concentrations (mean ± S.E.M.) of DHEAS (○), oestradiol-17-β (■), oestrone (▲) and oestrone sulphate (●) in maternal peripheral plasma measured serially up to the spontaneous onset of labour at term. The patients were of varying parity and do not include any for whom data are shown in figure 1. (Data of Turnbull et al., 1977 [37].)

Levels of plasma binding proteins and cytoplasmic receptors

The other possible modulator of the effects of progesterone and oestrogens, binding to intra- or extra-cellular binding proteins, has not been examined in detail. The plasma steroid-binding proteins, corticosteroid binding globulin (CBG) and sex hormone binding globulin (SHBG) bind approximately 40 and 80 percent of the circulating progesterone and oestradiol respectively, in late pregnancy (53, 54). Other proteins also bind these steroids, so that more than 90 percent of both is in the bound form. Since only the free (unbound) steroids are active, any changes in binding can alter the available active steroid concentration without any change in the total steroid concentration (which is what is usually measured by radioimmunoassay techniques). The greatest increase in SHBG in pregnancy occurs during the first two trimesters (54, 55). Levels of CBG also rise during gestation, but no major change has been reported in relation to the onset of labour.

Intracellular steroid-binding proteins (receptors) for oestradiol (56, 57), and progesterone (58) are present in human myometrium, but there appears to be no information available on their activities in the last trimester.

Summary of steroid changes preceding labour

The data reviewed above suggest that although there is a great deal of circumstantial evidence for a role for progesterone or oestradiol in the control of the onset of labour in man, it has not been possible to demonstrate consistent changes in the peripheral circulating concentrations of these steroids. It appears most likely that peripheral progesterone levels decrease during the last month of gestation in a large proportion of primigravid patients, but even in this group the finding does not apply in all cases. The same may be said of peripheral oestradiol levels. Measuring these hormones in uterine venous plasma is unlikely to demonstrate changes that are not seen systematically, in the absence of any alteration in metabolic clearance rate; in fact uterine venous concentrations in samples collected during surgery are liable to be misleading because of other effects, such as on uterine blood flow or hepatic clearance, which may be associated with both anaesthesia and stress.

In the absence of any consistent change in peripheral concentration of these steroids it is obviously important to investigate their local concentrations, and this has been recognized since the presentation of the local block hypothesis by Csapo (39, 40). No reliable data are available however on myometrial progesterone and oestradiol concentrations relative to the onset of labour. Although it is not possible to collect tissue at elective Caesarean sections *knowing at what time the patient would have gone into labour if untreated*, it would be helpful to measure myometrial progesterone concentrations in samples obtained at elective Caesarean section and at Caesarean section during labour, and, in order to control for effects of labour itself, at Caesarean section in induced labour. This approach has provided information on the possible role of umbilical plasma cortisol concentrations in the onset of labour (59, 37).

An alternative method of determining intrauterine levels of hormones is to measure them in amniotic fluid. Although this approach is hampered by possibly selective effects of metabolism by the amnion, which unlike other intrauterine tissues does not contain arylsulphatase (fig. 4) it has yielded useful data not only on steroids but also on levels of prostaglandins. It does not however point to a central role for progesterone or oestradiol in the onset of labour, though oestrone sulphate levels do rise in liquor, as well as in plasma, before term, suggesting an increase in total oestrogen synthesis during this period.

A number of oestrogens is present in maternal plasma during pregnancy, and although oestradiol-17β is the most active, it is by no means certain that oestrone and oestriol, the other major unconjugated oestrogens, are inactive. Both oestrone and oestriol will displace oestradiol-17β from the myometrial cytoplasmic oestrogen receptor (60) and both [^{3}H]oestrone and [^{3}H]oestradiol are found bound to the endometrial oestrogen receptor after infusion of [^{3}H]oestrone *in vivo* (61). Oestriol mimics oestradiol in its effect on uterine blood flow and uterine growth in sheep (62). Oestrone sulphate and the oestradiol sulphates are most likely to be converted to oestrone and oestradiol, and the high circulating levels of the conjugates may therefore represent potentially active oestrogens.

Target organs for progesterone and oestrogens

Possible changes in levels of progesterone and oestrogens have been discussed above in relation to peripheral blood and the myometrium, but it is by no means certain that the myometrium is the only target for the biological effects of these steroids, or indeed the most important one in terms of the onset of labour. Deanesly (63) found that after ovariectomy in guinea-pigs early in gestation the decidua was the first organ to display histological alterations attributable to progesterone withdrawal, and the decidua should also be considered a possible target in man. There are several reasons for considering the guinea-pig a good model for the endocrine control of human labour: it is a species in which progesterone administration has not been shown to reduce uterine contractility (64) and it does not display a marked reduction in placental progesterone production late in pregnancy (65). The fragile cells of the decidua have been considered a prime target for the abortifacient effects of intra-amniotic hypertonic saline in man (66, 67) and attention has recently been drawn to the decidua as a possible source of prostaglandins which may trigger labour at term (68, 69).

THE TIMING OF THE ONSET OF LABOUR: CERVICAL CHANGES DURING THE LAST TRIMESTER, AND A FACILITATORY ROLE OF PROGESTERONE AND OESTROGENS

The timing of the onset of labour is now known to be influenced by several factors. The marked diurnal rhythm in the time of the onset of labour, which occurs most frequently between midnight and 04.00 h, but seldom around mid-day (70, 71), implicates some acute controlling factor, probably maternal in origin. This diurnal rhythm seems unlikely to be related to the relatively minor variation in plasma oestradiol concentration ($\pm$ 12-15 percent about the mean) reported by Munson et al. (72) and Townsley et al. (73), which showed that levels peaked at 12 noon but were low at 12 midnight.

Also documented is the influence of changes in the shape and consistency of the cervix during the last 6-10 weeks gestation; patients with a ripe and dilating cervix are likely to deliver earlier than those in whom the cervix remains long and hard during the last trimester (74, 75). These cervical changes occur at a time when the uterus is becoming more active (displaying Braxton-Hicks contractions) and may be related to this increased contractility. They also occur at the time of the rise in peripheral and amniotic fluid oestrone sulphate levels, and it seems likely that there is a causative relationship between oestrogen concentrations and ripening of the cervix, which is probably mediated by prostaglandins. Systemic or locally administered prostaglandins or oestradiol cause the cervix to soften and dilate over a period of 8-12 h (76, 77, 78) and this treatment is becoming routine when induction of labour is indicated in patients with an unfavourable cervix (Calder, this volume). The degree of cervical ripeness and dilatation (Bishop score) near term is related to the concentration of prostaglandins E and F in amniotic fluid (Calder, this volume); levels of prostaglandin $F_{2\alpha}$ in amniotic fluid in turn correlate with amniotic fluid levels of oestrogen (37). There are therefore reasons for believing that amniotic fluid oestrogens are either important causally in the onset of labour, or reflect oestrogen levels in another more directly related tissue. No inverse relationship with progesterone has been established.

CONCLUSIONS

A large amount of information is now available on the roles of progesterone and oestrogens in controlling the time of the onset of labour in man, and although it is not possible to draw conclusions with such certainty as one can from studying the onset of parturition in animals, the following can be stated:

(a) Peripheral plasma concentrations of progesterone and oestradiol may be related to the onset of labour in some primigravidae, but they do not consistently change before parturition. Mean peripheral plasma concentrations of oestrone sulphate rise more consistently before term.

(b) Mean amniotic fluid concentrations of oestrone sulphate also rise before term.

(c) Oestrone sulphate in intrauterine tissues may be active by virtue of the wide distribution of arylsulphatase and 17β-oxidoreductase.

(d) Amniotic fluid or peripheral plasma concentrations of oestrogens may be related to the degree of cervical ripening and dilatation in late pregnancy, through an effect on prostaglandin levels.

(e) Any part played by progesterone or oestrogens is likely to be *permissive*, rather than *obligatory*, in the onset of labour. Decreasing levels of progesterone or increasing levels of oestrogens, whether acting locally or systemically, may lead to an earlier onset of labour, but are probably not involved in the acute control of the timing of parturition.

REFERENCES

1. Allen WM and Corner GW: Physiology of the corpus luteum: III. Normal growth and implantation of embryos after early ablation of the ovaries under the influences of extract of the corpus luteum. *Am J Physiol* 88, 340-346 (1929).
2. Liggins GC, Fairclough RJ, Grieves SA, Kendall JZ and Knox BS: The mechanism of initiation of parturition in the ewe. *Recent Prog Horm Res* 29, 111-150 (1973).
3. Currie WB and Thorburn GD: The fetal role in timing the initiation of parturition in the goat. In: *The Fetus and Birth*, Ciba Foundation Symposium no 47, Amsterdam, North-Holland, 1977, p. 49-66.
4. Anderson ABM, Flint APF and Turnbull AC: Mechanism of action of glucocorticoids in induction of ovine parturition: effect on placental steroid metabolism. *J Endocrinol* 66, 61-70 (1975).
5. Mann MR, Curet LB and Colas AE: Aromatizing activity of placental microsomal fractions from ewes in late gestation. *J Endocrinol* 65, 117-125 (1975).
6. Steele PA, Flint APF and Turnbull AC: Activity of steriod C-17,20 lyase in the ovine placenta: effect of exposure to foetal glucocorticoid. *J Endocrinol* 69, 239-246 (1976).
7. Steele PA, Flint APF and Turnbull AC: Increased utero-ovarian androstenedione production before parturition in sheep. *J Reprod Fertil* 46, 443-445 (1976).
8. Flint APF, Kingston JE, Robinson JS and Thorburn GD: Initiation of parturition in the goat: evidence for control by foetal glucocorticoid through activation of placental C_{21}-steroid 17α-hydroxylase. *J Endocrinol* 78, 367-378 (1978).
9. Flint APF, Anderson ABM, Steele PA and Turnbull AC: The mechanism by which foetal cortisol controls the onset of parturition in sheep. *Biochem Soc Trans* 3, 1189-1194 (1975).
10. Siiteri PK and MacDonald PC: Placental oestrogen biosynthesis during human pregnancy. *J Clin Endocr* 26, 751-761 (1966).
11. Lauritzen Ch: A clinical test for placental function using DHEA-sulphate and ACTH injections in the pregnant woman. *Acta Endocrinol* suppl 119, 188 (1967).

12. Korda AR, Challis JJ, Anderson ABM and Turnbull AC: Assessment of placental function in normal and pathological pregnancies by estimation of plasma oestradiol levels after injection of dehydroepiandrosterone sulphate. *Br J Obstet Gynaecol* 82, 656-661 (1975).
13. Klopper A and Billewicz W: Urinary excretion of oestriol and pregnanediol during pregnancy. *J Obstet Gynaecol Br Commonw* 70, 1024-1029 (1963).
14. Turnbull AC, Anderson ABM and Wilson GR: Maternal urinary oestrogen excretion as evidence of a foetal role in determining gestation at labour. *Lancet* 2, 627-629 (1967).
15. Beischer NA, Brown JB, Smith MA and Townsend L: Studies in prolonged pregnancy. II. Clinical results and urinary estriol excretion in prolonged pregnancy. *Am J Obstet Gynecol* 103, 483-495 (1969).
16. Sybulski S and Maughan GB: Maternal plasma oestradiol levels in normal and complicated pregnancies. *Am J Obstet Gynecol* 113, 310-315 (1972).
17. Csapo AI, Knobil E, van der Molen HJ and Wiest WG: Peripheral plasma progesterone levels during human pregnancy and labor. *Am J Obstet Gynecol* 110, 630-632 (1971).
18. Csapo AI: The 'See-Saw' theory of parturition. In: *The Fetus and Birth*, Ciba Foundation Symposium no 47, Amsterdam, North-Holland, 1977, p 159-195.
19. Haskins AL: The progesterone content of human placentas before and after the onset of labor. *Am J Obstet Gynecol* 67, 330-338 (1954).
20. Pinto RM, Fisch L, Schwarz RL and Montuori E: Action of oestradiol-17β upon uterine contractility and the milk-ejecting effect in the pregnant woman. *Am J Obstet Gynecol* 90, 99-114 (1964).
21. Pinto RM, Leon C, Mazzocco N and Scasserra V: Action of oestradiol-17β at term and at onset of labor. *Am J Obstet Gynecol* 98, 540-546 (1967).
22. Järvinen PA, Luukkainen T and Väistö L: The effect of oestrogen treatment on myometrial activity in late pregnancy. *Acta Obstet Gynecol Scand* 44, 258-264 (1965).
23. Larson JW, Hanson TM, Caldwell BV and Speroff L: The effect of oestradiol infusion on uterine activity and peripheral levels of prostaglandin F and progesterone. *Am J Obstet Gynecol* 117, 276-279 (1973).
24. Kelly JV: The effect of intravenous estrogens on uterine motility. *Am J Obstet Gynecol* 82, 1207-1210 (1961).
25. Klopper A and Dennis K: Effect of oestrogens on myometrial contractions. *Br med J 2*, 1157-1159 (1962).
26. Fuchs F and Stakemann G: Treatment of threatened premature labour with large doses of progesterone. *Am J Obstet Gynecol* 79, 172-176 (1960).
27. Klopper A and McNaughton M: Hormones in recurrent abortion. *J Obstet Gynaecol Br Commow* 72, 1022-1028 (1965).
28. Csapo, AI, de Sousa Filho MB, de Souza JC and de Souza O: Effect of massive progestational hormone treatment on the parturient human uterus. *Fertil Steril* 17, 621-636 (1966).
29. Csapo AI: Progestational therapy during pregnancy: an invitational symposium. *J Reprod Med* 3, 225-243 (1969).
30. Turnbull AC, Patten PT, Flint APF, Keirse MJNC, Jeremy JY and Anderson ABM: Significant fall in progesterone and rise in oestradiol levels in human peripheral plasma before the onset of labour. *Lancet* 1, 101-104 (1974).
31. Aitken EH, Preedy JRK, Eton B and Short RV: Oestrogen and progesterone levels in foetal and maternal plasma at parturition. *Lancet* 2, 1096-1099 (1958).
32. Short RV and Eton B: Progesterone in blood. III. Progesterone in peripheral blood of pregnant women. *J Endocrinol* 18, 418-425 (1959).
33. Llauro JL, Runnebaum B and Zander J: Progesterone in human peripheral blood before, during and after labor. *Am J Obstet Gynecol* 101, 867-873 (1968).
34. Yannone ME, McCurdy JR and Goldfein A: Plasma progesterone levels in normal pregnancy, labor and the puerperium. II. Clinical Data. *Am J Obstet Gynecol* 101, 1058-1061 (1968).

35. Rado A, Crystle CD and Townsley JD: Concentrations of estrogens in maternal peripheral plasma in late pregnancy, during labor and postpartum. *J Clin Endocrinol Metab* 30, 497-503 (1970).
36. Chew PCT and Ratnam SS: Serial levels of plasma oestradiol-17β at the approach of labour. *J Endocrinol* 71, 267-268 (1976).
37. Turnbull AC, Anderson ABM, Flint APF, Jeremy JY, Keirse MJNC and Mitchell MD: Human parturition. In: *The Fetus and Birth*, Ciba Foundation Symposium no 47, Amsterdam, North-Holland, 1977, p 427-452.
38. Dawood MY and Ratnam SS: Serum unconjugated estradiol-17β in normal pregnancy measured by radioimmunoassay. *Obstet Gynecol* 44, 194-199 (1974).
39. Csapo AI: Progesterone block. *Am J Anat* 98, 273-291 (1956).
40. Csapo AI: The luteo-placental shift, the guardian of pre-natal life. *Postgrad Med J* 45, 57-64 (1969).
41. Barnes AC, Kumar D and Goodno JA: Studies in human myometrium during pregnancy. V. Myometrial tissue progesterone analyses by gasliquid phase chromatography. *Am J Obstet Gynecol* 84, 1207-1210 (1962).
42. Runnebaum B and Zander J: Progesterone and 20α-dihydroprogesterone in human myometrium during pregnancy. *Acta Endocrinol suppl* 150 (1971).
43. Falk RJ and Bardin CW: Uptake of tritiated progesterone by the uterus of the ovariectomized guinea-pig. *Endocrinology* 86, 1059-1063 (1970).
44. Porter DG: The local effect of intrauterine progesterone treatment on myometrial activity in rabbits. *J Reprod Fertil* 15, 437-445 (1968).
45. Johansson EDB and Jonasson LE: Progesterone levels in amniotic fluid and plasma from women. *Acta Obstet Gynecol Scand* 50, 339-343 (1971).
46. Younglai EV, Etter SB and Pelletier C: Amniotic fluid progesterone and oestrogens in relation to length of gestation. *Am J Obstet Gynecol* 111, 833-839 (1971).
47. Gautray JP, Jolivet A, Dhem N, Vielh JP and Tajchner G: Réflexion sur le rôle du foetus dans le déclenchement du travail à terme: exploration du liquide amniotique. In: Avortement et Parturition Provoqués, Paris, Masson, 1974, p 227-238.
48. Murphy BEP, Patrick J and Denton RL: Cortisol in amniotic fluid during human gestation. *J Clin Endocrinol Metab* 40, 164-167 (1975).
49. Fencl M deM and Tulchinsky D: Total cortisol in amniotic fluid and fetal lung maturation. *N Engl J Med* 292, 133-136 (1975).
50. Sjövall J: Gas chromatographic determination of steroid sulphates in plasma during pregnancy. *Ann Clin Res* 2, 393-408 (1970).
51. Sjövall J: Gas chromatographic determination of steroid sulphates in plasma during pregnancy. *Ann Clin Res* 2, 393-408 (1970).
52. Sweat ML, Bryson MJ and Young RB: Metabolism of 17β-estradiol and estrone by human proliferative endometrium and myometrium. *Endocrinology* 81, 167-172 (1967).
53. Rosenthal HE, Slaunwhite WR and Sandberg AA: Transcortin: a corticosteroid-binding protein of plasma. X. Cortisol and progesterone interplay and unbound levels of these steroids in pregnancy. *J Clin Endocrinol Metab* 29, 352-367 (1969).
54. Tulchinsky D and Chopra IJ: Competitive ligand-binding assay for measurement of sex hormone-binding globulin (SHBG). *J Clin Endocrinol Metab* 37, 873-881 (1973).
55. Towler CM, Jandial V, Horne CHW and Bohn H: A serial study of pregnancy proteins in primigravidae. *Br J Obstet Gynaecol* 83, 368-374 (1976).
56. Wyss RH, Heinrichs WLeR and Hermann WL: Some species differences of uterine estradiol receptors. *J. Clin Endocrinol Metab* 28, 1227-1230 (1968).
57. Notides AC, Hamilton DE and Muechler EK: A molecular analysis of the human estrogen receptor. *J Steroid Biochem* 7, 1025-1030 (1976).
58. Jänne O, Kontula K, Luukkainen T and Vihko R: Estrogen-induced progesterone receptor in human uterus. *J Steroid Biochem* 6, 501-509 (1975).

59. Cawson MJ, Anderson ABM, Turnbull AC and Lampe L: Cortisol, cortisone and 11-deoxycortisol levels in human umbilical and maternal plasma in relation to the onset of labour. *J Obstet Gynaecol Br Commonw* 81, 737-745 (1974).
60. Notides AC, Hamilton DE and Rudolph JH: Estrogen-binding proteins of the human uterus. *Biochim Biophys Acta* 271, 214-224 (1972).
61. Siiteri PK, Ashby R, Schwarz B and MacDonald PC: Mechanism of estrogen action studies in the human. *J Steroid Biochem* 3, 459-470 (1972).
62. Clewell WH, Carson BA and Meschia G: Comparison of uterotrophic and vascular effects of estradiol-17β and estriol in the mature organism. *Am J Obstet Gynecol* 129, 384-388 (1977).
63. Deansely R: Retarded embryonic development and pregnancy termination in ovariectomized guinea-pigs: progesterone deficiency and decidual collapse. *J Reprod Fertil* 28, 241-247 (1972).
64. Porter DG, Yoshinaga K and Ford J: Progesterone levels, intraluminal pressure and electrical activity of the guinea-pig uterus. *J Endocrinol* 61, 255-263 (1974).
65. Challis JRG, Heap RB and Illingworth DV: Concentrations of oestrogen and progesterone in the plasma of non-pregnant, pregnant and lactating guinea-pigs. *J Endocrinol* 51, 333-345 (1971).
66. Brunk U and Gustavii B: Lability of decidual cells. In vitro effects of autolysis and osmotic stress. *Am J Obstet Gynecol* 115, 811-816 (1973).
67. Gustavii B and Brunk U: Lability of decidual cells. In vivo effects of hypertonic saline. *Acta Obstet Gynecol Scand* 53, 271-274 (1974).
68. Willman EA and Collins WP: The concentrations of prostaglandin E_2 and prostaglandin $F_{2\alpha}$ in tissues within the fetoplacental unit after spontaneous or induced labour. *Br J Obstet Gynaecol* 83, 786-789 (1976).
69. Gustavii B: Human decidua and uterine contractility. In: *The Fetus and Birth*, Ciba Foundation Symposium no 47, Amsterdam, North-Holland, 1977, p 343-353.
70. Shettles LB: Hourly variation in onset of labor and rupture of membranes. *Am J Obstet Gynecol* 79, 177-179 (1960).
71. Smolensky M, Halberg F and Sargent F: Chronobiology of the life sequence. In: *Advances in Climatic Physiology*, Tokyo, Igaku Shoin, 1972, p 281-318.
72. Munson AK, Yannone ME and Mueller JR: The diurnal pattern of 17β-oestradiol in pregnancy. *Acta Endocrinol* 69, 410-412 (1972).
73. Townsley JD, Dubin NH, Grannis GF, Gartman LJ and Crystle CD: Circadian rhythms of serum and urinary estrogens in pregnancy. *J Clin Endocrinol Metab* 36, 289-295 (1973).
74. Bishop EH: Pelvic scoring for elective induction. *Obstet Gynecol* 24, 266-268 (1964).
75. Anderson ABM and Turnbull AC: Relationship between length of gestation and cervical dilatation, uterine contractility and other factors during pregnancy. *Am J Obstet Gynecol* 105, 1207-1214 (1969).
76. Pinto RM, Rabow W and Votta RA: Uterine cervix ripening in term pregnancy due to the action of oestradiol-17β. *Am J Obstet Gynecol* 92, 319-324 (1965).
77. Calder AA, Hillier K and Embrey MP: Prostaglandin therapy for cervical ripening prior to induction of labour. In: *Advances in Prostaglandin and Thromboxane Research*. Vol. 2. New York, Raven Press, 1975, p 993.
78. Gordon AJ and Calder AA: Oestradiol applied locally to ripen the unfavourable cervix. *Lancet* 2, 1319-1321 (1977).

ENDOGENOUS PROSTAGLANDINS IN HUMAN PARTURITION

MARC J.N.C. KEIRSE

It is widely believed that the use of prostaglandins for termination of pregnancy and induction of labour would not have shown such meteoric expansion if it had not been founded on the firm conviction that a prostaglandin was the long-awaited missing link in parturitional physiology. Nevertheless, the mechanism controlling the onset of labour in women remains as uncertain today as it was when the prostaglandins were discovered more than 40 years ago. It is perhaps worth remembering, that prostaglandin made its entry into scientific writing at the same time and on the same page of the German weekly *Klinisch Wochenschrift* as another capital "p" of parturition, progesterone. Von Euler's paper (1), which ends with: *Die hier beschriebene äther- und wasserlösliche Substanz... wird vorläufig "Prostaglandin" genannt*, was printed immediately below a communication by Allen et al. (2) in which they had agreed *von jetzt ab... ausschliesslich den Namen "Progesteron" zu verwenden* for the hormone extracted from corporea lutea, previously known as progestin or luteosteron. Within a few years progesterone was virtually equated to parturition by the demonstration in rabbits that a withdrawal of progesterone terminated pregnancy whereas progesterone therapy maintained it. A few decades later and with a considerable amount of experimental data at hand its role in human parturition remains controversial (3; Flint, this volume). Prostaglandins were introduced into parturitional physiology some 30 years later (4) but their impact has been no less important.

If at present the role of progesterone in human parturition is still debated, it may be presumptuous to assume that one could correctly place the prostaglandins in the scheme of things. Indeed, it is likely that several of our current facts and concepts may need to be reconsidered within the next few years, in the light of new discoveries made in the field of general prostaglandin and thromboxane biochemistry or physiology.

In the sphere of parturition attention has been devoted almost exclusively to the prostaglandins E_2 (PGE_2) and $F_{2\alpha}$ ($PGF_{2\alpha}$). This constitutes an at least three-fold restriction in/of the prostaglandin field. Firstly, no attention is paid to other prostaglandin groups (fig. 1) most notably D prostaglandins, since evidence for the natural occurrence of the A, B, and C groups is still

M.J.N.C. Keirse et al. (eds.), Human Parturition, 101-142.

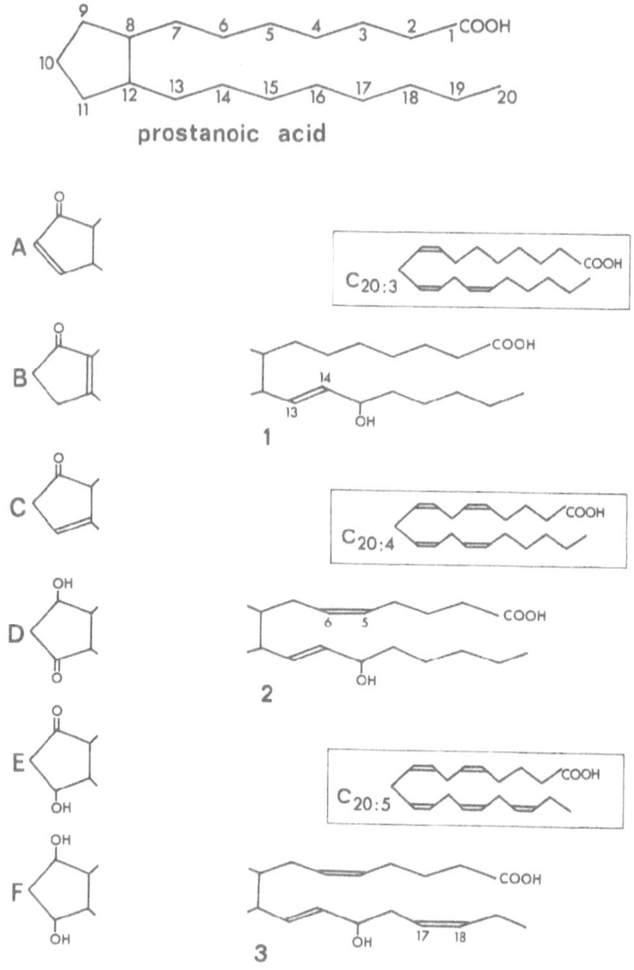

Fig. 1. Prostaglandin structure and nomenclature: prostaglandins are characterized by their cyclopentane ring (left) and the number of double bonds in the side chains (right). The inserts show the fatty acid precursors respectively for PG_1, PG_2 and PG_3 compounds.

controversial, certainly in man. Secondly, emphasis is placed upon the prostaglandins derived from arachidonic acid ($C_{20:4}$; fig. 1) at the expense of those derived from other fatty acids ($C_{20:3}$ and $C_{20:5}$; fig. 1). This is not entirely unwarranted as will be demonstrated below and indeed it is dubious whether other fatty acids contribute significantly to prostaglandin production in the human. The third restriction is perhaps the most important one particularly

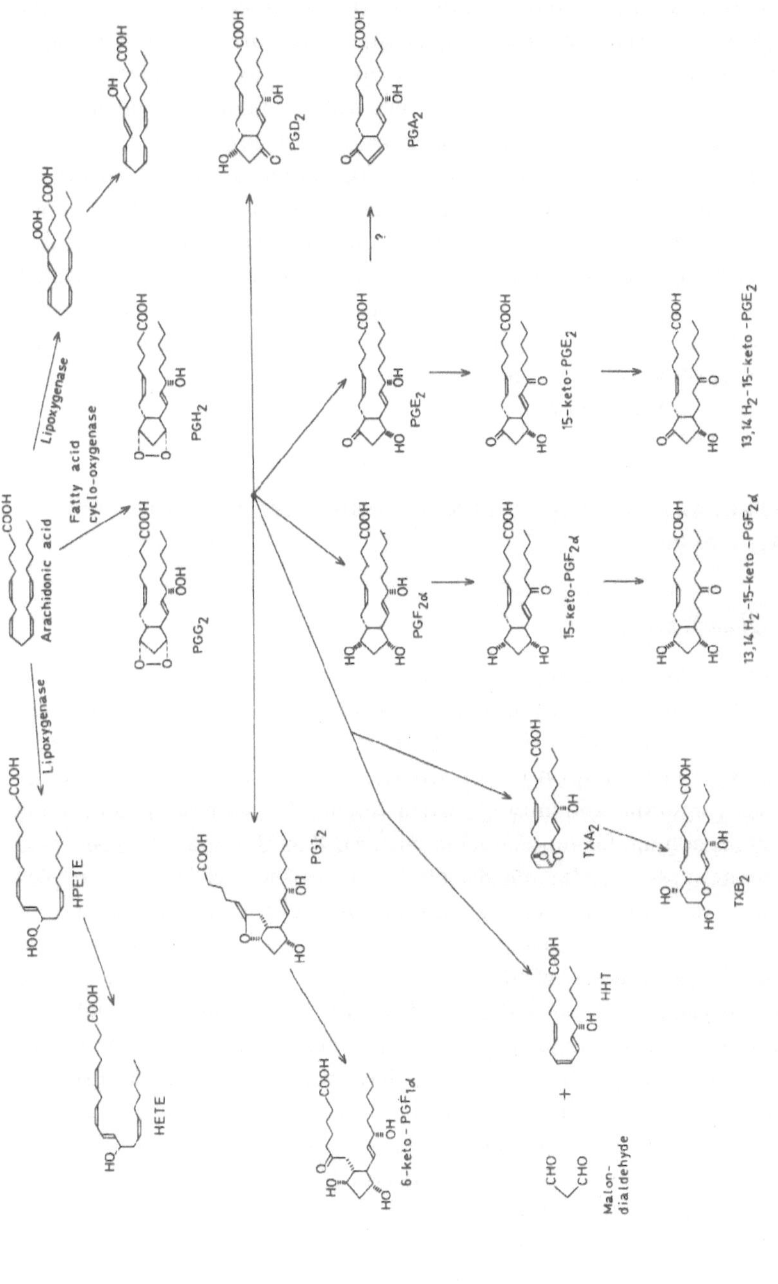

Fig. 2. Metabolism of arachidonic acid

since several authors (5-8) consider the liberation of arachidonic acid to be the major event in the control of prostaglandins and parturition. This restriction is illustrated in figure 2 which shows the major products formed from arachidonic acid by reactions which are to some extent analogous or identical to those which lead to the production of PGE_2 and $PGF_{2\alpha}$.

At present, evidence for the role of prostaglandins in human parturition includes: studies of their effect on uterine contractility (Thiery, this volume) and cervical ripening (Calder, this volume); inhibition of uterine activity and postponement of labour and delivery by administration of prostaglandin synthetase inhibitors (Wiqvist, this volume); and studies of their action at the cellular level. These aspects are not discussed here. In this article we examine whether and how human parturition is associated with an increase in endogenous prostaglandins.

PROSTAGLANDINS AND THEIR METABOLIC PATHWAYS IN INTRA-UTERINE TISSUES

Prostaglandin precursors

Endogenous prostaglandins are formed by enzymatic oxidation and cyclization of certain poly-unsaturated fatty acids. Since PGE_2 and $PGF_{2\alpha}$ are derived from arachidonic acid and PGE_1 and $PGF_{1\alpha}$ from dihomo-γ-linolenic acid, information on the distribution of these fatty acids may be of relevance for uterine and intra-uterine prostaglandin synthesis. Intra-uterine lipid stores contain far more arachidonic acid than dihomo-γ-linolenic acid (9). This applies to free fatty acids, fatty acids incorporated in phospholipids as well as to the total fatty acid composition. The relative abundance of arachidonic acid was a constant finding in all tissues investigated: umbilical cord, fetal membranes, placenta, myometrium and decidua. Arachidonic acid accounted for 7 to 20 percent of the free fatty acid composition, whereas hardly any dihomo-γ-linolenic acid was found in the free fatty acid fraction of the various tissues (9). Similar findings have been reported with respect to amniotic fluid (9-11), maternal plasma (12-14) and fetal plasma (12). These data may explain the predominance of prostaglandins of the '2' series (PGE_2 & $PGF_{2\alpha}$) over those of the '1' series (PGE_1 & $PGF_{1\alpha}$) noted in all studies which have specifically examined this question (15-17).

To be available as a precursor for prostaglandin biosynthesis arachidonic acid must be in non-esterified (or free) form. It has been suggested that the enzymatic release of free arachidonic acid, of which intracellular levels are generally believed to be very low, may be a controlling step in prostaglandin biosynthesis (18). Arachidonic acid can arise from a number of intracellular lipid pools such as triglycerides, cholesterol esters and phospholipids, and consequently there are a number of potential acylhydrolases capable of freeing arachidonic acid. Most of these have not been studied and attention has been directed mainly to the possible action of phospholipase A_2 in the control of prostaglandin biosynthesis. Well before it was discovered that prostaglandins are derived from fatty acids, Eliasson (19) had already observed that the addition of phospholipase A increased the formation of prostaglandins from vesicular glands *in vitro*. That this was due not to cleavage of prostaglandins but to that of their precursors has now become general knowledge. Evidence pertaining to this point was summarized by Flower and Blackwell (20) who, in a series of elegant experiments, confirmed that phospholipids are an important source of substrate for prostaglandin biosynthesis and that this source can be mobilized within the time span and under the conditions in which prostaglandin synthesis and release occurs. Equally as important however is their conclusion that substrate availability is not the only requirement for stimulation of prostaglandin biosynthesis. This point is of particular relevance since arachidonic acid serves as a precursor for a variety of other products than the prostaglandins E_2 and $F_{2}\alpha$ which have been implicated in human parturition (fig. 2). Research into these alternate routes of arachidonic acid metabolism within the pregnant uterus has merely begun, but already synthesis of thromboxane A_2 and prostacyclin (PGI_2) has been demonstrated respectively in umbilical cord vessels (21) and in placenta (22), whereas thromboxane B_2 and the prostacyclin metabolite, 6-keto-$PGF_{1}\alpha$, are also found in amniotic fluid (23, 24).

Evidence concerning the role of phospholipase in prostaglandin biosynthesis obtained in other tissues does not necessarily relate to uterine tissues, which in general show but low conversions of exogenous arachidonic acid into prostaglandins. Arachidonic acid is an essential fatty acid; it has a rather specialized turnover (25) and possibly a fairly selective transplacental transport (26) so that probably also supply of this fatty acid to the fetus should be considered. It should be noted in this respect that arachidonic acid accounts for a higher percentage of free fatty acids in the fetal than in the maternal circulation (12, 26).

All this indicates that the role of arachidonic acid in relation to pregnancy and parturition is an issue of great complexity. Equating arachidonic acid release to prostaglandin biosynthesis certainly must be an oversimplification.

Nevertheless the question of whether intra-uterine prostaglandin synthesis during parturition is controlled by the release of arachidonic acid from phospholipids has received a great deal of attention in recent years (5-8, 27, 28). It formed the key stone of Gustavii's lysosomal theory in which labour is likened to a delayed menstruation and in which leakage of lysosomal enzymes, including phospholipase A_2, in the decidua is ultimately responsible for prostaglandin synthesis and the initiation of labour (5, 29).

The importance of the lysosomal enzymes in the control of uterine prostaglandin production has been questioned by Batra and Bengtsson (6) who postulated that free fatty acids might be released by the ischaemia following myometrial contractions. However, evidence that prostaglandin synthesis in the pregnant uterus is specifically regulated by either of these mechanisms remains speculative. Also chorioamnion (27) and mainly the amnion (30) contain phospholipase A_2. Grieves and Liggins (30) found the highest phospholipase acitivities in decidua and amnion, whereas the activities of chorion and myometrium were substantially less (fig. 3).

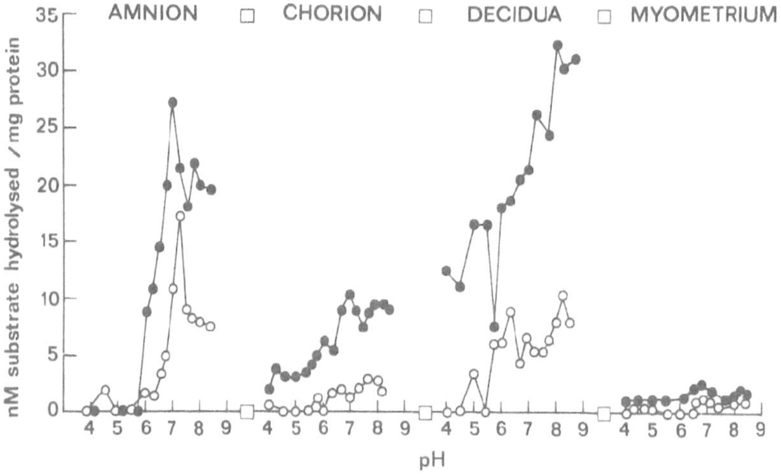

Fig. 3. Phospholipase A_2 activity in uterine tissues obtained at Caesarean section during labour in relation to pH. Phosphatidyl ethanolamine containing [^{3}H]-arachidonic acid at the *sn*-2 position was incubated at 37 °C with crude lysosomal fractions for 15 min (○) or 2 h (●). The amount of substrate hydrolyzed was calculated from the ratio of total counts in the reaction mixture to the counts in the purified fatty acid fraction.(Adapted from Grieves and Liggins [30].)

Although it is well known that there is a marked increase in free fatty acids in the circulation during labour (33, 34), it is dubious whether this is relevant to prostaglandin synthesis in the pregnant uterus. Schwarz et al. (31) found that the total fatty acid content of the fetal membranes contained a lower percentage of arachidonic acid during labour when compared to before labour. In the uterine decidua, which is also rich in arachidonic acid (9, 31), this percentage remained similar irrespective of whether or not labour had begun (31). These observations were interpreted as an indication of increased phospholipase activity in the fetal membranes during labour (31). Grieves and Liggins (30) however, found no differences in the *in vitro* phospholipase activity in the various tissues during labour (fig. 3) as compared to before labour. Filshie and Anstey (32) compared the concentrations of free and esterified arachidonic acid in various uterine tissues obtained by Caesarean section before or during labour. Concentrations of free arachidonic acid showed no significant changes with labour. The only significant difference in esterified arachidonic acid was found in the myometrium and this consisted of an increase rather than a decrease during labour. Hence there is no unequivocal evidence for an increase in either free arachidonic acid concentration or phospholipase activities in uterine tissues during as compared to before labour.

Prostaglandin biosynthesis

Biosynthesis of PGE_2 has been conclusively demonstrated by isotope dilution techniques in umbilical cord and fetal membranes but a significant formation of PGF was not observed in these experiments (9, 35). Biosynthesis of PGE_2 in the human umbilical cord is not limited to the umbilical vessels, for Jonsson et al. (36) demonstrated that the connective tissue produces prostaglandins in amounts comparable to those produced by the arteries. The same authors (36) also demonstrated that formation of PGE_2 exceeds that of PGE_1 and measurements of the amount of endogenous prostaglandins further confirmed that formation of PGE_2 exceeds that of PGF. According to Sykes et al. (37) prostaglandin synthesis in decidua and myometrium also yields mainly PGE, and is equally distributed between myometrium and decidua during late pregnancy. Kinoshita et al. (38) demonstrated prostaglandin biosynthesis in homogenates of decidua, chorion, amnion and placental villi. Contrary to Keirse and Turnbull (35) who found more prostaglandin synthesis in chorion than in amnion, they found the highest synthetase activity in amnion. However the experiments of Kinoshita et al. (38) did not allow for concomitant degradation of newly formed prostaglandins, which varies considerably between these tissues (35, 39).

Insufficient data are available at present to answer the question as to which of the various intra-uterine tissues has the highest biosynthetic potential *in vitro*. All tissues studied so far show very low conversion of exogenous arachidonic acid to prostaglandins, which on occasions may be difficult to even differentiate from non-enzymatic production (35). Changes in the biosynthetic potential in relation to the onset or the process of labour have not been reported. It is therefore impossible to reach firm conclusions with respect to the distribution of prostaglandin biosynthesis in the various intra-uterine tissues *in vivo*. However, enough evidence has become available to reemphasize our statement (35) that prostaglandins are so ubiquitous and some of the enzymes controlling their concentrations are so widely distributed throughout the pregnant uterus that the hypothesis that prostaglandin production could be confined to a single intra-uterine structure is likely to be an oversimplification.

Prostaglandin catabolism

The first evidence for prostaglandin catabolism in an intra-uterine tissue came from Nakano et al. (40) who, comparing the metabolic degradation of PGE_1 in a few tissue homogenates from 3 species, reported catabolism of PGE_1 by the human placenta. Jarabak (41) subsequently reported the partial purification of 15-hydroxy-prostaglandin dehydrogenase (15-PGDH) from the same tissue. Since then several studies have dealt with the purification and properties of placental 15-PGDH (42). Keirse and Turnbull (39) however showed that the placenta was not the only site and, in terms of enzyme activity per unit of weight, not even the most active site of prostaglandin catabolism within the pregnant uterus. Both 15-PGDH and 15-keto-prostaglandin-Δ^{13}-reductase were found to be widely distributed throughout the pregnant uterus early as well as late in gestation (39, 43). Their distribution in the term uterus followed the same pattern as that observed earlier in gestation. The highest 15-PGDH activities were found in the fetal membranes and placenta, followed by myometrium and decidua, whereas the lowest activity was observed in the umbilical cord (fig. 4). No prostaglandin catabolism was demonstrated in amniotic fluid or in umbilical venous blood. The membranes showed the highest 15-PGDH activity found in tissues from the pregnant uterus, but when membranes were separated into their components it was found that nearly all of the enzyme activity was located in the chorion, whereas amnion had a much lower 15-PGDH activity (fig. 5), which was not higher than that found in myometrium and decidua. The chorion which is of the same trophoblastic origin as the placenta therefore has the highest 15-PGDH activity per unit of weight of all intra-uterine tissues, catabolizing an average (n=6) of 430 nanomoles $PGF_{2\alpha}$/g chorion/min compared with 207 nanomoles $PGF_{2\alpha}$/g placenta/min (n = 44) under similar conditions (44, 45).

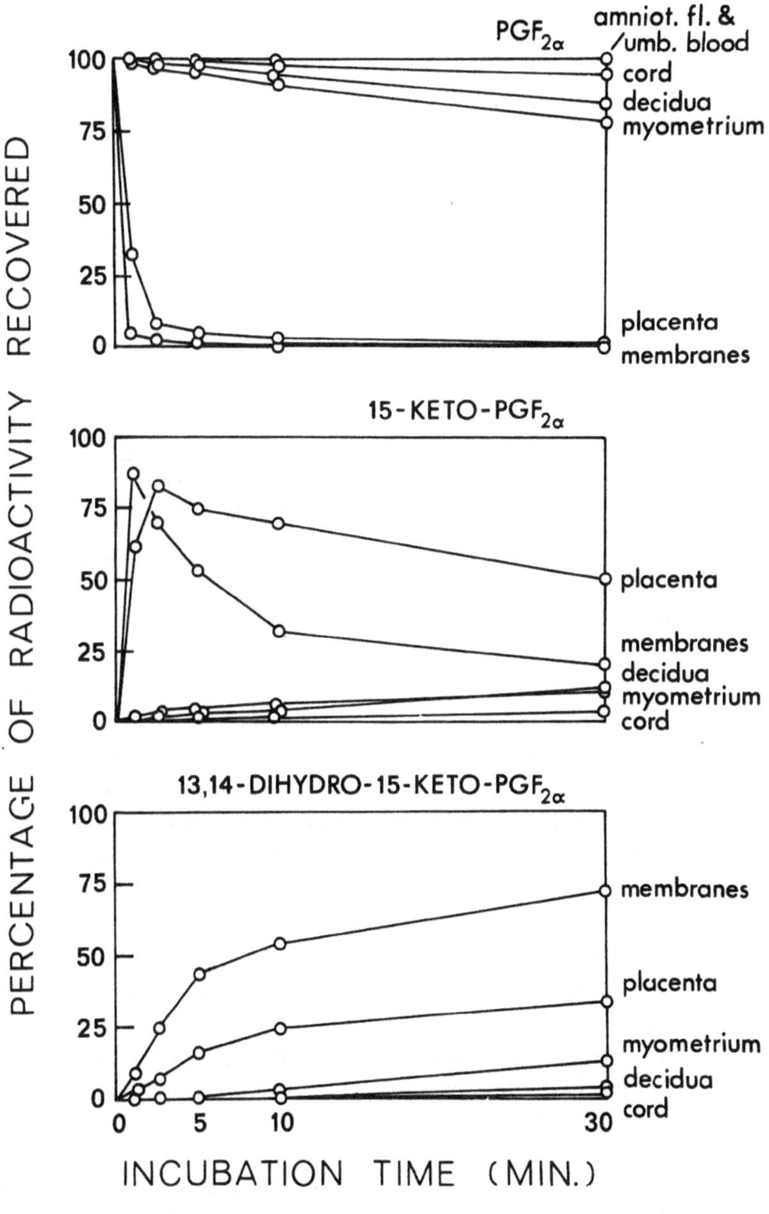

Fig. 4. Metabolism of ^3H-$PGF_{2\alpha}$in amniotic fluid, umbilical venous blood and homogenates of membranes, placenta, myometrium, decidua and umbilical cord, all obtained from the same patient at elective Caesarean section at term. Concentrations of $PGF_{2\alpha}$ used were 23 ng/ml blood or amniotic fluid and 900 ng/g tissue. Incubations were conducted at 37 °C in the presence of NAD^+ (2mM). Thin-layer chromatography was used for the separation of $PGF_{2\alpha}$ from its metabolites. (Adapted from Keirse and Turnbull [39].)

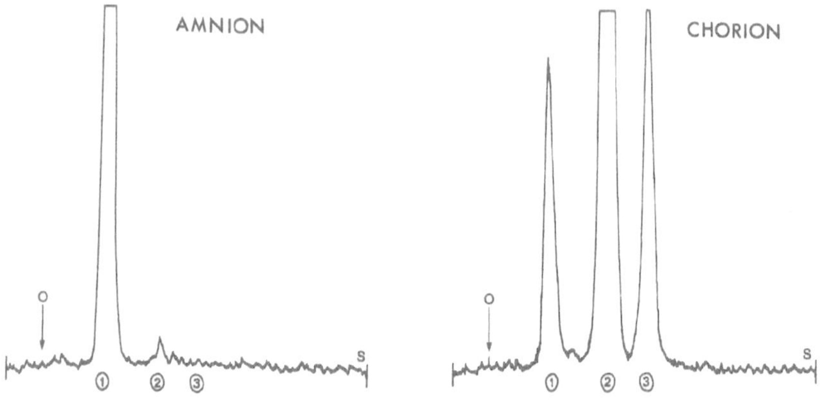

Fig. 5. Radiochromatogram scans of extracts of amnion and chorion subjected to thin-layer chromatography after 60 minutes incubation at 37°C with 200 ng ^{3}H-PGF$_{2\alpha}$/g tissue without addition of NAD. Authentic standards of PGF$_{2\alpha}$ (1), 15-keto-PGF$_{2\alpha}$ (2) and 13,14-dihydro-15-keto-PGF$_{2\alpha}$ (3) were run as references. Solvent system: chloroform-methanol-acetic acid-water (90 : 8 : 1 : 0.8, by vol; O : origin; S : solvent front; from Keirse and Turnbull [35]).

Throughout gestation, from 7 weeks onwards till term, tissue of trophoblastic origin, chorion and placenta, has a much higher 15-PGDH activity than the other intra-uterine structures (35, 39, 43). The high rates of 15-PGDH activity therefore appear to be a particular feature of trophoblastic tissue. Yet Alam et al. (46) noted severely depressed catabolism of PGE$_1$ in hydatidiform molar tissue, which is characterized by marked trophoblastic proliferation. Since the latter is avascular the high rate of catabolism in the placenta should perhaps be attributed to its high vascularity particularly since other tissues known to be rich in 15-PGDH such as lung, kidney, spleen and liver (47-49) have the same characteristic. However, this fails to explain why the relatively avascular chorion should be more active in prostaglandin catabolism than placental villous tissue. Although based on a semi-quantitative technique the observations on molar tissue (46) certainly suggest that 15-PGDH can be seriously altered under pathological conditions and depressed placental catabolism of PGE$_1$ has been observed also in pre-eclampsia (50). Schlegel et al. (51) noted that immature placentae obtained between 16 and 20 weeks gestation have lower 15-PGDH activity than do placentae obtained at term, and our own few data (9) tend to support this finding. These observations and animal evidence which showed that the cellular half-life of 15-PGDH is very short (52) suggest that prostaglandin degradation is an easily controllable step – a fact which may well be important for the modulation of prostaglandin concentrations near the time of parturition.

Keirse et al. (45) developed a quantitative assay for 15-PGDH in whole homogenates especially to examine whether 15-PGDH activity changes during parturition. Forty-four patients were studied either before labour, after spontaneous labour or after oxytocin-induced labour but no changes were observed. The 15-PGDH activity in placental homogenates ranged from 54 to 495 nmoles $PGF_{2}\alpha$/g placenta/min with no differences between the three groups (fig. 6). The 15-PGDH activity was not related either to differences in gestational age between 38 and 42 weeks, or to placental weight and birth-weight, and it was not markedly affected by the clinical use of prostaglandins for induction of labour at term. Using a semi-quantitative assay technique

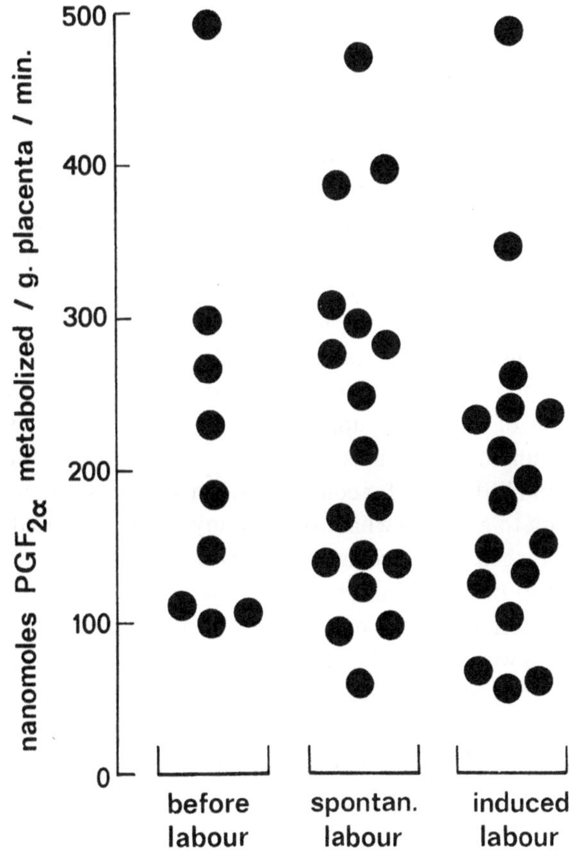

Fig. 6. 15-Hydroxy-prostaglandin dehydrogenase activity in human placentae obtained at elective Caesarean section before labour, and at vaginal delivery after spontaneous or oxytocin-induced labour. (Adapted from Keirse et al. [45]).

without the addition of co-factors, as a different approach, we (44) again found no differences in prostaglandin metabolism in either placenta or chorion in relation to labour in women. Although it is of course possible that *in vitro* techniques are insufficiently appropriate to examine the question of whether a decrease in prostaglandin catabolism is responsible for increasing prostaglandin concentrations during labour, it is interesting to note that the same group using the same technique could find such changes in sheep (53) but not in women (45). In this respect it should be realized that interspecies differences in the uterine metabolism of prostaglandins during pregnancy are considerable in both qualitative (distribution of the enzymes) and quantitative (enzyme activity) terms (54-56).

Prostaglandin concentrations

Karim (57) and Karim and Devlin (4), using a biological assay, first detected a mixture of PGE_1, PGE_2, $PGF_{2\alpha}$ and $PGF_{1\alpha}$ in umbilical cord vessels and decidua. The presence of PGE_2 and $PGF_{2\alpha}$, but not of PGE_1 or $PGF_{1\alpha}$, has since been confirmed in these as well as in other intra-uterine tissues (36, 58-62). In our opinion the measurement of prostaglandin concentrations in tissues from the pregnant human uterus contributes little, if anything, to the understanding of parturitional physiology. Indeed all tissue levels should be interpreted in the light of long established evidence (63) that prostaglandins are synthesized and released rapidly, in comparatively large quantities, upon simple distortion of cells. This applies to virtually all tissues studied but particularly to human tissues, for clinical and ethical requirements leave no room for ideal and little room for consistent methods of tissue collecting. It is therefore difficult to assess to what extent, if any, levels measured in uterine tissues reflect endogenous concentrations *in vivo*.

Only one group of investigators (61, 62) has dealt systematically with a whole range of uterine tissues and their results are summarized in table 1. PGE_2 and $PGF_{2\alpha}$ were detected by radioimmunoassay in all tissues studied. In the first of their studies (61), the highest concentrations were found in decidua, myometrium and cord, followed by the amnion, chorion and placenta. In contrast to findings of Karim (57), Karim and Devlin (4) and Pokoly and Jordan (59), the mean concentration of PGE_2 in all tissues was 27 to 518 percent higher than that of $PGF_{2\alpha}$. This is consistent with the data of Sykes et al. (37) Keirse and Turnbull (35), Jonsson et al. (36) and Mitchell et al. (64) which showed that formation of PGE takes precedence over that of PGF in uterine tissues. They further noted a significant rise in the concentration of prostaglandins in decidua and to a lesser extent in myo-

Table 1. The concentration of prostaglandins E_2 and $F_{2\alpha}$ in various tissues from the pregnant human uterus. (After Willman and Collins [61, 62].)

Tissue	Prostaglandin	Prostaglandin concentration (ng/g wet weight; mean ± S.D.)			
		at Caesarean section		at vaginal delivery after	
		before labor ($n = 9$)	during labor ($n = 8$)	spontaneous labor ($n = 6$)	induced labor ($n = 6$)
Placenta	PGE_2	10.4 ± 2.5	13.5 ± 5.3	17.8 ± 8.9	9.9 ± 3.2
	$PGF_{2\alpha}$	8.2 ± 3.4	9.6 ± 3.8	12.3 ± 5.7	8.5 ± 2.7
Umbilical cord	PGE_2	55.4 ± 8.8	55.8 ± 18.6	69.4 ± 29.9	31.5 ± 17.8
	$PGF_{2\alpha}$	10.7 ± 2.4	11.9 ± 4.1	15.0 ± 8.2	9.1 ± 4.2
Amnion	PGE_2	22.5 ± 12.7	47.7 ± 25.1	275.6 ± 153.6	61.6 ± 25.2
	$PGF_{2\alpha}$	9.8 ± 4.5	11.2 ± 5.5	28.9 ± 16.4	9.7 ± 8.8
Chorion	PGE_2	16.4 ± 6.3	18.6 ± 6.9	56.1 ± 20.4	36.2 ± 18.1
	$PGF_{2\alpha}$	5.4 ± 2.3	7.2 ± 5.8	12.5 ± 6.9	8.6 ± 5.8
Decidua	PGE_2	40.2 ± 17.8	107.6 ± 44.5	158.1 ± 54.1	92.8 ± 38.4
	$PGF_{2\alpha}$	15.4 ± 9.8	64.4 ± 35.3	51.5 ± 22.5	59.2 ± 19.7
Myometrium	PGE_2	41.9 ± 10.6	58.5 ± 26.5	—	—
	$PGF_{2\alpha}$	19.2 ± 7.2	32.6 ± 27.3	—	—

metrium and amnion at Caesarean section during labour when compared to before labour. Subsequently (62), they reported that PGE_2 concentrations are higher in placenta, umbilical cord and amnion but $PGF_{2\alpha}$ concentrations only in amnion after spontaneous labour when compared to oxytocin-induced labour. Consistent in both reports is the observation that prostaglandin levels are lowest in placenta and chorion. Hence the lowest concentrations were found in those tissues which have the highest 15-hydroxyprostaglandin dehydrogenase activities (39, 44). Since not only prostaglandin synthesis but also prostaglandin metabolism occurs rapidly (44), this further emphasizes the difficulties in interpreting prostaglandin levels in tissues and it may be anticipated that varying results will be published within the next few years. For example, contrary to the findings of Willman and Collins (table 1), Jonsson et al. (36) already reported that prostaglandin levels (PGE_2 equivalents) are substantially higher in umbilical cord obtained at vaginal delivery than in those obtained at Caesarean section.

The data of Mitchell et al. (64) using a totally different approach are not in agreement with those of Willman and Collins (table 1) either. These authors superfused tissues with a modified Krebs bicarbonate buffer and measured prostaglandin levels in the superfusate (table 2). Contrary to the data of

Table 2. Prostaglandin production by various tissues from the pregnant human uterus during tissue superfusion. (After Mitchell *et al.* [64].)

Tissue	Prosta-glandin	Prostaglandin concentration (ng/g dry weight/min; mean ± S.D.) in superfusates from tissues obtained	
		at Caesarean section before labour (n=10)	at vaginal delivery after spontaneous labour (n=10)
Placenta	PGE	2.8 ± 1.5	2.0 ± 1.2
	PGF	0.8 ± 0.8	0.7 ± 0.4
Amnion	PGE	9.6 ± 5.1	13.2 ± 7.0
	PGF	0.7 ± 0.6	0.8 ± 0.6
Chorion	PGE	3.1 ± 1.9	2.9 ± 1.5
	PGF	0.8 ± 0.6	0.5 ± 0.4
Decidua	PGE	2.5 ± 1.8	1.7 ± 0.8
	PGF	0.8 ± 0.8	0.5 ± 0.3

Willman and Collins (table 1) they found that production of PGE by amnion was several-fold greater than any other tissue whereas chorion also produced more than decidua (table 2). This indicates a marked PGE production in the fetal membranes and is consistent with the demonstration of prostaglandin biosynthesis in this tissue (35). However, the contribution of the amnion to prostaglandin production in the fetal membranes appears to be greater than would have been expected from the data of Keirse and Turnbull (35). There were no differences in prostaglandin production between tissues obtained after spontaneous vaginal delivery and those obtained at elective Caesarean section, but this – of course – does not necessarily apply to the *in vivo* situation.

PROSTAGLANDINS IN MATERNAL AND FETAL CIRCULATIONS DURING PREGNANCY AND PARTURITION

Maternal peripheral circulation

In the author's belief there is no place, in the study of the initiation or the mechanism of labour, for the measurement of primary prostaglandins in the peripheral circulation. However, assessment of the role of prostaglandins in human parturition has thus far relied heavily upon their quantification in the maternal peripheral circulation, and it is therefore pertinent to examine the available evidence. Numerous studies have dealt with this subject, particularly with PGF concentrations, in relation to pregnancy and labour and these are summarized in tables 3-5. Various trends have been described during pregnancy (table 3). Levels of PGF have, for instance, been found by some (65) to reach a maximum in the second trimester and by others to be significantly lower in the second trimester than in the first trimester (66) or to be lower in the second trimester than at any other time during pregnancy (67). Yet some authors (65, 67-70) report that the levels obtained in the third trimester of pregnancy are not statistically different from those obtained in non-pregnant women. It has been found that PGF levels are higher during labour than in pregnancy (67, 68, 71, 72) and increases in PGF concentration with the progression of labour have been demonstrated by some authors (68, 71-73) but not by others (74-76). Some authors (68, 73) have reported that PGF levels were higher in the late first stage of labour than in the second stage and at delivery, whereas others (71, 72) found the highest levels at delivery (table 4). Various trends in PGF concentration have further been noted with respect to the uterine contractions during labour and these are summarized in table 5.

When critically examined the data presented in tables 3-5 represent more than a high score of disagreement amongst various authors. Five years ago, it was already estimated from studies on the kinetics of prostaglandin metabolism (77), from daily urinary excretion rates of the major prostaglandin

Table 3. PGF levels in maternal peripheral venous blood (plasma or serum) during pregnancy before the onset of labour.

Authors	gestation period	PGF levels* (pg/ml)
Caldwell et al. (71)	1st trim.	600-900
Béguin et al. (80)	2nd trim.	0-400
Brummer (68)	28-40 wk	590 ± 510
Gutierrez-Cernosek et al. (65)	all	200-1850
	33-35 wk	340 ± 190
	37-41 wk	360 ± 150
Gillett et al. (96)	10-15 wk	400 ± 270
Brummer (66)	0-13 wk	620 ± 410
	14-26 wk	390 ± 470
	27-41 wk	450 ± 430
Patrono (97)	not stated	< 50-100
Van Orden and Farley (70)	3rd trim.	40-130
Challis and Tulchinsky (69)	7 wk-term	< 30-41
Challis et al. (86)	term	34 ± 40
Hennam et al. (67)	8-16 wk	29.6 ± 4.1
	17-20 wk	20.4 ± 4.7
	29-38 wk	26.7 ± 7.6
Shearman et al. (98)	16-20 wk	100-1500
Johnson et al. (91)	16-20 wk	26.3 ± 4.3
	⩾ 36 wk	27.1 ± 8.1
Pokoly and Jordan (59)	term	330 ± 245
Twomey et al. (99)	4-37 wk	0-2000
Zahradnik et al. (100)	term	180 ± 60
Kinoshita et al. (76)	term	3700 ± 2500

* Figures are means ± S.D. or range of values.

metabolites (78, 79) and on the basis of constant infusion of $PGF_{2\alpha}$ (80) that basal levels of $PGF_{2\alpha}$ in the peripheral circulation should be about 2 pg/ml (81). Even if, in view of the higher urinary excretion rate of the major PGF metabolite (82) higher levels could be expected during pregnancy and labour, these would still be well below any of the levels reported in tables 3-5. It is tempting to correlate the various trends in prostaglandin concentrations with changes in the plasma concentration of free fatty acids during pregnancy (14) and particularly with the sharp increase in circulating free fatty acids known to be associated with labour (33,34). Combined with the distinctive ability of blood platelets to synthesize prostaglandins, this may well account for the higher prostaglandin levels in peripheral maternal blood during labour. However, even then most of the data (tables 3-5) remain difficult to explain, which emphasizes the inherent difficulties in measuring and interpreting prostaglandin concentrations. The only conclusion therefore to be reached is

Table 4. PGF levels in maternal peripheral venous blood (plasma or serum) during labour.

Authors	Stage of labour, or cervical dilatation (cm) in 1st stage of labour	PGF levels* (pg/ml)
Karim (72)	1st	3380 (1500-8300)
	2nd	8040 (3600-22800)
	3rd	6360 (1900-21000)
Caldwell et al. (71)	1st	1200-3000
	2nd	3000-5000
Brummer (68)	1st	~ 240-4300
Brummer and Craft (73)	(0-4 cm)	~ 700
	(5-9 cm)	~ 1800
	2nd	~ 420
Craft et al. (87)	2nd	497 (125-860)
Patrono (97)	not stated	180-400
Challis et al. (86)	2nd	98 ± 87
Gréen et al. (74)	1st	~ 50-100
	2nd	
Hennam et al. (67)	not stated	33.1 ± 11.6
Hillier et al. (75)	1st	~ 260-1400
Johnson et al. (91)	1st	33.1 ± 11.6
	2nd	40.1 ± 17.6
Pokoly and Jordan (59)	1st + 2nd	290 ± 216
Zahradnik et al. (100)	(5 cm)	1300-3200
	(10 cm)	1200-5400
Kinoshita et al. (76)	1st	2000 ± 900
	2nd	1920 ± 1420

*Figures are means ± S.D. or range of values. Concentrations preceded by ~ are approximate, and were obtained from tabular or graphical material presented by the respective authors.

Table 5. Relationship between PGF concentrations in maternal peripheral venous plasma and uterine contractility during labour

Authors	PGF levels (pg/ml)	Author's comments
Karim (72)	<200-18000	appearance of $PGF_{2\alpha}$ precedes the uterine contraction
Jubiz et al. (84)	?	PGF maximum at the peak of the contraction
Sharma et al. (101)	< 75-427	maximum 15-45 s after the peak of the contraction
Challis et al. (86)	10-165	maximum 45-60 s after the peak of the contraction
Gréen et al. (74)	± 200	no relationship with the contraction
Johnson et al. (91)	35 ± 11 (S.D.)	no relationship with the contraction
Zahradnik et al. (100)	1200-5400	maximum 50 ± 8 s before the peak of the contraction

that these PGF levels in the peripheral circulation can hardly be interpreted as a measure of uterine prostaglandin production or as evidence for an involvement of prostaglandins in human parturition. Relatively few studies have dealt with concentrations of PGE in the maternal circulation during pregnancy and labour (59, 76, 83-85) but the data are no less confusing than those on PGF concentrations. It is not to be anticipated either that improvements in methodology and better assay techniques will bring us any further in this respect.

Umbilical circulation at birth

If study of prostaglandin concentrations in the maternal peripheral circulation fails to inform us on the involvement of prostaglandins in human parturition, it should be considered whether veins draining the pregnant uterus or the fetal circulation might yield more information. Both uterine venous blood and umbilical venous as well as arterial blood have been studied in this respect. Hertelendy et al. (83), for instance, reported PGE levels in umbilical venous plasma to average 1870 pg/ml but this was not confirmed by Keirse (9) who failed to detect PGE levels in excess of the lower limit of detection (1000 pg/ml) by gas liquid chromatography with electron-capture detection. PGF levels in the umbilical circulation have been studied by several investigators (59, 76, 86, 87) all of whom noted that arterial concentrations were sometimes higher and sometimes lower than venous concentrations. Challis et al. (86) and Craft et al. (87) found PGF levels to be higher in the fetal circula tion than in the maternal peripheral circulation, and interpreted this as indicating genuine prostaglandin production in the feto-placental unit. Yet, the absence of consistent differences between arterial and venous levels coupled with the marked metabolic capacity of fetal villous tissue (39) emphasize the inadequacy of this experimental approach for defining the site of prostaglandin production. The procedure for obtaining blood from umbilical arteries and vein is more complex than obtaining blood from a maternal antecubital vein, and it is done at a time when closure of the umbilical vessels, a process in which prostaglandins are thought to be involved (58, 88), occurs spontaneously without the added stimulus of manipulation. Furthermore, umbilical blood is relatively richer in both platelets (89) and arachidonic acid (12) than maternal blood. It is therefore dubious whether prostaglandin levels in umbilical plasma yield genuine information on intra-uterine prostaglandin synthesis.

The availability of better and more sensitive radioimmunoassays led Mitchell et al. (90) to recently re-examine some of these questions. Although they obtained lower prostaglandin levels than any of those reported above, their data have not helped our understanding of the value, if any, of prostaglandin concentrations in the umbilical circulation. In patients who had received epidural analgesia during labour, they (90) found no arterio-venous differences in the concentrations of either PGF, its major circulating metabolite or PGE. In patients who did not receive epidural analgesia, only levels of PGE schowed a statistically significant arterio-venous difference. Their data however, add another important point to the discussion and interpretation of prostaglandin levels in the umbilical circulation: the importance of the time interval between delivery of the baby and sampling. Indeed concentrations of PGE, PGF as well as the major circulating metabolite of PGF were found to rise continuously from the time of delivery of the baby (fig. 7). The authors offer no explanation for this finding and the fact that there are no dramatic changes after intervening cord clamping or placental delivery does not help to clarify the issue. However, this is well worthy of some further attention for its explanation may at once confirm that also prostaglandin concentrations in the umbilical circulation cannot correctly inform us on the role of these compounds in parturition (9).

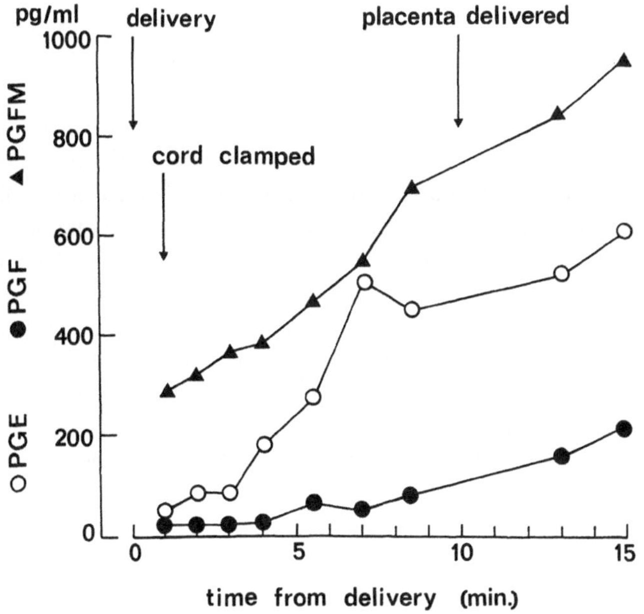

Fig. 7. Changes in the concentrations of PGE, PGF and 13,14-dihydro-15-keto-PGF in umbilical venous plasma after birth. (Adapted from Mitchell et al. (90)).

Uterine venous circulation

Studies of uterine venous blood have not been more helpful in this respect. Keirse and Flint (unpublished data, 1973) studying PGF concentrations in 40 samples of uterine venous plasma at Caesarean section found levels of 1.10 ± 0.23 ng/ml (mean ± S.E., n = 19) and 2.08 ± 0.42 ng/ml (n = 20), respectively, before the onset of labour and during labour. Although levels obtained during labour were higher ($p < 0.05$) than those obtained before labour it was concluded that conditions of collection and assay did not allow firm conclusions on the output of PGF from the pregnant uterus (9). Pokoly and Jordan (59) later reported PGE concentrations of 380 ± 110 pg/ml (mean ± S.E., n = 5) and PGF concentrations of 680 ± 270 pg/ml in uterine venous plasma before labour. They found no difference in either PGE or PGF concentrations between the few samples obtained before or during labour. Johnson et al. (91) reached the same conclusion with lower PGF levels, but reported, contrary to Pokoly and Jordan (59), that levels were higher in the uterine vein than in the maternal peripheral circulation. Careful analysis of these data in the light of findings reported in tables 3-5 does not allow any conclusion to be drawn with respect to either the production of prostaglandins by the pregnant uterus or their involvement in parturition. These data do show however, that the output of prostaglandins, particularly PGF, during labour is substantially lower in women than in other species such as sheep and goat (Mitchell, this volume; 92). This point may be of relevance in that it was shown (93) that the measurement of 13,14-dihydro-15-keto-PGF (PGFM) in the peripheral circulation can be used to monitor release of PGF from the uterus during parturition in sheep, there being a good correlation between PGFM levels in jugular venous plasma on the one hand and PGF levels in utero-ovarian venous plasma on the other. Such evidence is not available in the human and it would be wrong to infer that it applies to the human situation, in view of the differences in uterine venous PGF levels between these species. Furthermore, we (53-56, 94) and others (Mitchell, this volume) demonstrated several other differences between sheep and women in the responsiveness of the pregnant uterus to prostaglandins, in the quantity and in the distribution of prostaglandin catabolizing enzymes within the pregnant uterus.

Prostaglandin metabolites

It is clear that the physiology of pregnancy and parturition implies more than the mere presence of a pregnant uterus with its contents, whether it is contracting or not. Changes in the levels of prostaglandins or their metabolites in either the peripheral circulation or urine can therefore not be assumed to originate from the uterus unless this is proved to be the case. Indeed enzymes responsible for the synthesis or degradation of prostaglandins ate widely distributed among various organs in the body most of which may be amenable to changes during pregnancy or labour. Hence criticisms directed at the measurement of prostaglandins in the peripheral circulation as a means of studying the role of prostaglandins in labour, should be extended also to the study of metabolites. This applies to the study of Gréen et al. (74) who found that concentrations of PGFM in the maternal peripheral circulation increase during labour (fig. 8) as well as to that of Hamberg (82) who showed that the excretion of a major urinary metabolite of PGF is much higher during labour than in pregnancy. Mitchell et al. (95) showed that vaginal examination, sweeping of the membranes and rupture of the membranes all result in an

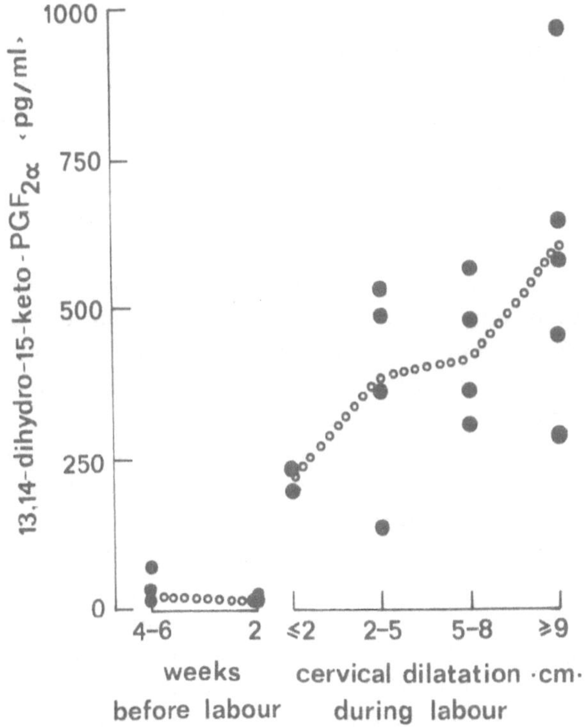

Fig. 8. Concentrations of 13,14-dihydro-15-keto-$PGF_{2\alpha}$ in maternal peripheral venous plasma during late pregnancy and labour. (Adapted from Gréen et al. [74].)

increase of PGFM in the peripheral maternal circulation. These data as well as those of Gréen et al. (74) and Hamberg (82) suggest that the levels of metabolites measured may to some extent reflect changes at the uterine level but they do not exclude a variety of other possibilities, e.g. changes in respiratory function. At present, it is therefore impossible to draw any scientifically valid conclusions on the role of prostaglandins in the initation of human labour from measurements made in either maternal or fetal circulations.

PROSTAGLANDINS IN AMNIOTIC FLUID DURING LATE PREGNANCY AND LABOUR

It is hardly conceivable that the relatively small amount of prostaglandins present in amniotic fluid plays a real role in uterine activation. Apart from a local cervical effect which they may possibly have when leaking through the cervix after rupture of membranes, the role of amniotic fluid prostaglandins in parturition surely must be minimal. Nevertheless concentrations of prostaglandins in amniotic fluid show an attractive feature in that neither synthesis nor degradation of prostaglandins take place in this fluid. *In vitro* incubation of amniotic fluid with a prostaglandin precursor, dihomo-γ-linolenic acid, does not result in creased levels of prostaglandins (9, 35) and neither is there a significant correlation between levels of arachidonic acid and those of PGF in amniotic fluid (102). Similarly incubation of amniotic fluid with labelled $PGF_{2\alpha}$ shows no inactivation (39; fig. 4). Although verification of these data by another group of investigators would be welcomed, it may presently be assumed that prostaglandins found in amniotic fluid originate from surrounding structures and represent the release and reabsorption resulting from prostaglandin production in the pregnant uterus. Both PGE_2 and $PGF_{2\alpha}$ have been identified in amniotic fluid (15, 16). Earlier (4, 103) and other (76, 104) reports which suggested the presence of appreciable amounts of PGE_1 and $PGF_{1\alpha}$ in amniotic fluid have not been confirmed by those who specifically examined this question using more appropriate methodology (15-17).

Although the prostaglandins (E_2 and $F_{2\alpha}$) measured and the actual levels of these compounds vary from one study to another, all studies are consistent in showing three trends which will be discussed in more detail below. Firstly all studies are consistent in showing that prostaglandin levels in amniotic fluid are lower in mid- pregnancy than at term (16, 17, 91, 105, 106). Secondly levels are higher during labour than before labour (4, 15, 16, 17, 75, 91, 105, 106, 107). Thirdly levels increase during labour (15, 16, 17, 75, 106, 107).

Before the onset of labour

Although it is generally agreed that PGF levels in amniotic fluid are lower in mid-pregnancy than at term, only Salmon and Amy (106) and Hibbard et al. (105), unlike other authors (16, 17), found a gradual rise in PGF concentrations with gestational ages from 36 weeks onwards. Mitchell et al (108) demonstrated that apparent contradictions between these studies may relate to sampling techniques. These authors found that amniotic fluid obtained by amniotomy contained significantly more PGF than that obtained by amniocentesis at comparable gestational ages. When samples obtained by amniotomy and by amniocentesis were considered separately, there was no significant increase in PGF concentrations with increasing gestational age (fig. 9).

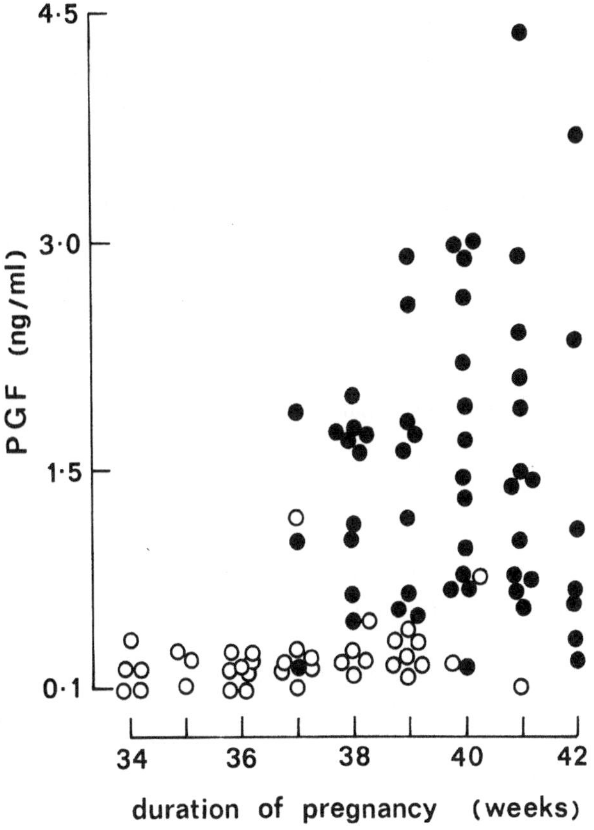

Fig. 9. Concentrations of PGF in amniotic fluid obtained by amniocentesis (○) or by amniotomy (●) before the onset of labour. (Adapted from Mitchell et al. [108].)

However, a significant increase in PGF concentrations appeared when amniocentesis and amniotomy samples were combined, and it is reasonable to assume that the frequency with which amniocentesis is performed decreases while that of amniotomy increases with advancing gestational age from 36 weeks. Although this may explain the findings of Hibbard et al. (105) it does not apply to the study of Salmon and Amy (106), since as asserted by Amy and Karim (109), these authors collected all samples obtained before labour by transabdominal amniocentesis. Dray and Frydman (17) found that not PGF concentrations but only PGE concentrations rose significantly between 35 and 36 weeks and that no further increases in the concentration of either compound occurred until term. However the increase reported by these authors is based on a mere 4 measurements ranging between 33 and 35 weeks and 4 more observations at 36 weeks so that further confirmation of these data is required. Hence there is presently no consensus of opinion as to whether prostaglandin concentrations increase during the last few weeks of pregnancy before the onset of labour. This does not signify that there is no such increase, for there are no data on serial measurements before the onset of labour and these may be necessary to overcome the effects of biological variations in both prostaglandin concentrations and length of gestation. In the rhesus monkey, Mitchell et al. (110) found a significant increase in the PGF concentrations in amniotic fluid during the last 10 days of pregnancy in all animals in which serial amniocenteses were performed. Furthermore, in human pregnancy the concentrations of the major circulating PGF metabolite, 13,14-dihydro-15-keto-PGF, in amniotic fluid obtained by amniocentesis show a small but significant increase over the 34 to 42 weeks' gestation period (108).

During labour

With the onset of labour there is a sharp increase in the concentrations of PGE_2 (15, 17) and $PGF_{2\alpha}$ (4, 16, 17, 75, 91, 105, 106, 107) in amniotic fluid (fig. 10).

During labour concentrations of both PGE_2 (15, 17) and $PGF_{2\alpha}$ (16, 17, 75, 106, 107) increase further in a statistically significant manner with progressing cervical dilatation (fig. 10). A similar increase in PGF concentrations as that seen during labour at term has been described during pre-term labour (111).

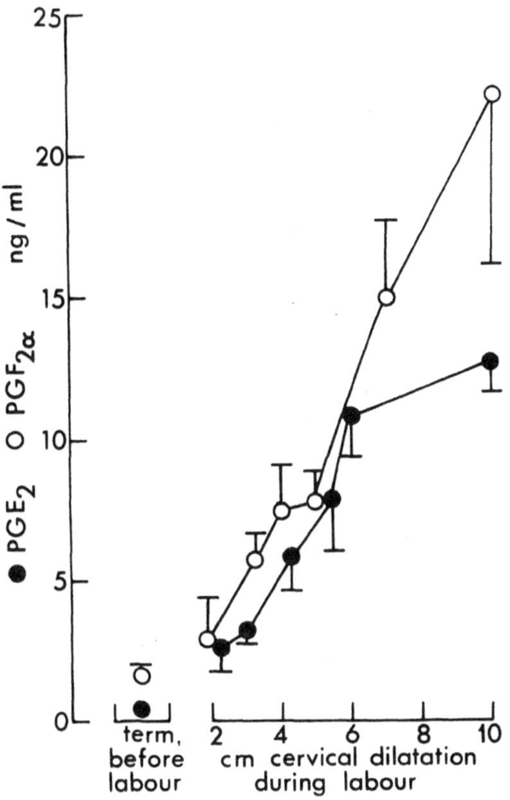

Fig. 10. Concentrations (mean ± S.E.M.) of PGE_2 and $PGF_{2\alpha}$ in amniotic fluid during late pregnancy and labour at term. (After data from Keirse and Turnbull (15) and Keirse et al. [16].)

REGULATION OF PROSTAGLANDIN CONCENTRATIONS IN THE PREGNANT UTERUS *IN VIVO*

In the preceding sections we have examined the available data on the production of prostaglandins in the pregnant uterus in relation to parturition. When summarizing we may conclude that the *prostaglandin generating system* – or *prostaglandin turnover* – in its entirety, ranging from the liberation of free arachidonic acid up to the catabolism of prostaglandins into relatively inactive products, can operate within the confines of the pregnant human uterus. Indeed, the prostaglandin precursor arachidonic acid (both in its free and in its bound form), enzymes which can liberate arachidonic acid, enzymes which transform arachidonic acid into prostaglandins as well as enzymes

Table 6. Distribution of prostaglandins and factors which may possibly regulate their concentration in tissues of the pregnant uterus.

	Amnion	Chorion	Decidua	Placenta	Myometrium	Umbilical cord	References
Compounds (measured *in vitro*)							
esterified arachidonic acid	+	+	+	+	+	+	9, 32
free arachidonic acid	+	+	+	+	+	+	9, 32
prostaglandin E_2	+	+	++	+	++	++	61, 62
prostaglandin $F_{2\alpha}$	+	+	++	+	++	+	61, 62
Enzyme activities *in vitro*							
phospholipase A_2	++	+	++		±		30
prostaglandin "synthetase"	+	+	+	±	+	+	35-38
15-hydroxy-prostaglandin dehydrogenase	+	++	+	++	+	+	35, 39

which catabolize prostaglandins are all widely distributed among the various intra-uterine tissues (table 6).

Evidence that the prostaglandin system *can* operate within the pregnant uterus does not necessarily signify that it actually *does* operate *in vivo* and in relation to parturition. No consistent changes were found in the various uterine tissues, in either arachidonic acid, phospholipase activity, prostaglandin biosynthesis or prostaglandin catabolism in relation to the onset or the process of labour. The measurement of prostaglandin concentrations in intra-uterine tissues and in maternal and fetal circulations has not helped to

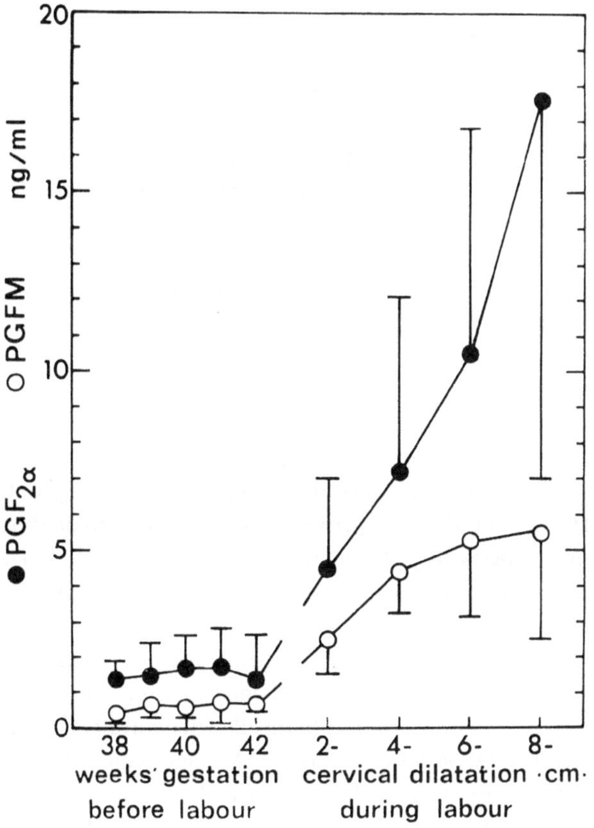

Fig. 11. Concentrations (mean ± S.D.) of $PGF_{2\alpha}$ and 13,14-dihydro-15-keto-$PGF_{2\alpha}$ in amniotic fluid obtained by amniotomy at term before the onset of labour and during labour. Means ± S.D. were calculated after distribution of all values according to gestational age before the onset of labour or to the degree of cervical dilatation between 2 and 10 cm during labour. The figure illustrates the three trends in prostaglandin concentrations before, at the onset of and during labour. (After data from Keirse et al. [16, 107] and Mitchell et al. [108].)

clarify the issue. On the other hand, the studies on amniotic fluid prove that the prostaglandin system is operational *in vivo*, and that it functions either differently or at a different level of activity before labour than at the onset of or during labour (fig. 11).

Before the onset of labour

Up to the onset of labour the prostaglandin system probably operates at a very low level. It is clear that prostaglandin levels at term are higher than in mid-pregnancy. On the other hand, changes in their concentration during the last few weeks of pregnancy are not marked enough to have been found by all authors. If there is – and the combined evidence suggests that there may well be – an increase in prostaglandin concentrations during the last few weeks of pregnancy, this is not due to a decrease in prostaglandin catabolism. Apart from the fact that no changes in prostaglandin catabolism could be demonstrated (44, 45), concentrations of 13,14-dihydro-15-keto-PGF (PGFM) in amniotic fluid show a small but significant increase during the last few weeks of pregnancy (108).

Several factors have been implicated in the control of intra-uterine prostaglandin synthesis prior to the onset of labour. So for instance reported Turnbull et al. (112) that, in amniotic fluid obtained by amniocentesis between 34 and 41 weeks, there was a significant relationship between concentrations of PGF and PGFM and those of oestradiol-17β. This correlation was limited to oestradiol and did not extend to oestrone sulphate, of which concentrations in amniotic fluid are approximately 10-fold higher than those of oestradiol (112). This does not provide much information on the control of prostaglandin synthesis for, although animal data suggest that oestrogen enhances prostaglandin production (113, 114), prostaglandins can stimulate placental synthesis of oestrogen *in vitro* (115, 116).

Gustavii (5, 29) suggested that hormonal alterations, e.g. increases in oestrogen and decreases in progesterone concentrations, are responsible for the labilization of lysosomes in decidual cells which are believed to be unusually fragile (117). Decidual cells obtained at Caesarean section at term but before the onset of labour indeed show marked degenerative changes (29). This would result in release of phospholipase A_2 into the cytoplasm of cells leading to an increasing availability of arachidonic acid and hence increasing prostaglandin synthesis in the decidua. Schwarz et al. (118) found binding of progesterone in lysosomal fractions of the fetal membranes and proposed that, as term approaches, the lysosomes have to compete with an increasing capacity for progesterone binding in the cytosol, which is particularly marked after 38 weeks (118). As a consequence the lysosomes would become more unstable and their contents would leak out, resulting in an enzymatic release of arachidonic acid in the fetal membranes (28, 31, 118).

Although these theories have much to recommend them (8), they have two major limitations. Firstly they do not take account of the wide distribution within the uterine environment of compounds and enzymes involved in prostaglandin synthesis and concentrate upon only one tissue, either the fetal membranes (28, 31, 118) or the decidua (5, 29) neither of which appear to be the site of action for the prostaglandins formed. The control of prostaglandin synthesis is generally believed to be effected at the junction between decidua and membranes and there is other evidence to support it (8, 35, 56, 108). The available data, however, do not allow us to limit our attention to only one of these tissues nor to exclude other intra-uterine tissues. For instance, it is worth noting that cervical tissue has not been mentioned yet as a possible site of uterine prostaglandin production. In the guinea pig at least, cervical tissue is as active as myometrial tissue in the catabolism of prostaglandins (Keirse, unpublished observations), and it is likely that the cervix is the site where, prior to the real onset of labour, prostaglandins show the effect which is most markedly relevant to the subsequent initiation of labour (119; Calder, this volume).

The second conceptual limitation of the studies of Gustavii (5, 29) and Schwarz et al. (28, 31, 118) is their assumption that the liberation of arachidonic acid from storage in phospholipids is the biochemical event which controls uterine prostaglandin synthesis *in vivo*. In a preceding section we have warned against the fallacies of equalizing arachidonic acid release with prostaglandin synthesis. In support of this assumption however, MacDonald et al. (7) found that injection of 300 to 1000 mg potassium arachidonate into the amniotic sac induces abortion in the second trimester of pregnancy, whereas another fatty acid, oleate, was inactive at these concentrations. In two subjects, the simultaneous ingestion of aspirin, a known prostaglandin synthetase inhibitor, prevented arachidonate-induced abortion. Although pharmacological data are not necessarily applicable to physiological events, this is a powerful argument which cannot be discarded. Yet in the rhesus monkey extra-amniotic administration of arachidonic acid does not terminate pregnancy or increase prostaglandin levels in amniotic fluid or maternal plasma (Robinson et al., this volume). Administration of PGE_2, on the other hand, in a dose which was only 2.5 percent that of arachidonic acid resulted in both termination of pregnancy and an increase in prostaglandin concentrations (Robinson et al., this volume). Although animal data cannot be extrapolated to man this raises a number of intriguing questions. Prostaglandin synthetase inhibitors are capable of inhibiting uterine contractility which is induced by other means than the administration of arachidonic acid. This approach therefore does not necessarily guarantee that administration of exogenous arachidonic acid stimulates prostaglandin synthesis and uterine activity in a direct manner. In our opinion it is necessary, if ethically possible, to repeat MacDonald's experiments (7) and to study the mechanism by which termination of pregnancy is achieved.

Gradual changes

The underlying factor to both facts and concepts concerning the control of prostaglandins prior to the onset of labour is that it is a gradual process. Apart from the fact that it may well be responsible for changes in cervical consistency and effacement (Calder, this volume) and for an increased sensitivity of the myometrium to other stimuli towards the end of pregnancy, little is known about it.

It may consist of a slow build up of prostaglandin production which, although virtually imperceptible, has such an effect on the myometrium (and possibly the cervix) that at a given moment in time – either by accumulating effects or by a lowering of thresholds – a minimal increase in prostaglandins is sufficient to account for the onset of labour. If this is the case, prostaglandin synthesis will, when sufficiently understood and accurately monitored, ultimately be able to inform us on the precise timing of the onset of labour. It is more likely however, that this gradual process should be interpreted as a maturation of enzyme systems. Occasionally and inadvertently it may cause small spikes of prostaglandin release which could be responsible for some of the changes observed, e.g. in cervical consistency and prostaglandin concentrations in amniotic fluid. However, this process would have little or no significance unless a particular extraneous stimulus leads to explosive prostaglandin production. In that case thorough knowledge and monitoring of the prostaglandin system will bring us no further in knowing exactly when labour will start. It will merely inform us as to how far preparations are under way and how severe the stimulus should be in order to make the most of these preparations.

Although we favour the latter mechanism, these two possibilities are not mutually exclusive. It is conceivable that a system designed to be self-accelerating can respond to a strong extraneous influence just as well as it can be envisaged that a proceeding maturational process ultimately requires but a very small stimulus in order to express itself.

Acute changes

That some stimuli can, at the end of pregnancy but preceding the onset of labour, acutely stimulate prostaglandin synthesis *in vivo* is well known. Mitchell et al. (108) observed a five-fold increase in the concentrations of PGF in amniotic fluid obtained by amniotomy as compared to that obtained by amniocentesis at similar gestational ages. Apart from the fact that it is known that prostaglandins are not stored in cells this cannot be interpreted as a mere release of prostaglandins but must include an activation of prostaglandin biosynthesis either in response to vaginal and cervical stimulation such as noted in sheep (114) or by disruption of the fetal membranes and decidua. Indeed also PGFM levels are found to be elevated at amniotomy but the increase with regard to levels obtained at amniocentesis is only two-fold and much lower than that of PGF (108).

Interestingly, a similar mechanism may also apply to levels of arachidonic acid, because MacDonald et al. (7) noted an eight-fold increase in the concentration of arachidonic acid during labour as compared to before labour. Amniotic fluid studied by these authors was collected by transabdominal amniocentesis, by transuterine amniocentesis at the time of Caesarean section, or by direct needle aspiration through the fetal membranes at the time of vaginal delivery or during labour. This indicates that all samples obtained before labour were obtained by amniocentesis whereas several if not all of those obtained during labour were obtained at amniotomy. This may well mean that the observed increase in arachidonic acid levels during labour (7) is not related to the initiation of parturition but to the effect of amniotomy. This would also correspond to the concepts of Gustavii (5, 29) and MacDonald's group (7, 27, 28, 31, 118) that disruption of the decidua and/or fetal membranes play an important role in arachidonic acid release. In the presence of a sufficiently mature prostaglandin generating system this may well be responsible for some of the acute effects on prostaglandin synthesis. Such a mechanism may perhaps even hold the explanation for a variety of clinical observations that, near term, labour can start in response to stimuli as artificial or spontaneous rupture of the membranes, infection of the fetal membranes or stripping the membranes from the adjacent decidua. The fact that several of these stimuli become more effective towards term may indicate that a certain maturational process is necessary for their effect.

Although it is not absolutely certain that amniotic fluid obtained by amniotomy contains more arachidonic acid than that obtained by amniocentesis, such a difference applies to several but not all of the products derived from it. Indeed levels of $PGF_{2\alpha}$, its metabolite (PGFM) and those of thromboxane B_2, the metabolite of thromboxane A_2, are higher at amniotomy (fig. 12). On

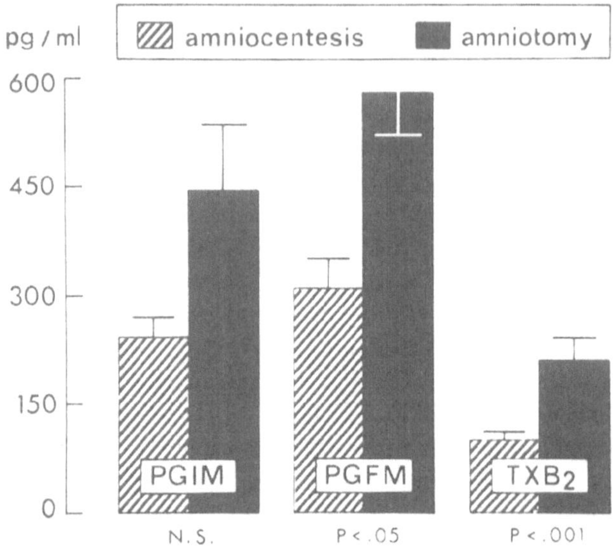

Fig. 12. Comparison between the concentrations (mean ± S.E.M.) of metabolites of PGI_2 (6-keto-$PGF_{1\alpha}$ PGIM), $PGF_{2\alpha}$(13,14-dihydro-15-keto-$PGF_{2\alpha}$ PGFM), and thromboxane A_2 (thromboxane B_2; TXB_2) in amniotic fluid obtained at amniotomy and at amniocentesis before the onset of labour. (After data from Mitchell et al. [23, 24, 108].)

the other hand there was no significant difference in the concentration of 6-keto-$PGF_{1\alpha}$, the metabolite of prostacyclin (PGI_2), between the amniocentesis and amniotomy samples (fig. 12).

Three main conclusions can be reached from the data discussed above. Firstly, the acute elevation of prostaglandin concentrations at amniotomy as compared to amniocentesis is not due to a decrease in prostaglandin catabolism. Therefore it must represent a genuine stimulation of prostaglandin synthesis. Secondly, to explain this effect on prostaglandin synthesis attention should be directed not only to the liberation of arachidonic acid but also to the enzymes which convert this compound into prostaglandins and perhaps mainly to those enzymes which differentiate formation of prostaglandins from that of prostacyclin or thromboxane A_2. Thirdly, if amniotomy can induce such a pronounced effect it must be conceivable that other stimuli may have a similar effect. Whether this implies that they can then also herald the spontaneous onset of labour is at present merely a matter of speculation.

The onset of labour

At and following the spontaneous onset of labour the prostaglandin generating system certainly is fully operational. Prostaglandin E and F concentrations measured as early as possible during spontaneous labour show marked increases when compared to before labour (fig. 10). This applies also to concentrations of PGFM (fig. 11) which again indicates that the increase in prostaglandin concentrations is not due to decreased catabolism. The fact that concentrations further rise during labour clearly indicates that this is not due to enhanced release but truly represents increased prostaglandin synthesis.

The all-important question is whether the increase in prostaglandin synthesis is the cause or the result of uterine contractility. From a clinical point of view this question appears to be neatly answered by the observations that administration of prostaglandins will induce uterine contractility (Thiery, this volume) whereas administration of prostaglandin synthetase inhibitors will inhibit it (Wiqvist, this volume). Pharmacological evidence, however, may not adequately answer physiological questions. Other evidence is more difficult to assess. Concentrations of PGF in amniotic fluid were found to be higher in early spontaneous labour than in early oxytocin-induced labour at similar stages of cervical dilatation (fig. 13). This observation was confirmed and extended by Hillier et al. (75) who showed that several hours of artificially stimulated uterine activity can be maintained before an increase in PGF occurs. We (107) later showed that PGF concentrations during early spontaneous labour are higher in patients whose labour progresses normally than in those who later require oxytocin therapy for failure to progress adequately in first stage labour (fig. 13). Although these combined data offer strong support for a postulated causal influence of prostaglandins in the mechanism of human parturition, a perfect answer to the question cannot be given. Indeed Hillier et al. (75) showed that after several hours of oxytocin infusion and from cervical dilatations of 4 to 5 cm onwards PGF levels increase steeply to reach values which at full cervical dilatation are not different from those observed at full dilatation during spontaneous labour. These results do not necessarily imply that increased prostaglandin levels are the result of uterine contractility. Several other possible explanations can be considered; e.g. oxytocin administration may, as demonstrated in sheep (Mitchell, this volume), also increase uterine prostaglandin synthesis in women. Probably the most important item is the fact that the increase in prostaglandin levels in induced labour appears to relate only to the acceleration phase of labour. Hence, the increased prostaglandin concentrations may well be a reflection of

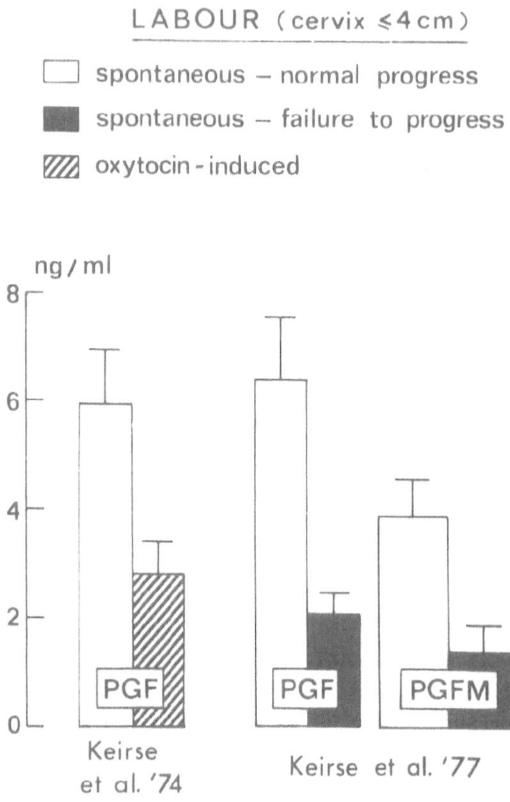

Fig. 13. Concentrations (mean ± S.E.M.) of PGF and 13,14-dihydro-15-keto-PGF (PGFM) in amniotic fluid during early labour in patients with normal spontaneous labour, with oxytocin-induced labour and with spontaneous labour which later required oxytocin therapy to correct dysfunctional uterine contractility. (After data from Keirse et al. [16, 107].)

the fact that induction of labour has succeeded in triggering the endogenous mechanism of parturition. This would be consistent with clinical observations that labour may proceed satisfactorily, when administration of oxytocin is greatly reduced or even withheld after the acceleration phase has been reached.

It is possible that our earlier data on PGE_2 concentrations in amniotic fluid (15) may need to be re-interpreted. In that study we found elevated PGE_2 levels in two out of twelve patients before the onset of clinical labour. Since one had 5 cm cervical dilatation and the other had been admitted in false labour previously the elevated PGE_2 levels were thought to be the consequence of uterine activity. In both patients however labour was then induced by simple amniotomy, which may possibly place a different emphasis on the cause-effect relationship between prostaglandin concentrations and the onset of labour.

Whether the onset of labour is also associated with increased liberation or increased concentrations of arachidonic acid has not unequivocally been demonstrated. Labour in general is associated with a marked increase in the levels of free fatty acids even in the maternal peripheral circulation (33, 34), though it is not certain if this also applies to concentrations of arachidonic acid which has a rather specialized turnover (25). As discussed above the results of MacDonald et al. (7) may relate more to differences between amniotomy and amniocentesis than to differences with the onset of labour, and they were not confirmed by Filshie and Anstey (32). Neverheless concentrations of thromboxane B_2 (23) and 6-keto-$PGF_{1}\alpha$ (24) in amniotic fluid are significantly higher during labour when compared to before labour. This may well indicate that the whole of the arachidonic acid cascade (120) starts to operate at a much higher level with the onset of labour.

During labour

With the further progression of labour there is a small but statistically significant increase in arachidonic acid concentrations in amniotic fluid (102). At this stage arachidonic acid concentrations show a 100-fold excess when compared to that of the prostaglandins (fig. 14), and there is no relationship between concentrations of arachidonic acid and those of either PGF or PGFM measured in the same samples. This indicates that – certainly at this stage – arachidonic acid or the release of arachidonic acid is unlikely to be the rate-limiting factor in uterine prostaglandin synthesis. As before labour there are no indications that the increase in prostaglandin concentrations should be attributed to a decrease in their catabolism, since concentrations of PGFM continue to rise (fig. 14) and the ratio between PGF and PGFM concentrations does not change (107). The ratio between PGF and PGFM was found to vary considerably between patients but a consistent pattern with respect to either the onset or the progress of labour was not observed. Hence, during labour the control of prostaglandin concentrations probably resides at the level of one or more of the enzymes which are responsible for the conversion of free arachidonic acid into prostaglandins. Consistent with this view is the fact that levels of thromboxane B_2 in amniotic fluid which are higher at amniotomy than at amniocentesis and higher during labour than before labour, do not further increase with the progression of labour (23), contrary to levels of arachidonic acid, PGE, PGF and PGFM (fig. 14). Neither do concentrations of the prostacyclin metabolite, 6-keto-$PGF_{1}\alpha$, which are also

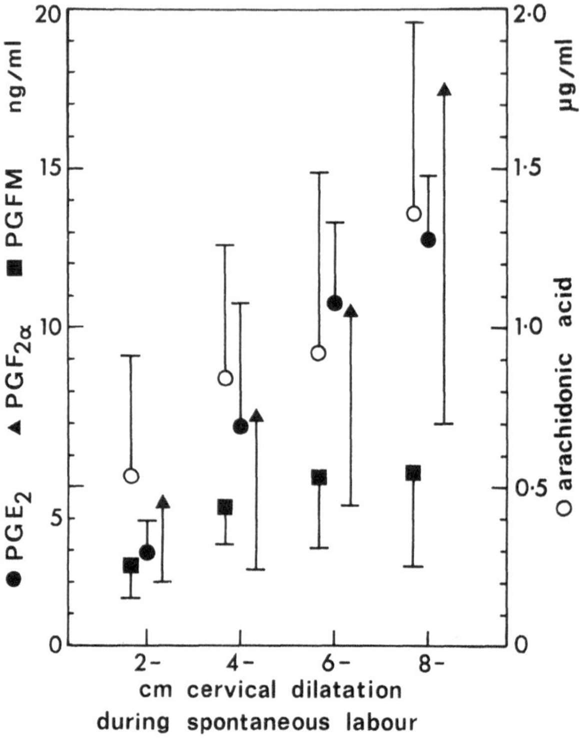

Fig. 14. Concentrations (mean ± S.D.) of free arachidonic acid, prostaglandin E_2, prostaglandin $F_{2\alpha}$ and 13,14-dihydro-15-keto-prostaglandin $F_{2\alpha}$ (PGFM) in amniotic fluid during spontaneous labour at term. Means ± S.D. were calculated after distribution of all values according to the degree of cervical dilatation between 2 and 10 cm. (After data from Keirse et al. [15, 16, 102, 107].)

higher during than before labour, increase with progressing cervical dilatation during labour (24). Furthermore, the results of Dray and Frydman (17) are difficult to explain if one assumes that arachidonic acid availability is the rate-limiting factor in prostaglandin synthesis during labour. When using serial measurements in the same subjects during labour, these authors found a reversal in the PGE/PGF ratio in amniotic fluid at some, though variable, stage of cervical dilatation. This and the other observations mentioned indicate that combined measurements of arachidonic acid and as many of its metabolic products as possible, may finally help to clarify how the control of prostaglandin concentrations in the pregnant uterus is executed.

ACKNOWLEDGMENT

I am grateful to Miss H. Wittenberg for typing the manuscript.

REFERENCES

1. Von Euler US: Über die spezifische blutdrucksenkende Substanz des menschlichen Prostata- und Samenblasensekretes. *Klin Wochenschr* 14, 1182-1183 (1935).
2. Allen WM, Butenandt A, Corner GW and Slotta KH: Zur Nomenklatur des Corpus luteum-hormons, *Klin Wochenschr* 14, 1182 (1935).
3. Csapo AI: The 'see-saw' theory of parturition. In: *The Fetus and Birth*, Ciba Foundation Symposium no 47, Amsterdam, Elsevier/Excerpta Medica/North-Holland 1977, p 159-195.
4. Karim SMM and Devlin J: Prostaglandin content of amniotic fluid during pregnancy and labour. *J Obstet Gynaecol Br Commonw* 74, 230-234 (1967).
5. Gustavii B: Labour: a delayed menstruation? *Lancet* 2, 1149-1150 (1972).
6. Batra S and Bengtsson LP: Mechanism for increased production of prostaglandins in labour. *Lancet* 1, 1164-1165 (1976).
7. MacDonald PC, Schultz FM, Duenhoelter JJ, Gant NF, Jimenez JM, Pritchard JA, Porter JC and Johnston JM: Initiation of human parturition. I. Mechanism of action of arachidonic acid. *Obstet Gynecol* 44, 629-636 (1974).
8. Liggins GC, Forster CS, Grieves SA and Schwartz AL: Control of parturition in man. *Biol Reprod* 16, 39-56 (1977).
9. Keirse MJNC: Studies on prostaglandins in relation to human parturition. *D Phil Thesis*, University of Oxford, 1975.
10. Das SK, Foster HW, Adhikary PK, Mody BB and Bhattacharyya DK: Gestational variation of fatty acid composition of human amniotic fluid lipids. *Obstet Gynecol* 45, 425-432 (1975).
11. Singh E J and Zuspan FP: Amniotic fluid lipids in normal human pregnancy. *Am J Obstet Gynecol* 117, 919-925 (1973).
12. Hansen AE, Wiese HF, Adam DJD, Boelsche AN, Haggard ME, Davis H, Newsom WT and Pesut L: Influence of diet on blood serum lipids in pregnant women and newborn infants. *Am J Clin Nutr* 15, 11-19 (1964).
13. Quinto P, Bottiglioni F and Flamigni C: Metabolic studies in healthy pregnant women. *J Obstet Gynaecol Br Commonw* 74, 544-555 (1967).
14. McDonald-Gibson RG, Young M and Hytten FE: Changes in plasma non esterified fatty acids and serum glycerol in pregnancy. *Br J Obstet Gynaecol* 82, 460-466 (1975).
15. Keirse MJNC and Turnbull AC: E prostaglandins in amniotic fluid during late pregnancy and labour. *J Obstet Gynaecol Br Commonw* 80, 970-973 (1973).
16. Keirse MJNC, Flint APF and Turnbull AC: F prostaglandins in amniotic fluid during pregnancy and labour. *J Obstet Gynaecol Br Commonw* 81, 131-135 (1974).
17. Dray F and Frydman R: Primary prostaglandins in amniotic fluid in pregnancy and spontaneous labor. *Am J Obstet Gynecol* 126, 13-19 (1976).
18. Kunze H and Vogt W: Significance of phospholipase A for prostaglandin formation. *Ann N Y Acad Sci* 180, 123-125 (1971).
19. Eliasson R: Studies on prostaglandin. Occurrence, formation and biological actions. *Acta Physiol Scand* 46, suppl 158, 1-73 (1959).
20. Flower RJ and Blackwell GJ: The importance of phospholipase A_2 in prostaglandin biosynthesis. *Biochem Pharmacol* 25, 285-291 (1976).

21. Tuvemo T, Strandberg K, Hamberg M and Samuelsson B: Maintenance of the tone of the human umbilical artery by prostaglandin and thromboxane formation. In: *Advances in prostaglandin and thromboxane research*, Samuelsson B and Paoletti R (eds), vol 1, New York, Raven Press, 1976, p 425-428.
22. Myatt L and Elder MG: Inhibition of platelet aggregation by a placental substance with prostacyclin-like activity. *Nature* 268, 159-160 (1977).
23. Mitchell MD, Keirse MJNC, Anderson ABM and Turnbull AC: Thromboxane B_2 in amniotic fluid before and during labour. *Br J Obstet Gynaecol* 85, 442-445 (1978).
24. Michell MD, Keirse MJNC, Brunt JD, Anderson ABM and Turnbull AC: Concentrations of the prostacyclin metabolite, 6-keto-prostaglandin $F_{1\alpha}$, in amniotic fluid during late pregnancy and labour. *Br J Obstet Gynaecol* 86, 350-353, 1979.
25. Hagenfeldt L, Hagenfeldt K and Wennmalm A: Turnover of plasma free arachidonic and oleic acids in men and women. *Horm Metab Res* 7, 467-471 (1975).
26. Robertson AF and Sprecher H: A review of human placental lipid metabolism and transport, *Acta Paediatr Scand*, suppl. 183, 1-18 (1968).
27. Schultz FM, Schwarz BE, MacDonald PC and Johnston JM: Initiation of human parturition. II. Identification of phospholipase A_2 in fetal chorioamnion and uterine decidua. *Am J Obstet Gynecol* 123, 650-653 (1975).
28. Schwarz BE, Schultz FM, MacDonald PC and Johnston JM: Initiation of human parturition, IV. Demonstration of phospholipase in the lysosomes of human fetal membranes. *Am J Obstet Gynecol* 125, 1089-1092 (1976).
29. Gustavii B: Release of lysosomal acid phosphatase into the cytoplasm of decidual cells before the onset of labour in humans. *Br J Obstet Gynaecol* 82, 177-181 (1975).
30. Grieves S and Liggins GC: Phospholipase A activity in human and ovine uterine tissues. *Prostaglandins* 12, 229-241 (1976).
31. Schwarz BE, Schultz FM, MacDonald PC and Johnston JM: Initiation of human parturition. III. Fetal membrane content of prostaglandin E_2 and $F_{2\alpha}$precursor. *Obstet Gynecol* 46, 564-568 (1975).
32. Filshie GM and Anstey MD: The distribution of arachidonic acid in plasma and tissues of patients near term undergoing elective or emergency caesarean section. *Br J Obstet Gynaecol* 85, 119-123 (1978).
33. Burt RL: Plasma nonesterified fatty acids in normal pregnancy and the puerperium. *Obstet Gynecol* 15, 460-464 (1960).
34. Nelson GH; Serum nonesterified fatty acid levels in human pregnancy as determined by various titration procedures. *Am J Obstet Gynecol* 92, 202-206, (1965).
35. Keirse MJNC and Turnbull AC: The fetal membranes as a possible source of amniotic fluid prostaglandins. *Br J Obstet Gynaecol* 83, 146-151 (1976).
36. Jonsson CE, Tuvemo T and Hamberg M: Prostaglandin biosynthesis in the human umbilical cord. *Biol Neonate* 29, 162-170 (1976).
37. Sykes JAC, Williams KI and Rogers AF: Prostaglandin production and metabolism by homogenates of pregnant human deciduum and myometrium. *J Endocrinol* 64, 18P-19P (1975).
38. Kinoshita K, Satoh K and Sakamoto S: Biosynthesis of prostaglandin in human decidua, amnion, chorion and villi. *Endocrinol Japon* 24, 343-350 (1977).
39. Keirse MJNC and Turnbull AC: Metabolism of prostaglandins within the pregnant uterus. *Br J Obstet Gynaecol* 82, 887-893 (1975).
40. Nakano J, Montague B and Darrow B: Metabolism of prostaglandin E_1 in human plasma, uterus and placenta, in swine ovary and in rat testicle. *Biochem Pharamacol* 20, 2512-2514 (1971).
41. Jarabak J: Human placental 15-hydroxyprostaglandin dehydrogenase. *Proc Nat Acad Sci USA* 69, 533-534 (1972).
42. Hansen HS: 15-Hydroxyprostaglandin dehydrogenase. A review. *Prostaglandins* 12, 647-679 (1976).

43. Keirse MJNC, Williamson JG and Turnbull AC: Metabolism of prostaglandin $F_{2\alpha}$ within the human uterus in early pregnancy. *Br J Obstet Gynaecol* 82, 142-145 (1975).
44. Keirse MJNC, Hanssens MCAJA, Hicks BR and Turnbull AC: Prostaglandin metabolism in placenta and chorion before and after the onset of labour. *Eur J Obstet Gynecol Reprod Biol* 6, 1-5 (1976).
45. Keirse MJNC, Hicks BR and Turnbull AC: Prostaglandin dehydrogenase in the placenta before and after the onset of labour. *Br J Obstet Gynaecol* 83, 152-155 (1976).
46. Alam N, Clary P, Shade AR and Russell PT: Absence of prostaglandin E_1 metabolism in hydatidiform mole. *Am J Obstet Gynecol* 119, 1131-1132 (1974).
47. Ännggård E, Larsson C and Samuelsson B: The distribution of 15-hydroxy-prostaglandin dehydrogenase and prostaglandin-Δ^{13}-reductase in tissues of the swine. *Acta Physiol Scand* 81, 396-404, 1971.
48. Samuelsson B, Granström E, Gréen K and Hamberg M: Metabolism of prostaglandins. *Ann N Y Acad Sci* 180, 138-163 (1971).
49. Keirse MJNC, Hicks BR and Kendall JZ: Fetal and maternal metabolism of prostaglandin $F_{2\alpha}$ in the guinea pig *Eur J Obstet Gynecol Reprod Biol* 9, 265-271, 1979.
50. Alam NA, Clary P and Russell PT: Depressed placental prostaglandin E_1 metabolism in toxemia of pregnancy. *Prostaglandins* 4, 363-370 (1973).
51. Schlegel W, Demers LM, Hildebrandt-Stark HE, Behrman HR and Greep RO: Partial purification of human placental 15-hydroxyprostaglandin dehydrogenase: kinetic properties. *Prostaglandins* 5, 417-433 (1974).
52. Blackwell GJ, Flower RJ and Vane JR: Rapid reduction of prostaglandin 15-hydroxy-dehydrogenase activity in rat tissues after treatment with protein synthesis inhibitors. *Br J Pharmacol* 55, 233-238 (1975).
53. Keirse MJNC, Mitchell MD and Flint APF: Changes in myometrial and placental 15-hydroxy-prostaglandin dehydrogenase with ovine parturition: production of prostaglandin metabolites in vitro and in vivo. *J Reprod Fert* 51, 409-412 (1977).
54. Keirse MJNC, Hicks BR and Turnbull AC: Metabolism of prostaglandin F-2α in fetal and maternal cotyledons of sheep. *J Reprod Fertil* 46, 417-420 (1976).
55. Keirse MJNC, Hicks BR and Turnbull AC: Comparison of intra-uterine metabolism of prostaglandin $F_{2\alpha}$ in ovine and human pregnancy. *J Endocrinol* 67, 24P-25P (1975).
56. Keirse MJNC, Hicks BR, Kendall JZ and Mitchell MD: Comparison of intrauterine prostaglandin metabolism during pregnancy in man, sheep and guinea pig. *Eur J Obstet Gynecol Reprod Biol* 8, 195-203 (1978).
57. Karim SMM: The identification of prostaglandins in human umbilical cord. *Br J Pharmacol Chemother 29*, 230-237 (1967).
58. Hillier K: Occurrence and actions of some prostaglandins in human umbilical and placental blood vessels. *Ph D Thesis*, University of London, 1970.
59. Pokoly TB and Jordan VC: Relation of steroids and prostaglandin at vaginal delivery and Cesarean section. *Obstet Gynecol* 46, 577-580 (1975).
60. Demers LM and Gabbe SG: Placental prostaglandin levels in pre-eclampsia. *Am J Obstet Gynecol* 126, 137-139 (1976).
61. Willman EA and Collins WP: Distribution of prostaglandin E_2 and $F_{2\alpha}$ within the foetoplacental unit throughout human pregnancy. *J Endocrinol* 69, 413-419 (1976).
62. Willman EA and Collins WP: The concentrations of prostaglandin E_2 and prostaglandin $F_{2\alpha}$ in tissues within the foetoplacental unit after spontaneous or induced labour. *Br J Obstet Gynaecol* 83, 786-789 (1976).
63. Bennett A, Friedmann CA and Vane JR: Release of prostaglandin E_1 from the rat stomach. *Nature* 216, 873-876 (1967).
64. Mitchell MD, Bibby J, Hicks BR and Turnbull AC: Specific production of prostaglandin E by human amnion in vitro. *Prostaglandins* 15, 377-382 (1978).
65. Gutierrez-Cernosek RM, Zuckerman J and Levine L: Prostaglandin $F_{2\alpha}$ in sera during human pregnancy. *Prostaglandins* 1, 331-337 (1972).

66. Brummer HC: Serum $PGF_{2\alpha}$ levels during human pregnancy. *Prostaglandins* 3, 3-5 (1973).
67. Hennam JF, Johnson DA, Newton JR and Collins WP: Radioimmunoassay of prostaglandin $F_{2\alpha}$ in peripheral venous plasma from men and women. *Prostaglandins* 5, 531-541 (1974).
68. Brummer HC: Serum $PGF_{2\alpha}$ levels during late pregnancy, labour and the puerperium *Prostaglandins* 2, 185-194 (1972).
69. Challis JRG and Tulchinsky D: A comparison between the concentration of prostaglandin F in human plasma and serum. *Prostaglandins* 5, 27-31 (1974).
70. Van Orden DE and Farley DB: Prostaglandin $F_{2\alpha}$ radioimmunoassay utilizing polyethylene glycol separation technique. *Prostaglandins* 4, 215-233 (1973).
71. Caldwell BV, Burstein S, Brock WA and Speroff L: Radioimmunoassay of the F prostaglandin. *J Clin Endocrinol Metab 33*, 171-175 (1971).
72. Karim SMM: Appearance of prostaglandin $F_{2\alpha}$ in human blood during labour. *Br med J* 4, 618-621 (1968).
73. Brummer HC and Craft IL: Prostaglandin $F_{2\alpha}$and labour. *Acta Obstet Gynecol Scand* 52, 273-275 (1973).
74. Gréen K, Bygdeman M, Toppozada M and Wiqvist N: The role of prostaglandin $F_{2\alpha}$in human parturition. Endogenous plasma levels of 15-keto-13,14-dihydro-prostaglandin $F_{2\alpha}$ during labour. *Am J Obstet Gynecol* 120, 25-31 (1974).
75. Hillier K, Calder AA and Embrey MP: Concentrations of prostaglandin $F_{2\alpha}$ in amniotic fluid and plasma in spontaneous and induced labours. *J Obstet Gynaecol Br Commonw* 81, 257-263 (1974).
76. Kinoshita K, Satoh K and Sakamoto S: Prostaglandin $F_{2\alpha}$and E_1 in plasma and amniotic fluid during human pregnancy and labor. *Endocrinol Japon* 24, 155-162 (1977).
77. Granström E: On the metabolism of prostaglandin $F_{2\alpha}$in female subjects. Structures of two metabolites in blood. *Eur J Biochem* 27, 462-468 (1972).
78. Hamberg M: Inhibition of prostaglandin synthesis in man. *Biochem Biophys Res Commun* 49, 720-726 (1972).
79. Hamberg M; Quantitative studies on prostaglandin synthesis in man. II. Determination of the major urinary metabolite of prostaglandins $F_{1\alpha}$ and $F_{2\alpha}$. *Anal Biochem* 55, 368-378, (1973).
80. Béguin F, Bygdeman M, Gréen K, Samuelsson B, Toppozada M and Wiqvist N: Analysis of prostaglandin $F_{2\alpha}$ and metabolites in blood during constant intravenous infusion of prostaglandin $F_{2\alpha}$ in the human female. *Acta Physiol Scand* 86, 430-432 (1972).
81. Samuelsson B: Quantitative aspects of prostaglandin synthesis in man. *Adv Biosci* 9, 7-14 (1973).
82. Hamberg M: Quantitative studies on prostaglandin synthesis in man. III. Excretion of the major urinary metabolites of prostaglandins $F_{1\alpha}$ and $F_{2\alpha}$ during pregnancy. *Life Sci* 14, 247-252 (1974).
83. Hertelendy F, Woods R and Jaffe BM: Prostaglandin E levels in peripheral blood during labor, *Prostaglandins* 3, 223-227 (1973).
84. Jubiz W, Frailey J, Child C and Bartholomew K: Physiologic role of prostaglandins of the E (PGE), F (PGF) and AB (PGAB) groups. Estimation by radioimmunoassay in unextracted human plasma. *Prostaglandins* 2, 471-487 (1972).
85. Whalen JB, Clancey CJ, Farley DB and Van Orden DE: Plasma prostaglandins in pregnancy. *Obstet Gynecol* 51, 52-55 (1977).
86. Challis JRG, Osathanondh R, Ryan KJ and Tulchinsky D: Maternal and fetal plasma prostaglandin levels at vaginal delivery and Caesarean section. *Prostaglandins* 6, 281-288 (1974).
87. Craft IL, Scrivener R and Dewhurst CJ: Prostaglandin $F_{2\alpha}$ levels in the maternal and fetal circulation in late pregnancy. *J Obstet Gynaecol Br Commonw* 80, 616-618 (1973).

88. Tuvemo T, Strandberg K, Hamberg M and Samuelsson B: Formation and action of prostaglandin endoperoxides in the isolated human umbilical artery. *Acta Physiol Scand* 96, 145-149 (1976).
89. Foley ME, Clayton JK and McNicol GP: Haemostatic mechanisms in maternal, umbilical vein and umbilical artery blood at the time of delivery. *Br J Obstet Gynaecol* 84, 81-87 (1977).
90. Mitchell MD, Brunt J, Bibby J, Flint APF, Anderson ABM and Turnbull AC: Prostaglandins in the human umbilical circulation at birth. *Br J Obstet Gynaecol* 85, 114-118 (1978).
91. Johnson DA, Manning PA, Hennam JF, Newton JR and Collins WP: The concentration of prostaglandin $F_{2\alpha}$ in maternal plasma, foetal plasma and amniotic fluid during pregnancy in women. *Acta Endocrinol* 79, 589-597 (1975).
92. Currie WB, Wong MSF, Cox RI and Thorburn GD: Spontaneous or dexamethasone-induced parturition in the sheep and goat: changes in plasma concentrations of maternal prostaglandin F and foetal oestrogen sulphate. *Mem Soc Endocrinol* 20, 95-118 (1973).
93. Mitchell MD, Flint APF and Turnbull AC: Plasma concentrations of 13, 14-dihydro-15-keto-prostaglandin F during pregnancy in sheep. *Prostaglandins* 11, 319-329 (1976).
94. Keirse MJNC, Patten PT, Anderson ABM, Turnbull AC, Johns A, Wooster M and Pickles VR: Pregnant sheep myometrium responds to prostaglandins in vitro but not in vivo. *Int Res Commun Syst* 73-4, 8-5-1- (1973).
95. Mitchell MD, Flint APF, Bibby J, Brunt J, Arnold JM, Anderson ABM and Turnbull AC: Rapid increases in plasma prostaglandin concentrations after vaginal examination and amniotomy. *Br med J* 2, 1183-1185 (1977).
96. Gillett PG, Kinch RAH, Wolfe LS and Pace-Asciak C: Therapeutic abortion with the use of prostaglandin $F_{2\alpha}$. A study of efficacy, tolerance, and plasma levels with intravenous administration. *Am J Obstet Gynecol* 112, 330-338 (1972).
97. Patrono C: Radioimmunoassay of prostaglandin $F_{2\alpha}$ in unextracted human plasma. *J Nucl Biol Med* 17, 25-29 (1973).
98. Shearman RP, Lyneham RC, Walsh JC, Itzkowic D and Shutt DA: Electroencephalographic changes after intraamniotic prostaglandin $F_{2\alpha}$ and hypertonic saline. *Br J Obstet Gynaecol* 82, 314-317 (1975).
99. Twomey SL, Bernett GE and Drewes PA: Serum prostaglandin $F_{2\alpha}$ levels during normal pregnancy. *Clin Biochem* 8, 60-61 (1975).
100. Zahradnik HP, Geisthövel F, Weitzell R and Breckwoldt M: Prostaglandin-F-Spiegel im menschlichen Plasma während der späten Schwangerschaft und während der Wehentätigkeit, *Geburtshilfe Frauenheilkd* 36, 710-714 (1976).
101. Sharma SC, Hibbard BM, Hamlett JD and Fitzpatrick RJ: Prostaglandin $F_{2\alpha}$ concentrations in peripheral blood during the first stage of normal labour. *Br Med J* 1, 709-711 (1973).
102. Keirse MJNC, Hicks BR, Mitchell MD and Turnbull AC: Increase of the prostaglandin precursor, arachidonic acid, in amniotic fluid during spontaneous labour. *Br J Obstet Gynaecol* 84, 937-940 (1977).
103. Karim SMM: Identification of prostaglandins in human amniotic fluid, *J Obstet Gynaecol Br Commonw* 73, 903-908 (1966).
104. Singh EJ and Zuspan FP: Content of amniotic fluid prostaglandins in normal, diabetic and drug-abuse human pregnancy. *Am J Obstet Gynecol* 118, 358-361 (1974).
105. Hibbard BM, Sharma SC, Fitzpatrick RJ and Hamlett JD: Prostaglandin $F_{2\alpha}$ concentrations in amniotic fluid in late pregnancy. *J Obstet Gynaecol Br Commonw* 81, 35-38 (1974).
106. Salmon JA and Amy JJ: Levels of prostaglandin $F_{2\alpha}$ in amniotic fluid during pregnancy and labour. *Prostaglandins* 4, 523-533 (1973).

107. Keirse MJNC, Mitchell MD and Turnbull AC: Changes in prostaglandin F and 13,14-dihydro-15-keto-prostaglandin F concentrations in amniotic fluid at the onset of and during labour. *Br J Obstet Gynaecol* 84, 743-746 (1977).
108. Mitchell MD, Keirse MJNC, Anderson ABM and Turnbull AC: Evidence for a local control of prostaglandins within the pregnant human uterus. *Br J Obstet Gynaecol* 84, 35-38 (1977).
109. Amy JJ and Karim SMM: Prostaglandins and other oxytocic substances in amniotic fluid. In: *Amniotic fluid – research and clinical application*, Fairweather DVI and Eskes TKAB (eds), 2nd ed., Amsterdam, Elsevier/North-Holland, 1978, p 321-345.
110. Mitchell MD, Patrick JE, Robinson JS, Thorburn GD and Challis JRG: Prostaglandins in the plasma and amniotic fluid of rhesus monkeys during pregnancy and after intrauterine fetal death, *J Endocrinol* 71, 67-76 (1976).
111. Tamby Raya RL, Salmon JA, Karim SMM and Ratnam SS: F prostaglandin levels in amniotic fluid in premature labour, *Prostaglandins* 13, 339-348 (1977).
112. Turnbull AC, Anderson ABM, Flint APF, Jeremy JY, Keirse MJNC and Mitchell MD: Human parturition. In: *The Fetus and Birth.* Ciba Foundation Symposium no 47, Amsterdam Elsevier/Excerpta Medica/North-Holland, 1977, p 427-452.
113. Liggins GC, Fairclough RJ, Grieves SA, Kendall J and Knox BS: The mechanism of initiation of parturition in the ewe. *Recent Prog Horm Res* 29, 111-150 (1973).
114. Flint APF, Anderson ABM, Patten PT and Turnbull AC: Control of utero-ovarian venous prostaglandin F during labour in the sheep: acute effects of vaginal and cervical stimulation. *J Endocrinol* 63, 67-87 (1974).
115. Alsat E and Cédard L: The stimulatory action of the prostaglandins on the production of oestrogens by the human placenta perfused in vitro. *Prostaglandins* 3, 145-153 (1973).
116. Lehmann WD: Der Einfluss von Prostaglandin $F_{2\alpha}$ und beta-adreneger Substanzen (Th 1165a) auf die Steroidbiosynthese der Placenta. *Arch Gynäkol* 217, 251-261 (1974).
117. Brunk U and Gustavii B: Lability of human decidual cells. In vitro effects of autolysis and osmotic stress, *Am J Obstet Gynecol* 115, 811-816 (1973).
118. Schwarz BE, Milewich L, Johnston JM, Porter JC and MacDonald PC: Initiation of human parturition. V. Progesterone binding substance in fetal membranes. *Obstet Gynecol* 48, 685-689 (1976).
119. Conrad JT and Ueland K: Reduction of the stretch modulus of human cervical tissue by prostaglandin E_2. *Am J Obstet Gynecol* 126, 218-223 (1976).
120. Ramwell PW, Leovey EMK and Sintetos AL: Regulation of the arachidonic acid cascade. *Biol Reprod* 16, 70-87 (1977).

INFLUENCING UTERINE CONTRACTILITY WITH OXYTOCIN

ALEXANDER C. TURNBULL

The role of oxytocin in human parturition has puzzled physiologists and clinicians alike during the greater part of this century. Whereas its physiological role may still be enigmatic (Swaab and Boer, this volume) its pharmacological effects on uterine smooth muscle have been known for many years. Intravenous oxytocin administration remains the favoured method of inducing effective uterine contractility in late human pregnancy.

It may therefore be timely to consider some of the concepts which form the basis of the use of oxytocin for stimulating uterine contractions and to outline some practical points concerning its application in human pregnancy. In this chapter it is not proposed to enter into debate on the pros and cons of induction of labour, although it is fully realized that rational use of a drug requires careful consideration of the indications for its administration.

OXYTOCIN SENSITIVITY IN PREGNANCY

Oxytocin stimulates increased uterine contractility but this is only of clinical value during the last few weeks of human pregnancy when uterine activity increases before the spontaneous onset of labour and oxytocin becomes capable of stimulating contractions strong enough to cause progressive cervical dilatation and delivery of the baby. The main indications for using oxytocin in human pregnancy, therefore, are induction of labour at term and augmentation of slow dysfunctional labour of spontaneous onset.

During the greater part of pregnancy the uterus is remarkably insensitive to oxytocin. In contrast to the ability of prostaglandins to induce uterine contractility at virtually all stages of pregnancy (1), the clinical usefulness of oxytocin is more limited. Oxytocin is not effective for induction of abortion or pre-term labour, nor to empty the uterus in pregnancies complicated by hydatidiform mole. In the presence of intra-uterine fetal death or serious fetal abnormality oxytocin is of little value unless there is already some spontaneous uterine contractility or a ripe cervix. Even at full term, oxytocin

M.J.N.C. Keirse et al. (eds.), Human Parturition, 143-153.

may fail to induce effective and progressive labour if the uterus is insensitive to oxytocin and the cervix long and closed.

The sensitivity of the uterus to oxytocin seems to be related to the level of spontaneous contractility. In early and mid-pregnancy the uterus is remarkably quiescent as measured by changes in amniotic fluid pressure (2) although there is some electrical activity throughout pregnancy (Van Leeuwen et al., this volume). In general, there is but little response of the pregnant uterus *in vivo* to oxytocin infusion before 20 weeks of gestation (fig. 1). Beyond 20 weeks there is an increase in oxytocin sensitivity (fig. 1) at about the same time as the spontaneous contractility of the uterus increases (2).

Although many authors have found an increase in oxytocin sensitivity near term (3, 4), there is a wide scatter of activity indicating considerable individual variation in uterine response to oxytocin (5). This might be an expression of differences in the degree of activation of the mechanisms which control the initiation of labour. On the other hand, neither the spontaneous nor oxytocin-induced contractility is able to foretell the imminence of the onset of labour (5). The greater the uterine activity in late pregnancy, the more the dilatation

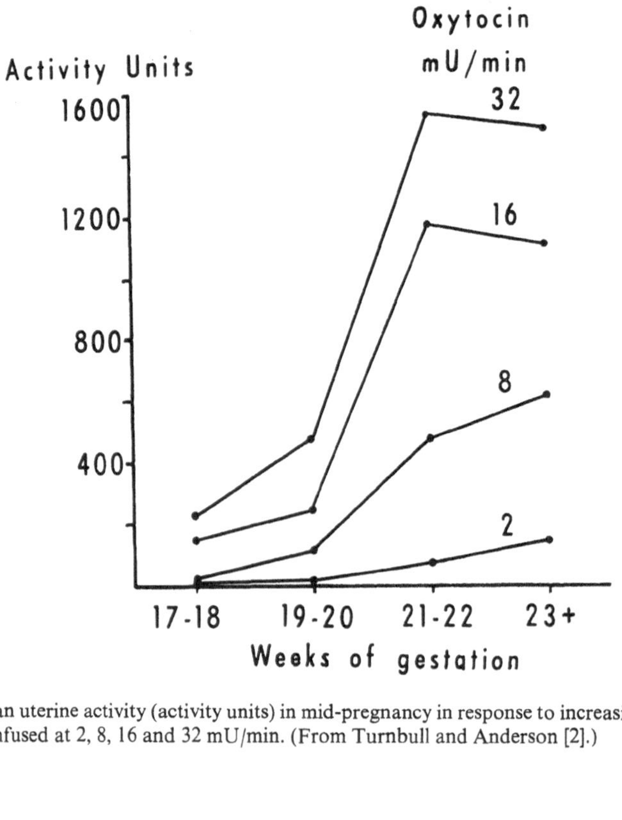

Fig. 1. Mean uterine activity (activity units) in mid-pregnancy in response to increasing doses of oxytocin infused at 2, 8, 16 and 32 mU/min. (From Turnbull and Anderson [2].)

and effacement of the cervix (6), and there is no doubt that the latter is very important as an indicator of the effectiveness of oxytocin in inducing labour (Calder, this volume). The practical implications of the above findings are that the response of the uterus to oxytocin increases in late pregnancy, that this response relates to cervical ripeness, but most importantly that uterine sensitivity to oxytocin differs greatly from woman to woman.

ROUTES OF ADMINISTRATION

Since oxytocin is a circulating hormone intravenous infusion is the most natural and usual route of administration. Buccal administration is possible but is generally considered to carry a risk of inducing uterine hypertonus. If used at all, the dose regime advocated by Chalmers and Moorhouse (7) should probably not be exceeded; this provides about one-sixth of the doses advocated in earlier publications.

Although oxytocin can be administered effectively by means of a standard, gravity-fed, intravenous infusion set, a motor-driven, positive-pressure infusion pump has a greater safety margin with regard to reliable regulation of the infusion rate. It is not influenced by the pressure in the arm vein which greatly influences the rate of a gravity-fed infusion. Many varieties of motor-driven infusion pumps are commercially available.

DOSE REGIMES

Induction of labour

The infusion of oxytocin requires first the *initiation* of effective uterine contractions and then the *maintenance* of uterine activity at a level adequate for normal progression of first and second stage labour and delivery of the baby in good condition. Since the dose of oxytocin required to initiate labour depends on the oxytocin sensitivity of the uterus, and since this can differ so much from case to case, a wide dose range of oxytocin has to be deployed. Once labour is established the oxytocin sensitivity of the uterus increases and less oxytocin may be required to maintain labour than to initiate it.

Maintenance of labour once established can thus be achieved with quite a low oxytocin dose. Beazley et al. (8) have shown with induced labour that progress after 5 cm cervical dilatation can be maintained by approximately 7 mU oxytocin/min. This finding may be related to the findings of my Oxford colleagues Hillier, Calder and Embrey (9) that in oxytocin induced labour the concentration of F prostaglandins in amniotic fluid begins to increase only when cervical dilatation reaches about 4 to 5 cm. In spontaneous labour by contrast amniotic fluid prostaglandin levels seem to have increased early in labour although they also increase further as the cervix dilates (10).

The realization that the effect of oxytocin on the uterus in late pregnancy varied greatly from patient to patient (fig. 2) led Turnbull and Anderson (11) to advocate a regime of "oxytocin titration" which started with a low dose of oxytocin (1 or 2 mU/min) but increased the dose steadily every 15 or 30 min until effective uterine contractions were induced. The end point of this escalating oxytocin "titration" was effective labour, the dose of oxytocin itself was not the vital consideration. Induction was only considered successful if

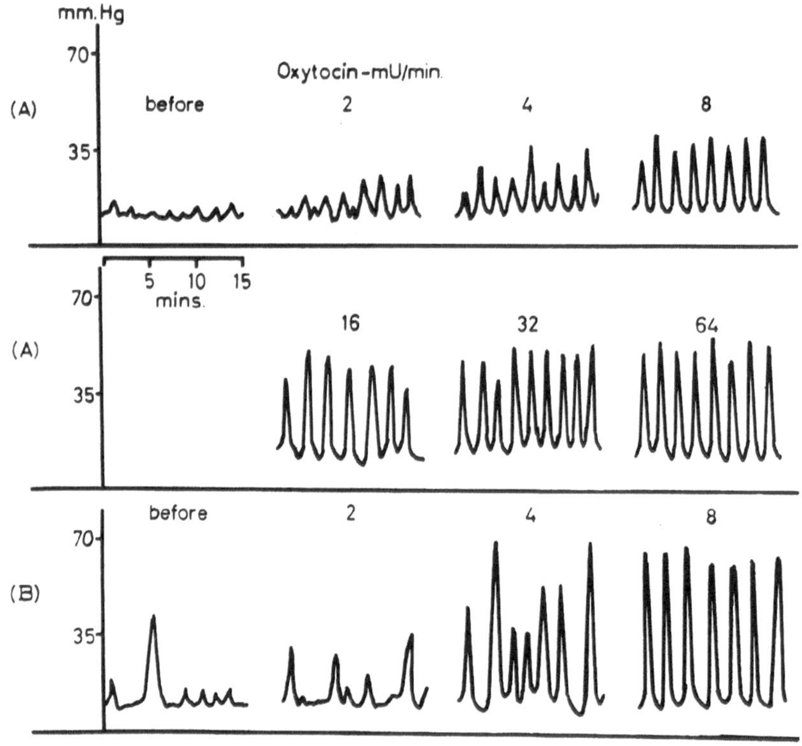

Fig. 2. Sections of amniotic fluid pressure records in two patients with different sensitivity to oxytocin.

Patient (A) required 64 mU/min oxytocin to stimulate uterine contractions of comparable intensity (mm Hg) to that produced in patient (B) by 8 mU/min oxytocin. (From Turnbull and Anderson [11].)

progressive labour and delivery was achieved on the first attempt, because if amniotomy has been performed and oxytocin infusion has to be continued for a second day the rapidly increasing potential risk of intra-uterine infection represents failure even if it does not become clinically apparent.

In the Aberdeen Maternity Hospital, from 1964, this regime of oxytocin titration was used, 12 h on average after low amniotomy, for all cases requiring induction of labour and was also used to accelerate established labour of spontaneous onset in which progress was abnormally slow, judged by the failure of the cervix to dilate in a normal progression. In these cases, the old concept of hypotonic and hypertonic inertia was found to be fallacious.

The results compared with those in previous years (12, 13) showed a notable reduction in induction-delivery intervals, and duration of labour (almost 90 percent of primigravidae now being delivered within 24 h). Caesarean section for a "failed induction" disappeared and the incidence of Caesarean section for prolonged dysfunctional labour was reduced by 50 percent. In cases where section was required, the decision to proceed could be made much earlier in labour, when the condition of both mother and baby was satisfactory. The incidence of uterine infection, and of fetal distress during labour, were reduced and perinatal mortality fell to its lowest level (18 per 1000) in 1966. Puerperal infection was reduced and puerperal psychosis following Caesarean section disappeared. Uterine rupture occurred in only one of the 1500 cases in which oxytocin titration was used, and this was a patient in her 12th pregnancy, who made a good recovery following hysterectomy. Although it could be debated whether the improvement in results related to the change in the regime for oxytocin administration and it is recognized that only in the context of a randomised clinical trial could such a conclusion be reached, the favourable clinical experience with this regime led us to believe that the new policy represented an advance in the clinical management of labour induction. Previously, failure to induce labour had usually meant that oxytocin infusion had failed to stimulate any clinically detectable uterine contractions, often leading to Caesarean section because of prolonged delay alone or delay complicated by uterine infection. Even many of the "successful" inductions required repeated oxytocin infusions, with 16 percent of all oxytocin infusions failing to induce labour on the first attempt, an unpleasant and frightening experience for most patients (11).

Augmentation of labour

Once labour has begun spontaneously, the oxytocin sensitivity of the uterus is increased even when labour is complicated by uterine dysfunction and progress is slow. This complication is mainly found in primigravid labour and Turnbull and Anderson (11, 12) demonstrated the great efficiency with which this slow progress can be accelerated by using intravenous oxytocin in the same way as for induction. Starting at a low level the dose is increased to whatever is required to produce strong contractions and progressing cervical dilatation without causing fetal distress. Regular assessment of cervical dilatation is essential for the early diagnosis of dysfunction. Graphing cervical dilatation as a "partogram" indicates if there is a need for oxytocin, and when there is, in assessing its effectiveness. Using oxytocin titration to augment dysfunctional labour in Aberdeen between 1964 and 1966 reduced the incidence of Caesarean section for dysfunctional labour by 50 percent and made possible delivery of 90 percent of primigravidae within 24 h of the onset of labour (13). Subsequently, O'Driscoll (14, 15) in Dublin has used such an approach extensively and delivers the great majority of primigravidae in his care within eight hours of admission. O'Driscoll and his colleagues stress that uterine rupture is almost unknown in primigravidae and that disproportion is also an over-diagnosed complication in primigravidae, abnormal progress being mainly due to poor uterine function. In the primigravida with a normal cephalic presentation poor progress in labour is therefore best treated by intravenous oxytocin administration. In most cases, stimulating effective uterine contractions brings about progressive cervical dilatation and vaginal delivery (14, 15).

AUTOMATIC OXYTOCIN INFUSION SYSTEMS

As a result of the extensive clinical experience with oxytocin infusion described earlier, it was clear that if an automatic system for induction of labour could be designed in which the dose of oxytocin would be regulated by the strength and frequency of the uterine contractions, this could be a useful new development.

The basic difficulty inherent in the concept of the uterus itself regulating the rate of oxytocin infusion is that uterine contractility is a relatively slow phenomenon, while, by contrast, the effect of oxytocin on the uterus is extremely rapid when it is injected intravenously. Fortunately however, the level of uterine contractility resulting from a constant rate of infusion of oxytocin soon stabilises, and although an increase in the rate of infusion is quickly followed by an increment in contractility, this again stabilises at a higher level within a relatively short time (16, 17, 18). The development and operation of an automatic infusion system for oxytocin has been described by

Francis et al. (16) and by Turnbull (17). This electronic system automatically regulates the rate at which an intravenous infusion of oxytocin is administered in accordance with the strength and frequency of the contractions of the uterus. The feed-back system depends on accurate measurement of uterine activity, obtained by direct recording of amniotic fluid pressure. This equipment did not, however, have a mechanism for reducing the rate of oxytocin infusion once labour had become established and there were worries expressed (20) that over-stimulation of the uterus might occur. These worries have been overcome by recent modification of the automatic system (Induction and Monitoring System, Type MM2, Pye Dynamics Ltd.). The MM2 limits the rate of infusion of oxytocin by reference to the proportion of the total time for which the intra-uterine pressure exceeds the placental blood pressure (about 20 mm Hg). The oxytocin dose rate is programmed to increase progressively over a period of about two hours until contractions are established at a level which is deemed to be safe in relation to the blood supply to the fetus. Maintenance of contractions at this level is regulated by the automatic system which is capable of progressively lowering the oxytocin infusion rate and even switching it off altogether if the uterine contractions effectively cause labour to progress.

Another type of oxytocin infusion equipment has been developed by Steer and his colleagues (19) based on his hypothesis (18) that oxytocin-induced labour has a stable phase during which uterine activity is largely independent of the oxytocin infusion rate. The equipment measures electronically the area under the intra-uterine pressure curve by means of an intra-uterine catheter coupled to a pressure transducer and recorder. This system detects the change from the incremental to the stable phase of labour so that the lowest dose of oxytocin can be selected which will produce optimal uterine activity. It was found that in a group of women with induced labour lasting less than five hours there was no increase in uterine activity above an oxytocin infusion rate of 12 mU/min; no increase above 18 mU/min in another group when labour lasted more than five hours.

Both these systems infuse oxytocin continuously to induce effective uterine contractions but since oxytocin release in labour probably occurs in a series of spurts (21), Pavlou et al. (22) investigated the efficacy of intermittent oxytocin administration in the induction of labour using the Cardiff Infusion System (16, 17). Compared with results in a group of women receiving continuous oxytocin, the pulsed oxytocin regime gave similar induction-delivery intervals, a significantly lower total dose of oxytocin but a much higher maximum dose rate (64 mU/min in over half the pulsed group compared with no patient in the continuous group requiring more than 32 mU/min). Thus, attempting to mimic the physiological spurt release of oxytocin does allow induction of labour to be achieved with a lower total dose of oxytocin than in controls although the latest modification of the Cardiff Infusion system described earlier (MM2) will, in most cases, infuse less oxytocin *in toto* than the pulsed regime.

In one of the earlier papers on induction of labour by Turnbull and Anderson (23) it was suggested that no more than 12 to 15 h should elapse following amniotomy before oxytocin infusion was started to induce labour. This was based on the finding that if amniotomy alone was going to successfully induce labour it would do so within 12 to 15 h in 90 percent of patients (fig. 3). Over the years it has become increasingly common in clinical practice, in the UK at least, not to wait for the onset of labour after amniotomy, but to rupture the membranes and start the oxytocin infusion almost simultaneously. It should be remembered, however, that amniotomy is a simple and fairly effective method of inducing labour in late pregnancy, particularly when the cervix is favourable (23) and not all patients require oxytocin in addition.

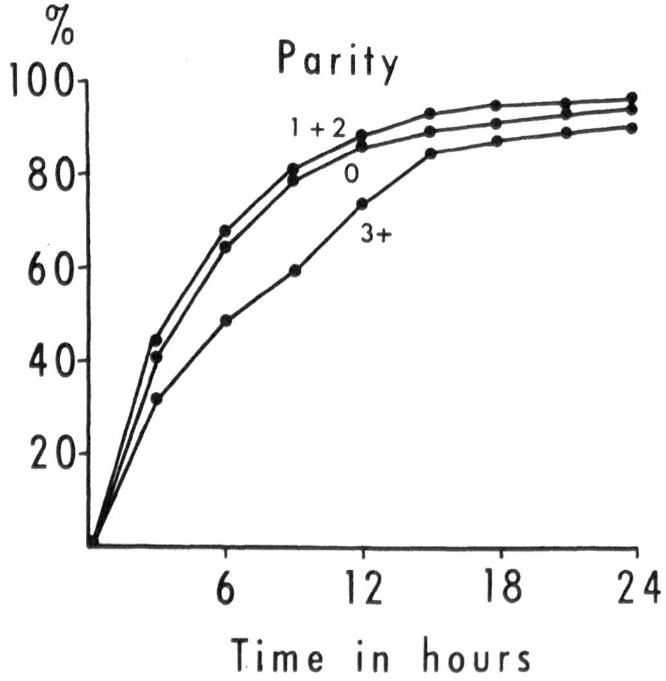

Fig. 3. Cumulative percentage of patients of parity 0, 1 and 2, and greater than 3 in whom labour was induced successfully within 24 h of amniotomy. (From Turnbull and Anderson [23].)

There has been debate on whether the use of intravenous oxytocin infusion for induction of labour can be considered a physiological procedure. According to Chard (24) an infusion rate of 2 to 8 mU/min in late pregnancy would yield plasma levels not in excess of 10 μU/ml, given the known half-life and volume of distribution of the hormone. Measurement of endogenous oxytocin concentrations in venous plasma during spontaneous labour gave peak levels of 2 to 5 μU/ml and never exceeded 12.5 μU/ml (25). Thus, the physiological levels of oxytocin during spurt release into the circulation are, in general, not very different to those achieved by an oxytocin infusion of 2 to 8 mU/min, the dose range which is effective for induction of labour in a large percentage of women at term. Although Chard (26) has argued that the use of oxytocin for induction of labour must be regarded as a pharmacological procedure, and we would agree, measurements of circulating concentrations of oxytocin do not in general support that statement. On the other hand, induction of labour by continuous administration of oxytocin will not mimic the physiological situation if the hormone is released in spurts although it is debatable in clinical practice whether oxytocin administered as a series of spurts is any more physiological, given that circulating concentrations of the hormone may not be as important as what happens at the target organ i.e. the myometrium.

DANGERS OF OXYTOCIN

Both mother and fetus can be put at risk by oxytocin over-dosage causing excessive uterine activity and hypertonus. In the mother complications range from unnecessarily painful contractions to precipitate delivery and even uterine rupture, particularly in multiparae in whom oxytocin should always be used with the greatest caution. In the fetus uterine hypertonus can cause hypoxia, damage from unduly rapid delivery or even death. Maternal oxytocin administration seems to increase the incidence of neonatal jaundice although the evidence is contradictory and the problem rarely serious. Oxytocin can also cause maternal complications because of its anti-diuretic action which increases with the dose; at 45 mU/min the effect is equal to vasopressin. If given in high dose and with large volumes of dilute dextrose solution, water intoxication can develop with generalised hypertonus, fits and unconsciousness, a potentially lethal complication. There is evidence that the risk of convulsions relates to the degree of hyponatraemia, the critical value for plasma sodium concentrations probably being 120 to 125 mmol/l. It seems that these low sodium concentrations can occur after as little as 4 l of dextrose solution in association with high dose oxytocin infusions (27).

CONCLUSIONS

If labour is to be induced, or to be augmented, it should be done with efficiency and safety. Excellent results can be obtained if oxytocin is commenced at a low dose and gradually escalated until effective contractility is initiated. The oxytocin dose range needed for induction of labour is usually between 4 and 16 mU oxytocin/min although occasionally a rate as high as 32 mU/min may be needed. Careful monitoring of uterine contractility and fetal heart rate is always important but particularly with high dose rates. Awareness of the anti-diuretic properties of oxytocin is also important.

The fact that the dose of oxytocin is determined by the level of uterine contractility led to the development of self-regulating infusion equipment, described by Turnbull (17). That system has now been further developed so that the onset of labour is initiated in a more gradual way and the oxytocin dose reduced to the lowest level possible once labour has been established.

REFERENCES

1. Embrey MP: *Prostaglandins in reproduction.* London, Churchill, 1975.
2. Anderson ABM and Turnbull AC: Spontaneous contractility and oxytocin sensitivity of the human uterus in mid-pregnancy. *J Obstet Gynaecol Br Commonw* 75, 271-277 (1968).
3. Smyth CN: Uterine irritability. The concept and its clinical applications, exemplified by the oxytocin sensitivity test. *Lancet* 1, 237-239 (1958).
4. Theobald GW: The choice between death from post-maturity or prolapsed cord and life from induction of labour. *Lancet* 1, 59-65 (1959).
5. Turnbull AC and Anderson ABM: Uterine contractility and oxytocin sensitivity during human pregnancy in relation to the onset of labour. *J Obstet Gynaecol Br Commonw* 75, 278-288 (1968).
6. Anderson ABM and Turnbull AC: Relationship between length of gestation and cervical dilatation, uterine contractility and other factors during pregnancy. *Am J Obstet Gynecol* 105, 1207-1214 (1969).
7. Chalmers JA and Moorhouse HM: Further experience with buccal oxytocin. *J Obstet Gynaecol Br Commonw* 73, 59-66 (1966).
8. Beazley JM, Banovic I and Feld MS: Maintenance of labour. *Br Med J* 2, 248-250 (1975).
9. Hillier K, Calder AA and Embrey MP: Concentrations of prostaglandin $F_{2\alpha}$ in amniotic fluid and plasma in spontaneous and induced labours. *J Obstet Gynaecol Br Commonw* 81, 257-263 (1974).
10. Keirse MJNC, Flint APF and Turnbull AC: F prostaglandins in amniotic fluid during pregnancy and labour. *J Obstet Gynaecol Br Commonw* 81, 131-135 (1974).
11. Turnbull AC and Anderson ABM: Induction of labour Part II: Intravenous oxytocin infusion. *J Obstet Gynaecol Br Commonw* 75, 24-31 (1968).
12. Turnbull AC and Anderson ABM: Induction of labour Part III: Results with amniotomy and oxytocin "titration". *J Obstet Gynaecol Br Commonw* 75, 32-41 (1968).
13. Anderson ABM, Turnbull AC and Baird D: The influence of induction of labour on Caesarean section rate, duration of labour and perinatal mortality in Aberdeen primigravidae between 1938 and 1966. *J Obstet Gynaecol Br Commonw* 75, 800-811 (1968).

14. O'Driscoll K, Jackson RJA and Gallagher JT: Active management of labour and cephalopelvic disproportion. *J Obstet Gynaecol Br Commonw* 77, 385-389 (1970).
15. O'Driscoll K, Stronge JM and Minogue M: Active management of labour. *Br Med J* 3, 135-137 (1973).
16. Francis JG, Turnbull AC and Thomas FF: Automatic oxytocin infusion equipment for induction of labour. *J Obstet Gynaecol Br Commonw* 77, 594-602 (1970).
17. Turnbull AC: An automatic oxytocin infusion system for the induction of labour. In: *Avortement et parturition provoqués*, Bosc MJ, Palmer R and Sureau Cl (eds), Paris, Masson et Cie, 1974, p 257-265.
18. Steer PJ, Little DJ, Lewis NL, Kelly MCME and Beard RW: Uterine activity in induced labour. *J Obstet Gynaecol Br Commonw* 82, 433-441 (1975).
19. Woolfson J, Steer PJ, Bashford CC and Randall NJ: The measurement of uterine activity in induced labour. *J Obstet Gynaecol Br Commonw* 83, 934-937 (1976).
20. Neves dos Santos LM, Odendaal HJ, Crawford JW and Henry MJ: Investigation of some problems associated with the Cardiff infusion pump. *Br J Obstet Gynaecol* 83, 225-228 (1976).
21. Gibbens D, Boyd MRH and Chard T: Spurt release of oxytocin during human labour. *J Endocrinol* 53, liv-lv (1972).
22. Pavlou C, Barker GH, Roberts A and Chamberlain GVP: Pulsed oxytocin infusion in the induction of labour. *Br J Obstet Gynaecol* 85, 96-100 (1978).
23. Turnbull AC and Anderson ABM: Induction of labour Part I. Amniotomy. *J Obstet Gynaecol Br Commonw* 74, 849-854 (1967).
24. Chard T: Oxytocin. In: *Clinical neuroendocrinology*, Martini L and Besser GM (eds), New York, Academic Press, 1977, p 569-583.
25. Gibbens GLD and Chard T: Observations on maternal oxytocin release during human labor and the effect of intravenous alcohol administration. *Am J Obstet Gynecol* 126, 243-246 (1976).
26. Chard T: The physiology of labour and its initiation. In: *Benefits and hazards of the new obstetrics*, Chard T and Richards M (eds), London, Spastics International Medical Publications, 1977, p 72-82.
27. Morgan DB, Kirwan NA, Hancock KW, Robinson D and Ahmad S: Water intoxication and oxytocin infusion. *Br J Obstet Gynaecol* 84, 6-12 (1977).

INDUCTION OF LABOR WITH PROSTAGLANDINS

MICHEL THIERY

This decade has witnessed the publication of numerous reports on the induction of labor with prostaglandins. That they are effective oxytocic compounds has become general knowledge. Classification of the available data is by no means easy because several factors must be taken into consideration, such as length of gestation, indication for the induction, type of prostaglandin used, dose and route of administration, etc. A review of all published material is therefore hardly possible and perhaps of little relevance in the context of this book. Furthermore, several recent reviews have dealt with the various aspects of the induction of labor with prostaglandins such as effectiveness, routes of administration, perinatal effects, etc. (1-8). Rather than reiterate these, the present chapter deals with the practical aspects of using prostaglandins for the induction of labor and intends to be a guideline rather than an exhaustive enumeration of data.

COMPARATIVE PHARMACOLOGY: OXYTOCIN VS. PROSTAGLANDINS

The *uterine* response to prostaglandins is comparable to that of oxytocin but there are a number of divergences which may be of importance to the clinician. The same is true for the *systemic* effects of these two types of compounds, some of which are responsible for characteristic side-effects whereas others may contra-indicate their administration, at least in certain types of patients.

Uterine (local) effects

1. In practice, the uterotonic effect of oxytocin is virtually limited to the *term* uterus. In contrast, both the non-pregnant and the pregnant myometrium respond readily to prostaglandins. In the non-gravida and during the first two trimesters of gestation, myometrial sensitivity to prostaglandins is comparable, whereas during the last trimester of pregnancy uterine receptivity probably increases. Consequently, unlike oxytocin, rather small doses of

M.J.N.C. Keirse et al. (eds.), Human Parturition, 155-164.

prostaglandins are effective for the induction of pre-term labor, a property which has proved to appeal to obstetricians attempting to interrupt pregnancies before term or/and in the presence of an unfavorable cervix.

2. The clinician should be aware that around term the individual *myometrial sensitivity* to a prostaglandin is highly variable. Nonetheless, it is generally accepted that in the same gravida the limits between intravenous (I.V.) dose levels that will trigger normal uterine contractility and those that will grossly overstimulate the myometrium are much more narrow than is found to be the case with I.V. oxytocin. Consequently, the risk of uterine hyperstimulation is even greater with I.V. prostaglandins than with I.V. oxytocin. This is the reason why most of those who have used prostaglandins consider recording of the fetal heart rate and uterine contractility mandatory when a prostaglandin is administered for the induction of labor in women with a viable fetus. Moreover, to deliver the desired dose level accurately an electric infusion pump should be used instead of the usual gravity-fed devices.

3. The natural prostaglandins have a shorter *plasma half-life* than oxytocin and more than 90% of the drug administered will be inactivated by a single passage through the lungs. This of course is not the case for synthetic prostaglandin analogs which are not inactivated by the tissue enzymes. Consequently, compared to the uterine effect produced by natural prostaglandins, the effect of the corresponding analogs is more protracted and more intense, which makes analogs unsuited for induction of labor in the presence of a viable fetus. In contrast, the *biological half-life* of natural prostaglandins is significantly longer than that of oxytocin. Indeed, as may be inferred from tocographic recording, it may take up to an hour after the prostaglandin infusion has been cut off before any considerable decrease of uterine activity is recorded. This may be due to the fact that the infused PG triggers the release of endogenous oxytocin and/or increases the myometrial sensitivity to oxytocin. Whatever the explanation of the phenomenon, it might be wise to choose a longer interval between consecutive increases in dose levels when using a prostaglandin. Furthermore, since stopping the infusion in the presence of uterine hyperstimulation may often be insufficient to reduce uterine activity effectively, it would be sound policy in these circumstances to administer a β-mimetic to the mother.

4. An important property of prostaglandins is that they act *locally*, i.e. directly on the sites where they are synthesized. The clinical implications of this characteristic are immense, in that they have made it possible,

by delivering the oxytocic compound directly to the uterus, to use much smaller effective doses and therefore to reduce specific side-effects very considerably.

5. Both PGE_2 and $PGF_{2\alpha}$ are not greatly inactivated within the *digestive tract*. Consequently, effective uterine stimulation can also be obtained by giving the prostaglandin by the oral and the buccal routes. In fact, for elective labor induction the oral route has become the most widely used alternative to I.V. infusion.

Systemic effects

1. Probably the most important difference between oxytocin and natural prostaglandins is the absence of *antidiuretic activity* in the latter. Therefore, prostaglandins are superior for the induction of patients with hypertensive states and chronic heart or renal disease. If the need for high dosages of oxytocin is anticipated, our preference would be to use prostaglandins rather than run the risk of producing water retention.

2. High doses of $PGF_{2\alpha}$ have been reported to induce clinical *bronchoconstriction*, but asthmatic attacks do not seem to have been reported at the doses used for labor induction even in patients with a bronchial disease. For intra-amniotic $PGF_{2\alpha}$ used for inducing midtrimester abortion, one group of investigators has reported *convulsions and EEG alterations*. However, these reports have not been confirmed by others and we have clearly shown that PGE_2 is certainly not an epileptogenic drug. We have not found changes in *intraocular pressure* during the induction of labor with I.V. $PGF_{2\alpha}$ either. The *sickling phenomenon* has been induced *in vitro* with PGE_2 in erythrocytes of women having the trait or suffering from the disease but $PGF_{2\alpha}$ lacks this effect. Consequently, there might be some point in systematically replacing prostaglandins by oxytocin when treating patients with bronchial disease, glaucoma or sickle cell anemia.

Combined use of prostaglandin and oxytocin

When these two classes of oxytocics are administered simultaneously their uterotonic effects summate. This is of importance because the clinician should know that he can exploit this phenomenon, especially when high prostaglandin doses are needed. Indeed, when oxytocin and a prostaglandin are combined, the dosage of the latter drug can be drastically reduced, which will result in a much lower incidence and severity of gastro-intestinal side effects.

Some investigators suspect that infused prostaglandins trigger the release of oxytocin from the maternal pituitary. Although this phenomenon is not fully proven, it would mean that when oxytocin is administered after a prostaglandin infusion or – to put it in a more general way – to a woman who is under the influence of a prostaglandin, one should be aware that uterine overstimulation might occur.

LABOR INDUCTION WITH PROSTAGLANDINS

Only two *natural* prostaglandins are currently used for this indication: PGE_2 and $PGF_{2\alpha}$. Initially, technical problems were encountered with respect to the stability of PGE_2, and the elimination of these difficulties caused considerable delay in the clinical assessment of this compound. During the last few years, however, PGE_2 has largely replaced the firstcomer $PGF_{2\alpha}$. The reason for this preference is not entirely clear, but some investigators believe that equipotent doses of $PGF_{2\alpha}$ produce more side-effects that PGE_2. Other natural prostaglandins have been investigated, but for the induction of labor our knowledge about compounds such as PGE_1, $PGF_{1\alpha}$, and PGA_1 is still sketchy. *Synthetic analogs*, on the other hand, have not been used to induce labor, except in cases of fetal demise or anomaly, for which they are extremely effective.

Prostaglandins can be given by a variety of *routes*, but for induction of labor only three of these are currently in use: the I.V. route, the oral or buccal route, and the extra-amniotic route. As for oxytocin there is a real risk of uterine hyperstimulation if the subcutaneous or intramuscular route is used. In addition, natural prostaglandins elicit severe pain at the injection sites. Injection of a prostaglandin directly into the wall of the uterus or into the cervix – a radical treatment for hypotonic postpartum haemorrhage – is painless and well tolerated. With the vaginal route, resorption is unpredictable and the maternal side effects are often severe.

The intravenous route

As for oxytocin, the best results are obtained in combination with amniotomy. The prostaglandin is infused in escalating doses, making use of a pump. The initial dose level (0.1 μg/min PGE_2 or 1.0 μg/min $PGF_{2\alpha}$) is stepped-up progressively which can be done by adding a constant increment or by doubling consecutive doses until labor is established. There is no maximum level. The infusion is then maintained until the delivery or for an hour after the expulsion of the placenta to prevent postpartum haemorrhage. Unless myometrial hyperstimulation, abnormal fetal heart rate patterns, or disturbing maternal side-effects occur, the same rate of prostaglandin is infused although during the stage of accelerated dilatation the dose level can usually be decreased. As already indicated, labor induction should be conducted under monitor control, because the margin between the effective dose and the dose causing uterine hypertonus is fairly narrow.

PGE_2 is about ten times more potent than $PGF_{2}\alpha$, but when infused in adequate doses both compounds are equally effective and – we believe – equally well tolerated by mother and fetus. If the inducibility prospects are favorable and there is no cephalopelvic disproportion, almost 100 percent of the women are delivered within 24 h and with mean induction-delivery intervals usually shorter than 7 h. Thus, for the *elective* induction of labor, the efficacy of I.V. prostaglandins is of the same order as that of I.V. oxytocin. However, prostaglandins are *not superior* and will cause some specific side-effects, such as gastro-intestinal upset and, at the site of infusion, transient venous erythema. These side-effects are of minimal severity and they do definitely not require the interruption of drug administration.

The oral and buccal routes

Because of the unacceptable rate of gastro-intestinal side-effects caused by oral $PGF_{2}\alpha$, only PGE_2 is used. The oral administration of escalated doses of PGE_2 (for example 0.5 mg, doubled every 30 min, until adequate uterine activity is obtained, or a maximum single dose of 3.0 mg) is more efficacious than that of a fixed dose (for example 0.5 mg at intervals of 30 to 60 min). The best results with PGE_2 tablets have been reported in parous women with a favorable cervix and after rupture of the membranes. Under these conditions, the procedure is just as successful as I.V. oxytocin or prostaglandin. However, in nulliparae and in subjects with an unfavorable cervix, oral PGE_2 is less effective.

A few investigators, including ourselves, have assessed the oromucosal (buccal) route for the administration of PGE_2. The conclusion is that when the same protocol is used as for oral PGE_2, the efficacy and safety of the method are also comparable.

The extra-amniotic route

Extra-amniotic infusion of a *solution* of PGE_2 via a transcervically inserted catheter is highly efficacious, safe, and causes no maternal side-effects. The drug is titrated, the initial dose rate (0.33 μg/min) being increased by 0.17 μg/min every 15 min until adequate uterine work is produced. This technique is particularly indicated in women with an unfavorable cervix or those carrying a fetus in breech presentation or in cases of unengaged cephalic presentation, because the membranes can be kept intact. After amniotomy, further administration via the same route is possible if care has been taken not to displace the catheter. Otherwise, I.V. oxytocin or PGE_2 can be given.

The use of a single extra-amniotic injection of 0.5 mg PGE_2 suspended in a *viscous gel* for prelabor ripening of the cervix is discussed elsewhere (Calder, this volume). It will suffice to mention here that when applied to women with a ripe or an almost ripe cervix, this method will induce labor in most cases. We have shown that with an equipotent dose (5 mg) of $PGF_{2\alpha}$ in gel results are comparable to those obtained with PGE_2.

* * *

Thus, the three routes proposed for the administration of prostaglandins are *complementary*. When applied correctly, they are perinatally safe. Possibly, uterine hypertonus may be encountered somewhat more frequently with I.V. prostaglandins than with I.V. oxytocin, but overstimulation is definitely less frequent with oral and extra-amniotic PGE_2. In the absence of or after prompt correction of hypertonus, the perinatal outcome is comparable to that of spontaneous or oxytocin-induced labor. Maternal acid-base equilibrium and the usual laboratory parameters in the blood and urine, utero-placental blood flow, and placental function, are not affected during labor induction with a prostaglandin. Moreover, no difference is found in the fetal heart rate patterns, fetal and neonatal acid-base equilibrium, Apgar scores, neonatal course, and psychomotor development of the infant up to 3 years of age. Finally, the use of PGE_2 in labor is not followed by an increased incidence of neonatal hyperbilirubinemia.

THERAPEUTIC (NON-ELECTIVE) INDUCTION

Most of what has been said up to now, applies to the elective induction of labor but the problem becomes much more complicated when we consider non-elective or therapeutic inductions. The main reasons for this are that candidates for non-elective induction are characterized (1) by poor inducibility features; (2) relative fetal immaturity or excessive gestational age; and (3) the presence of any one of a variety of fetal or maternal problems. To further complicate matters, in most cases several of these factors are present. The combination of an unripe cervix with a diminished fetal reserve makes induction particularly difficult and more hazardous than in elective cases, and the obstetrician will have to decide whether the individual fetus is capable of sustaining the prolonged stress of labor. If not, delivery should be by the abdominal route. When induction is chosen, close monitoring of maternal and fetal functions is mandatory and facilities must be constantly and instantly available in case cesarean section becomes acutely indicated.

Placental insufficiency and maternal pathology

In cases where placental function and/or maternal pathology indicate termination of the pregnancy (such as maternal hypertensive and cardiovascular diseases, diabetes, iso-immunization, intra-uterine growth retardation, prolonged gestation, etc.) preference is given to the I.V. route, which permits accurate drug titration. If induction prospects are favorable prostaglandins and oxytocin are equally good. However, in patients with a pre-existent cardiovascular, hypertensive, or renal disease, dose levels of oxytocin should preferably not exceed 16mU/min. In hypertensive gravidae a specific untoward effect of I.V. PGE_2 on fetal oxygen homeostasis has been postulated on theoretical grounds. So far, however, clinical results have not corroborated the increased risk of fetal hypoxia. In difficult cases, on the other hand, prostaglandins are probably superior to oxytocin in terms of the absence of an antidiuretic effect, the overall success rate, and the shorter duration of labor. Here, the prostaglandin can be given via the I.V. or extra-amniotic route, amniotomy being performed as soon as practicable. If the cervix is extremely unfavorable, the induction should be preceded by cervical ripening.

Premature rupture of the membranes

After 34-36 weeks of gestation, premature rupture of the ovular sac is treated by induction of labor. If the cervix is ripe, I.V. oxytocin or prostaglandins are given. Confronted with an unripe cervix, I.V. prostaglandin is more efficacious and safer for the mother (water intoxication).

Fetal death or malformation

In cases of severe fetal malformation or intra-uterine death the problem is entirely different, because here one can practically ignore the passenger. For this indication, prostaglandins given by the I.V. or the extra-amniotic route have proved to be very effective. One should probably caution against the use of the intra-amniotic route, because it seems to have occasionally led to massive resorption of the injected prostaglandin through the devitalized fetal membranes, leading to severe systemic effects or hyperstimulation and even rupture of the uterus. Intravaginal PGE_2 (20 mg every 3 h) has been shown to be very effective, but the gastro-intestinal side-effects produced were often severe. Oxytocin, even in very high doses, is of limited efficacy and may cause water intoxication. Whatever method of termination of pregnancy is chosen, in cases of long-standing fetal death disseminated intravascular coagulation must first be excluded or corrected by the I.V. administration of heparin (5,000 U/4 h) for 2 to 3 days.

Breech presentation

In case of breech presentation, the extra-amniotic infusion of a solution of PGE_2 is highly successful. A single dose of 0.3-0.5 mg PGE_2 in gel instilled into the extra-ovular space is supreme in ripening the cervix or triggering labor immediately. For the management of breech presentation, the possibility of using the extra-amniotic route is a precious acquisition, because it permits a delay of amniotomy, thus reducing the risk of cord prolapse.

Disproportion and following uterine surgery

Neither a previous lower segment cesarean section (in the absence of disproportion) nor the suspected existence of borderline cephalo-pelvic disproportion (in the absence of a scarred uterus) constitute an absolute contraindication for induction. In these cases either I.V. prostaglandin or oxytocin can be used. Of course, labor must be closely monitored and epidural analgesia refrained from – at least in women who have been sectioned – in order not to mask the clinical signs of impending uterine rupture.

After removal of a cervical stitch, fibrosis is usually found around the suture tract. This should be allowed to soften spontaneously, before induction is considered at all.

A history of classical (corporeal) cesarean section, hysterotomy (second-trimester abortion, fibroids), or a Strassman-type operation is an absolute contra-indication for vaginal delivery and, consequently, for induction of labor.

CONCLUSIONS

The picture which emerges from the tremendous amount of clinical work on labor induction with prostaglandins may tentatively be summarized in a few points:

1. For elective induction of labor, both I.V. $PGF_{2\alpha}$ and PGE_2 are effective, well tolerated, and safe provided these compounds are handled properly. However, I.V. prostaglandins are *not* superior to I.V. oxytocin for this indication.
2. If inducibility prospects are favorable (ripe cervix, parous patient) oral PGE_2 is an alternative to I.V. prostaglandins.
3. The fact that prostaglandins adequately stimulate the unfavorable uterus as well, gives these drugs a considerable advantage over oxytocin.
4. Local application of prostaglandins has opened new clinical possibilities. Labor induction by extra-amniotic infusion of prostaglandins is effective, safe, and perfectly well tolerated by the mother. If the cervix is unfavorable, the same method can still be applied. However, prelabor ripening with extra-amniotic prostaglandins in viscous gel offers a valuable simplification.
5. For a number of therapeutic inductions (breech and floating cephalic presentation, intrauterine death or severe malformation) prostaglandins administered by various routes have given excellent results. Other characteristics of prostaglandins (such as the absence of water retention) may be beneficial in case of difficult induction or with certain types of maternal pathology.

REFERENCES

1. Amy JJ and Thiery M: Labor – spontaneous and induced. In: *Clinical perinatology*, Aladjem S, Brown AK and Sureau C (eds), 2e édition, Saint Louis, Mosby, 1979 (in press).
2. Embrey MP: *The prostaglandins in Human Reproduction*. London, Churchill, 1975.
3. Embry MP: Oxytocics and the uterus. In: *Scientific Foundations of Obstetrics and Gynaecology*, Philipp E, Barnes J and Newton M (eds), London, W. Heinemann, 1977, p 798-810.
4. Embrey MP and Hillier K: Prostaglandins in Reproduction. In: *Recent Advances in Obstetrics and Gynaecology*, Stallworthy J and Bourne G (eds), London, Churchill, 1977, p 75-104.
5. Thiery M: Elective induction of labor at term with oxytocin and prostaglandins. Technique

and fetal and maternal effects. In: *Avortement et Parturition provoqués*, Bosc MJ, Palmer R and Sureau C (eds), Paris, Masson, 1974, p 267-287.
6. Thiery M and Amy JJ: Induction of labour with prostaglandins. In: *Advances in Prostaglandin Research. Prostaglandins and Reproduction*, Karim SMM (ed), Lancaster MTP, 1975, p 149-228.
7. Thiery M and Amy JJ: *Spontaneous and induced labor: two roles for the prostaglandins.* In: Obstetrics and Gynecologic Annual, vol. 6, Wynn RM (ed), New York, Appleton-Century-Crofts, 1977, p 127-171.
8. Thiery M and Amy JJ: Perinatal effects of natural prostaglandins used for labor induction. In: *Advances in Prostaglandin and Thromboxane Research*, Vol 4, Coceani F and Olley PM (eds), New York, Raven Press, 1978, p 307-324.

INHIBITION OF UTERINE CONTRACTILITY WITH β-MIMETIC DRUGS

TOM K.A.B. ESKES AND GERARD G.M. ESSED

Delivery too early in pregnancy and its consequences for neonatal mortality and morbidity is one of the major issues in obstetrics. Since the mechanism of human parturition is a complicated and multifactorial process, there has been a wide search for drugs capable of inhibiting uterine contractility and possibly able to delay labor.

The uterine inhibitory effects of ether and halothane (fluothane) have been known for some time but treatment of long duration was impossible. Analgesic drugs or benzodiazepines were not active. Progesterone was able to maintain pregnancy only in animals in which pregnancy is dependent upon a functioning corpus luteum. In a double-blind study Fuchs et al. (1) were unable to demonstrate the efficacy of progesterone in the maintenance of human pregnancy. Recently however some evidence for a lengthening of pregnancy by the administration of 17α-hydroxy-progesterone was published (2). In 1962 catecholamines and especially β-mimetic drugs were introduced in obstetrics. Since then a variety of such substances showing strong uterine inhibitory effects have been developed. In the USA in particular intravenous ethanol is advocated for the lengthening of pregnancy in cases of early labor (3). Also prostaglandin synthetase inhibitors especially indomethacin should be mentioned as more recent uterine inhibitors (4). The effect of magnesium sulfate is rather short-lasting. Recently however magnesium sulfate and alcohol were compared for the prevention of pre-term labor (5). In this study magnesium sulfate was the better agent. Diazoxide proved to be effective *in vitro* and *in vivo* (6, 7).

PHARMACOLOGY OF β-MIMETIC DRUGS

Progress in chemical synthesis made it possible to change the molecular structure of catecholamines. Especially the introduction of large alkyl groups to the amino group and changes in the catechol group caused shifts in the action-spectrum. Two different effects were discovered, those of norepinephrine (α-adrenergic) and those of isopropylnorepinephrine or

M.J.N.C. Keirse et al. (eds.), Human Parturition, 165-187.

Table 1. A differentiation in the effects of nor-epinephrine, epinephrine and isuprel.

organs	nor-epinephrine and epinephrine α-receptors, α-sympatho-mimetic actions	epinephrine and isuprel β-receptors, β-sympatho-mimetic actions
vascular system, heart	myocardial ectopic excitation	myocardial contraction -augmentation, cardiac acceleration
muscular vessels	slight decrease in blood flow, vasoconstriction	strong increase in blood flow, vasodilation (trophic function)
brain vessels (human)	decrease in blood flow, vasoconstriction	increase in blood flow, vasodilation
splanchnic area	strong decrease in blood flow, vasoconstriction (regulation of blood pressure)	slight increase in blood flow (trophic function?)
splenic capsule	contraction (regulation of blood pressure)	
renal vessels	strong decrease in blood flow (regulation of glomerular blood flow and diuresis)	
cutaneous vessels	strong decrease in blood flow, vasoconstriction (temperature regulation)	slight increase in blood flow (trophic function?)
pilomotor response	contraction, raising of hairs (temperature regulation)	
bronchial tree		bronchial relaxation
intestine	relaxation of intestinal smooth muscle	
ureter	contraction	
vas deferens	contraction	
uterus	excitation, uterine contractions (depending on condition of uterus, promoted by estrogens)	inhibition of uterine contractions
dilatormuscle of iris	contraction (mydriasis)	
membrana nictitans	contraction	
carbohydrate metabolism	increase blood-sugar level (glycogenolysis liver)	increase blood-sugar level (glycogenolysis muscle)
fat metabolism	mobilization of fat (shift from depots to liver)	

isuprel (β-adrenergic). Epinephrine possesses both effects (table 1).

Ahlquist (8) postulated two types of adrenergic receptors named α- and β-adrenergic receptors. β-adrenergic drugs are especially capable of inhibiting uterine contractions. The working mechanism is considered to be a stimulation by β-receptors of the enzyme adenylcyclase in the cell membranes. This enzyme converts adenosinetriphosphate (ATP) into 3-5′-adenosinemonophosphate (cyclic AMP). Cyclic AMP is an activator of phosphorylase implicated in glycolysis (fig. 1). This form of energy promotes active sodium transport giving hyperpolarization of muscle cells and muscle relaxation. Lands (9) found that the β-receptors in different organs were not stimulated equally. New drugs like ritodrine (Prepar®) and fenoterol (Partusisten®) especially stimulate the β-receptors in the uterus, bronchial tree and striated muscle, being called β-2-receptors. Isoprenaline stimulates also β-1-receptors in heart blood vessels and lipokinesis.

The half-lives of various β-adrenergic drugs differ. Real catecholamines are characterized by a hydroxy-group in the ortho- and metaposition and a mono-amino group. They are inactivated by the enzymes catechol-o-methyltransferase (COMT) and mono-amino-oxidase (MAO). Epinephrine and isoprenaline have a short half life of approximately 3 min. Changes in the

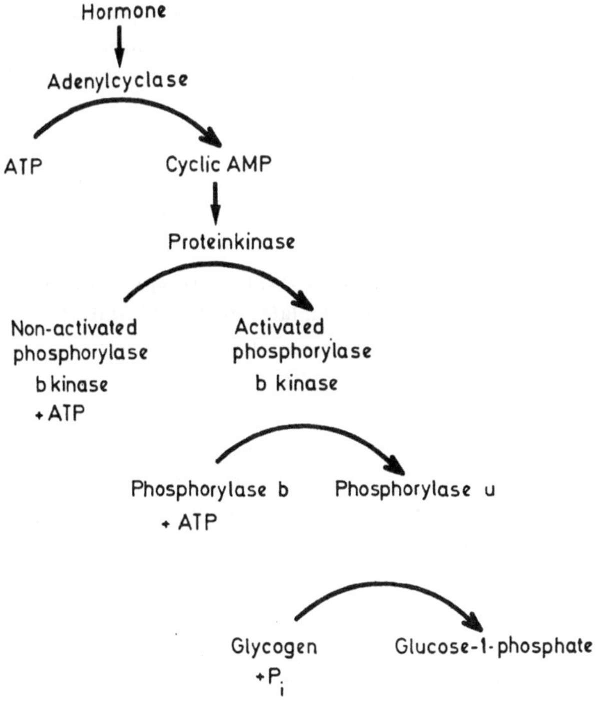

Fig. 1. Schematic representation of β-adrenergic stimulation.

catechol group and the longer nitrogen chain prevent enzymatic inactivation. The half life of substances as ritodrine and fenoterol is therefore longer than that of the real catecholamines. This property should be taken into account in clinical practice.

The working mechanism of β-adrenergic drugs was reviewed by Weidinger and Wiest (10). The effect of catecholamines on uterine activity in animals varies considerably from one species to another. Grüber (11) could state: "Certainly no single organ in the body has been studied as thoroughly by experimenters with more conflicting results and opinions..." In the cat a difference was even found between the pregnant and non-pregnant state with catecholamines being respectively stimulators and inhibitors of contractility. Partly these data are conflicting because of methodological differences *in vitro* (bath fluids, isometric *versus* isotonic recording) or *in vivo* (balloon *versus* open-tip catheters). The different effects of catecholamines on the uterus of animals can be seen, for instance, in the possibility to stop labor in the event of impending danger (e.g. deer, horse, etc.). Epinephrine can then be seen as a "hormonal receptor" inhibitor (or stimulator). Norepinephrine can be considered as a sympathetic neurotransmitter. In this context it appears that the human lost at least the last possibility because of the absence of adrenergic neural fibres, in the myometrium (12).

Only those studies of the action of β-adrenergic drugs on the pregnant human uterus will be mentioned which have used adequate methods of recording uterine activity i.e. intra-uterine pressure. Epinephrine could inhibit uterine activity in the human but gave a "rebound phenomenon" after stopping the infusion (13). Further derivatives of epinephrine did not show this rebound effect and were also used later in clinical trials. For fenoterol no pharmacokinetic data in terms of blood levels of the parent drug appear to be available. In the study of Buchelt and Rominger (14) plasma levels of the sum of the drug and its metabolites are available. These are extensively metabolized to pharmacologically inactive products and so of little clinical interest. For salbutamol (15) ritodrine (16) and terbutaline (17) assay methods of adequate sensitivity and accuracy are available to perform pharmacokinetic studies. The significance of these half-lives for instance in oral administration manifests itself in a repeated dosage schedule. After a single oral dose of ritodrine, an effective half-life of about two hours can be estimated, but when three dosages are given at eight-hour intervals, the effective half-life doubles. The plasma levels of all three drugs are much lower with oral than with parenteral administration (16). This effect is due to the drug being extensively metabolized during its intestinal absorption or its first passage through the liver. The metabolic conversion from β-adrenergic drugs to sulphuric or glucuronic esters mainly takes place in the intestinal mucosa. The preference for the parenteral route of administration to block uterine activity is therefore not surprising.

CLINICAL TRIALS IN PRE-TERM LABOR

Methodology of pharmacological studies

The problem of proving that an agent which inhibits uterine contractions is also capable of stopping labor is the fact that in some women with pre-term labor these contractions disappear without any treatment at all. Therefore the only way to assess this is a carefully designed study using randomization with control groups and statistical evaluation. To judge published reports on such "treatment" one has to consider the "Ten commandments of clinical trials" (table 2) which should be fulfilled before definite proof of a certain pharmacological effect of a drug is so evident that withdrawal of that drug is unethical. In our opinion the study should be prospective including a written protocol with a limited and well-defined question to be answered. Some drugs do not permit a complete double-blind set-up, because side effects of the drug hypothesized to be effective break the protocol. This is the case with β-mimetics because of maternal tachycardia. The best form of randomization is the so-called envelope system with a careful description as to what should be done with the individual patient, the so-called allocated randomized trial. Doses and routes of medication should be mentioned. Some form of control of drug taking has to be found, especially in outpatient studies with oral treatment. The correct reasons for inclusion or

Table 2. The "ten commandments" for clinical trials.

1.	prospective
2.	double blind
3.	randomized
4.	allocated
5.	doses and routes of medication
6.	other medication or measures
7.	pharmacokinetics (drug levels)
8.	patients included
9.	patients excluded
10.	proper statistics

Table 3. Clinical trials judged according to the "ten commandments".

Criteria	Drugs used in the various studies (referred to between brackets) and fulfilment of criteria				
	Ritodrine (56)	Ritodrine *vs.* Librium (57)	Terbutaline (58)	Ritodrine *vs.* Alcohol (59)	Ritodrine *vs* Ritodrine + Indomethacin (18)
Prospective	+	+	+	+	+
Double blind	+ ?	–	+ ?	–	+
Randomized	+	+	+	+	+
Allocated	+	–	–	+	–
Medication	+	+	+	+	+
No other measures	+	–	–	–	–
Drug levels	–	–	–	–	–
Included	+	+	+	+	+
Excluded	–	+	+	+	+
Statistics	+	+	+	+	+
Total +	8 or 7	6	7 or 6	7	7

exclusion in the trial should be stated, and finally proper statistics should be used considering age, parity and obstetrical groups as separate items. It goes without saying that means and standard deviations are only allowed in figures representing a Gaussian distribution. If not, data are best represented by medians and range, using non-parametric tests such as Wilcoxon and Pearson's correlation coefficients to calculate statistically significant differences.

Along this line of ten commandments we will discuss the several clinical trials on β-adrenergic drugs and their effects on early labor. Five studies are selected from the literature which are judged to be sufficient to urge the use of β-adrenergic drugs when early labor is threatening, because that treatment does lengthen the duration of pregnancy (table 3). Recently a double-blind prospective study was carried out by Gamissans et al. (18) which compared ritodrine and placebo to ritodrine and indomethacin suppositories and suggested that the latter treatment was significantly better in prolonging pregnancy ($p < 0.05$). Serious neonatal problems or effects on the ductus Botalli in the ritodrine-indomethacin group were not observed.

Definition of success

Richter (19) pointed out that no satisfactory evaluation of success could be obtained by analyzing only the time gained by treatment. In his formula the gestational age at the onset of treatment is considered (table 4). Baumgarten and Grüber (20) described the tocolytic index. The obstetrical situation at the beginning of the treatment was given a score which takes into account

Table 4. Estimation of the effect of long-term β-mimetic drugs by means of the prolongation index. (From Richter, 1977 [19].)

Formula:

$$PI = \frac{\Delta t}{t_0} \cdot 100$$

t_0 = gestational age at onset of uterine relaxant treatment

Δt = lag time between onset of treatment and delivery

Example:

t_0 = 25 weeks

Δt = 10 weeks

$$PI = \frac{10}{25} \cdot 100 = 40$$

factors as uterine contractions, ruptured membranes, bloody show and cervical dilatation (table 5). Essed et al. (21) found the tocolytic index to be of value in the clinical judgement of the prognosis of treatment (table 6).

Table 5. Tocolytic index. (From Baumgarten and Grüber, 1973 [20].)

	0	1	2	3	4
uterine contr.	0	irregular	regular	—	—
ruptured membranes	0	—	high	—	low
"show"	0	×	—	—	—
bloody discharge	0	—	×	—	—
dilatation	0	1 cm	2 cm	3 cm	≥ 4 cm

Table 6. Correlation between tocolytic index (20) and prolongation index (19) in 372 consecutive patients treated for threatening early labor. (From Essed et al., 1978 [21].)

Tocolytic index	Median prolongation index	No of patients	Statistical differences (Mann-Whitney U-test)
5	1	50	
			$p < 0.001$
4	7	51	
			$p < 0.005$
3	15	74	
			not significant
2	16	118	
			$p < 0.005$
1	26	79	

UTERINE BLOOD FLOW DURING β-ADRENERGICS

The recorded reactions of the maternal cardiovascular system (22) suggest an increase in utero-placental blood flow (table 7). Since there are no reliable and reproducible techniques of measuring uteroplacental flow in women we have to rely – for the time being – on animal studies, particularly those which are not influenced by the use of anaesthetic agents. Such a model can be found in the "chronic animal preparation" of sheep and monkey (23, 24). Brennan et

Table 7. Uterine blood flow during β-adrenergic treatment.

Species	Methodology	Drug	Results	Authors
Sheep	Electromagnetic flow probes	Salbutamol	Increase	Brennan et al., 1977 (25)
		Fenoterol	Increase	Ehrenkranz et al., 1976, 1977 (60, 61).
		Ritodrine	Decrease	Brennan et al., 1977 (25)
Monkey	Radioangiography	Metaproterenol	Increase	Wallenburg et al., 1973 (28)
Human	Thermistor (cervix)	Ritodrine	Increase	Brettes et al., 1976 (26)
	113 M Indium	Fenoterol	Increase	Lippert et al., 1976 (27)
		Orciprenaline	Increase	Rondinelli et al., 1974 (63)
		Ritodrine	Increase	Janish et al., 1974 (64)
		Fenoterol	Increase	

al. (25) demonstrated in the chronic sheep preparation with electromagnetic flow probes an increased uterine vascular resistance during ritodrine infusion and a decreased uterine vascular resistance with salbutamol and fenoterol. Despite this marked reduction of uterine blood flow and maternal acidaemia with ritodrine, fetal acid-base status was "improved" at the end of the six hours infusion. Brettes et al. (26) investigated in a "double-blind" cross-over study the effect of ritodrine intravenously on uterine blood flow, using an intrauterine thermistor probe inserted into the anterior lip of the cervix in late human pregnancy. The differences in response to ritodrine and placebo were statistically significant. The authors suggest an increase of uteroplacental blood by ritodrine. It has to be stressed however, that a thermistor probe inserted into the cervix at best measures local blood flow and this may not reflect total uterine blood flow nor placental perfusion. Lippert et al. (27) studied the action of fenoterol (Berotec®) on human placental, myometrial and cardiac blood pools using 113m Indium injected intravenously. In eight cases with oxytocin-induced labor, fenoterol produced an increase in placental and myometrial pools with corresponding decrease of the cardiac pool. Wallenburg et al. (28) performed placental radio-angiography in 13 lightly anaesthetized pregnant rhesus monkeys. Intravenous infusion of metaproterenol accelerated the intervillous spurts due to vasodilatation.

FETAL EFFECTS DURING PREGNANCY

β-Adrenergic drugs do cross the placental barrier in sheep (29) and monkeys (30). The fetal heart frequency increases in the human (31) (32), suggesting placental passage and the presence and activity of fetal β-receptors. The increase of 10-20 beats/min is probably concomitant with an increase of fetal cardiac output (33). De Haan et al. (30) studied the influence of Th 1165-a (Partusisten®) in acute experiments in six pregnant rhesus monkeys. The maternal heart rate increased, arterial blood pressure decreased somewhat, pulse pressure increased. The fetal heart frequency did not increase. In three animals uteroplacental fetal bradycardia occurred after the infusion (fig. 2). In none of the experiments was there an improvement in the fetal acid-base balance. Nochimson et al. (34) found no significant changes in fetal heart action in 10 women in labor infused with ritodrine at 150 μg/min. The effects of terbutaline on mother and fetus were evaluated by Caritis et al. (35) in eight near-term pregnant baboons. Significant suppression of postoperative spontaneous and oxytocin augmented uterine activity was achieved with infusion rates of 0.36 and 0.56 μg/min respectively. Maternal and fetal blood pressure

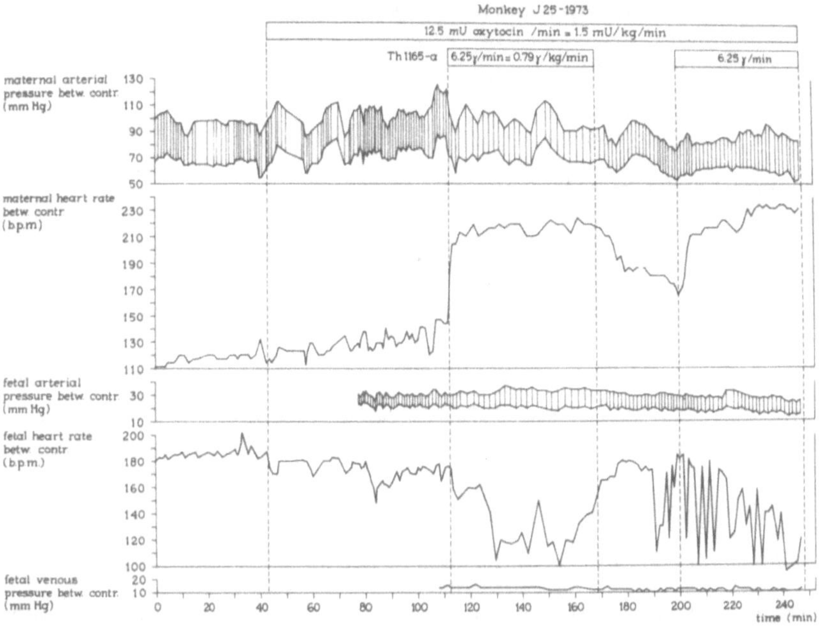

Fig. 2. Effect of Th 1165a on maternal and fetal heart rate and arterial pressure in a rhesus monkey. (From De Haan et al. [30].)

and acid-base states as well as fetal heart rate were unaffected but a mild maternal tachycardia was observed. Both maternal and fetal blood glucose levels were increased.

INTRAPARTUM TOCOLYSIS WITH β-MIMETICS

With increasing clinical experience with β-mimetic agents in obstetrics, these drugs have been used more frequently for indications other than the suppression of early labor. Important examples of this include their supposed beneficial effect upon placental blood flow in E.P.H. gestosis, or when a rapid but short-lasting relaxation of the uterus is desired during labor. Several indications for intrapartum tocolysis have been suggested. These are summarized in table 8. Relaxation of the uterus may be a life-saving temporizing method until caesarean section can be performed in case of impending rupture of the uterus.

When feto-pelvic disproportion is diagnosed in a breech presentation with

Table 8. Indications for intrapartum tocolysis with β-mimetics.

I.	Intrapartum fetal distress
	1. umbilical cord complications
	2. excessive uterine activity
	3. placental insufficiency
	4. supine hypotensive syndrome
II.	Impending rupture of the uterus
III.	External or internal version
IV.	Before cesarean section to avoid further engagement of a breech
V.	Manual removal of the placenta complicated by a contraction ring
VI.	Manual reposition of an inversion of the uterus

a high degree of cervical dilatation, tocolysis while awaiting abdominal delivery may be helpful. Most important from a quantitative point of view, however, is the administration of β-mimetics in case of intrapartum fetal distress.

Treatment of fetal distress with β-mimetic agents

Uterine contractions at any time may reduce or even totally arrest blood flow in the pregnant uterus and intervillous space of the placenta by compression of the intramyometrial blood vessels, (36) and thus can be an asphyxial stress for the fetus. Because of the recovery time between contractions these periodic decreases in uterine blood flow do not necessarily lead to severe fetal hypoxia and acidosis. However, in cases of abnormally intense uterine motility, the feto-maternal exchange can be diminished to such an extent that the fetal pO_2 and pH must decrease. Even normal uterine activity during labor may affect the fetus in the same way when materno-fetal exchange is hampered, for reasons such as umbilical cord complications or placental insufficiency. Considering these facts, it seems rational to try to improve deteriorating fetal condition in these circumstances by diminishing uterine activity.

The first report on treatment of intrapartum fetal distress came from South America when Caldeyro-Barcia et al. (37) described 2 cases of fetal distress with normal uterine contractions. After tocolysis (orciprenaline intravenously), late decelerations disappeared and the pH of the fetal capillary blood rose to normal values. Schmidt and Hirdes reported on 60 caesarean sections for fetal or mixed fetal-maternal indication. Half of the patients were alternatively treated prior to the operation with fenoterol (Partusisten®; 0.08-0.1 mg). A significant difference was found between the treated and untreated patients, in the pH of umbilical venous blood, the fenoterol group being less acidotic (7.22 ± 0.08 *vs.* 7.29 + 0.08). With a considerably lower dose of the same substance, Künzel et al. (39) found a significant rise in pO_2 during normal labor but no alteration in pH of mother or fetus.

Another approach to influence the fetal oxygenation and fetal acid-base status in normal labor was made by Humphrey et al. (40). They studied 35 women in the second stage, specifically excluding patients with clinical signs of fetal distress. In a double blind controlled study, women were given either a placebo or 1.5 μg/kg/min ritodrine (Prepar®) i.v. or 3.0 μg/kg/min ritodrine i.v. A progressive fall in pH, pO_2 and oxygen saturation was seen in the fetal blood of the control group whereas in the ritodrine groups these changes were abolished or even reversed. In general, the improvements were more pronounced in the group of patients treated with the larger dose.

Kastendiek et al. (41) found in 14 patients with established fetal acidosis in the second stage of labor not only a significant rise of pH and base excess following a 50 μg bolus of fenoterol i.v. followed by an infusion of 2.5 μg/min for 15 min, but also a correlation between the severity of the acidosis and the rise of pH and base excess. Gamissans et al. (42, 43) demonstrated a significant improvement of fetal acidosis of hypoxic origin after intravenous administration of a contraction inhibiting dose of ritodrine (Prepar®) to women at the end of the first or during the second stage of labor. Another report came from Lipshitz (44), who treated six patients with severe fetal distress intrapartum with a 10 μg intravenous bolus of hexoprenaline (Ipradol®) as a temporizing measure before instrumental delivery. In all cases a rapid improvement of the fetal heart rate and a rise in the fetal pH was observed, reflecting an improvement in the fetal condition probably due to the reversal of the aggravating factors which had caused the fetal distress.

The first trials of intrapartum treatment of fetal distress with β-mimetic agents were carried out with continuous infusion of the drug. Recently, there has been a tendency to use an "one shot" therapy, for a bolus injection seems to be a convenient and rapid method of stopping (excessive) uterine activity for a limited period of time. In our department we have modified the bolus treatment by injecting the β-mimetic agent slowly over a period of several minutes. In our experience such an approach causes immediate cessation of uterine activity with less maternal cardiovascular side effects than a bolus injection of the same total dose.

Mechanisms of action of β-mimetic agents in the treatment of fetal distress

Whether intrapartum administration of β-mimetics in cases of fetal distress may be considered as curative treatment depends largely upon the cause of fetal distress. Several of the causal factors are reversible. Excessive uterine contractility can be reduced by intravenous administration of tocolytic agents. A decrease of the uterine blood flow due to a supine hypotension will easily be cured by turning the women on their side. Although in many instances umbilical cord compression can be effectively relieved by changes in the position of the mother, the recovery time for the fetus may be shortened by simultaneous complete relaxation of the uterus. A true knot in the cord, partial abruption of the placenta or severe placental insufficiency as a cause of fetal jeopardy, however, will certainly limit the effect of uterine inhibiting agents in increasing fetal pO_2 and pH. In such cases, the use of these drugs should be regarded as a temporizing measure only and should not lead to postponement of delivery.

Whatever the reasons of fetal asphyxia, and whether the etiologic factors are reversible or not, the rate of progression of the fetal hypoxia is enhanced by uterine contractions. Therefore, rapid deterioration of the fetus will be avoided or at least minimized by prompt, complete relaxation of the uterine muscle.

Because of the reduction of blood flow in the uterus and intervillous space during contraction of the myometrium (36), relaxation of the muscle must be considered a major contributing factor in the process of intra-uterine fetal recovery after tocolytic treatment. This applies even more when excessive uterine motility is present.

The influence on uterine and placental blood flow was discussed above.

β-mimetic stimulation results in an increased glycogenolysis in liver and muscles and, as a consequence, a raised plasma glucose level both in mother and fetus (43, 45). This increase in blood glucose level could be beneficial to the fetus in distress, as long as the fetus maintains a certain degree of oxygenation. In fetal hypoxia however this very carbohydrate load will have a deleterious effect on fetal brain structures probably as a result of the markedly higher extent to which lactic acid accumulates in brain tissue in a hyperglycemic state (46, 47).

Because of the lack of glucose-6-phosphatase in muscle cells glycogenolysis in muscle will lead to production of lactic acid, much of which diffuses into the blood stream, from which it is largely removed by the liver and reconverted to glycogen or glucose. The net effect however will be an increase in the maternal level of lactic acid. This results in a slight metabolic acidosis which will also affect the fetus because of the placental transfer of lactate (47). Moreover the lipolytic action of these agents will also contribute to a fall in maternal pH and base excess.

Administration of the drug

To achieve prompt suppression of unwanted uterine activity for a limited period of time, the β-mimetic agent can be given either intravenously or in aerosol form. The effect of an intravenous bolus injection of the drug is more rapid than that of an equivalent dose administered as a timed infusion. Equivalent bolus doses are 25-50 μg of fenoterol, 3-6 mg of ritodrine and 100-200 μg of salbutamol (44).

Because of compression of pelvic vessels in the supine position, bolus injections are preferably administered with the patient in the lateral position. An infusion of glucose (5 percent), recording of heart rate and blood pressure are recommended and an antagonist should be available.

The cardiovascular effect may be neutralized by the intravenous administration of propranolol which antagonizes also the tocolytic activity or practolol which antagonizes more selectively the cardiovascular effects. Oxytocics antagonize only the tocolytic action of β-mimetics.

METABOLIC EFFECTS

The metabolic effects of β-adrenergic drugs were reviewed by Weidinger and Wiest (48) and Weidinger and Mohr (49). β-adrenergic drugs stimulate adenylcyclase in liver and muscles leading to a higher production of glucose by glycogenolysis. The end product is an increase in blood glucose levels despite an increase in insulin secretion. When treatment with β-adrenergic drugs is continued, glucose levels can normalize. The end product of glycolysis in muscle is lactate. Lactate concentrations in the blood do increase during infusion of β-adrenergic drugs. Cyclic AMP activates lipase that liberates free fatty acids from triglycerides. Also the glycerol content of the serum increases. Potassium levels in serum can decrease during β-adrenergic treatment by a shift of potassium from the extra- to intracellular compartment. Glucose tolerance can be appreciably impaired when ritodrine is given intravenously (50). Insulin responses were not decreased. β-stimulated glycogenolysis causes a significant rise of blood glucose concentrations. Glucose is increasingly metabolized to lactate. During the first 30 min of infusion of fenoterol in healthy gravidae in the third trimester a highly significant fall of serum potassium occurred probably due to an increase of insulin. A rapid recovery of potassium levels was seen after stopping the infusion. The highly significant decrease of base excess and pH reflects a metabolic acidosis caused by lipolysis and ketonaemia. There is a partial respiratory compensation as indicated by decreased pCO_2 and increased pO_2. Lipolytic hydrolysis of triglycerides leads to a rapid increase of free glycerol and free fatty acid concentrations (51). The deterioration of the glucose tolerance is evident shortly after the administration of β-adrenergic drugs but cannot be observed after chronic administration (52).

INDICATIONS AND CONTRA-INDICATIONS

For the time being the diagnosis of pre-term labor is a clinical diagnosis based upon the presence of painful uterine contractions, bloody show and progressive cervical dilatation. In each case factors that contribute to pre-term labor have to be considered, as well as a thorough investigation of fetal well-being. The question should be answered whether the fetus is better off in a neonatal unit than in utero. The indications for uterine inhibition are summarized in table 9.

Table 9. Indications for uterine inhibition with β-mimetics.

I.	Excessive uterine activity
	1. spontaneous hypertonus
	2. drug-induced hypertonus
	3. partial placental abruption
	4. polyhydramnios and drainage
II.	Threatening pre-term labor
III.	Excessive uterine activity by:
	1. external version
	2. internal version
	3. intra-abdominal surgery during pregnancy
	4. uterine surgery during pregnancy (myomectomy, cerclage, etc.)
IV.	Fetal distress

Contra-indications are always relative and can be judged to be more or less serious. In thyroid disease administration of β-adrenergic drugs can be dangerous due to an already existing higher sympathetic tone. Combination with other drugs such as chronically used antihypertensive drugs or general anaesthesia with fluothane may be dangerous (extrasystoles, fibrillation, asystole). Monoamine oxidase inhibitors are used for the treatment of some psychiatric disorders. Their presence will modify the metabolism of β-agonists. The asthmatic patient who already uses β-adrenergic drugs may be at risk from a paradoxical response to excess beta-stimulation. Recently Kubli (53) has warned against the combined use of adrenergic drugs and corticosteroids, sometimes used to stimulate fetal lung maturity. In Germany four cases of maternal death could be attributed to this combination, death occurring by pulmonary oedema and heart failure. Infections with high fever change the endogenous levels of catecholamines. Antibiotic treatment is more appropriate than β-adrenergic drugs. Nevertheless in urinary tract infections with slight temperature elevations and uterine contractions the administration of β-adrenergic drugs can be helpful.

Premature rupture of the membranes forms a separate entity. On the one hand this is the ideal group to test the ability of uterine inhibitory drugs to arrest pre-term labor, on the other there is a risk of intra-uterine infection. If the fetus has no chance of survival outside the uterus because of the duration of pregnancy and/or lecithin concentration in amniotic fluid, inhibition seems indicated. Dystrophia myotonia (syndrome of Curschmann Steinert) is considered a contra-indication for β-mimetic drugs because of increasing symptoms of myotonia. In cases of severe pre-eclampsia the maternal and/or fetal condition can deteriorate rapidly. Stimulation of labor then seems to be a better choice. In diabetes careful control of blood glucose levels is needed. Heart disease and especially disturbances of conductance form a relative contra-indication. Electrocardiograms taken before and during treatment are a wise precaution. The administration of β-adrenergic drugs in cases of placenta praevia can mask symptoms of shock because of the resulting tachycardia. In cases of placental abruption β-adrenergic drugs are only indicated when placental reserve guarantees continuing fetal well-being. The relationship between uterine activity and the maternal coagulation syndrome is not clear. Some believe that the hypertonic and hypercontractile uterus forces intra-uterine material into the maternal circulation. Others believe that this hypertonus prevents entry of thromboplastic material into the maternal circulation (54).

Fetal growth retardation if associated with a deficient uteroplacental circulation could increase the risk of intra-uterine death and hence might be regarded as a contra-indication for β-adrenergic treatment. It might be unwise to interfere with the endogenous trigger for labor and delivery since this may be protective for the fetus and prevent its intra-uterine demise. Fetal distress can also be regarded as a relative contra-indication because as soon as the diagnosis is established by fetal cardiogram and blood-gas analysis, it seems wise to terminate pregnancy or labor. An exception can be made for rapid inhibition of uterine activity during labor by an intravenous bolus injection as described above, in preparation for caesarean section during the second phase of labor. Furthermore, the acid base status of the fetus showed improvement when intravenous ritodrine was used in the second stage of labor (40).

Table 10. Measured blood loss at delivery in patients between 28-38 weeks gestation from a consecutive series of 3363 patients (1975-1976). (Placental anomalies were excluded; in none of the groups was there a significant difference between treated and control patients.)

Group	No. of patients	Blood loss (ml)	
		median	range
All patients			
treated	112	295	50-1800
control	221	300	50-2150
2nd stage < 30 min			
treated	87	250	50-1800
control	174	250	50-2150
2nd stage > 30 min			
treated	25	320	50-1050
control	47	300	50-2000
Multiple pregnancies excluded			
treated	98	255	50-1800
control	206	270	50-2150

Although the fear of increased blood loss post partum after prolonged treatment with β-adrenergic drugs may be justified, we found no differences in measured blood loss post partum between patients treated with β-mimetics and a control group. Table 10 gives the median and range of measured blood loss after vaginal delivery in patients treated with β-mimetics compared with untreated patients with gestational ages between 28 and 38 weeks and without placental anomalies out of a consecutive series of 3363 patients. No significant differences were found between both groups (Mann Whitney U-test) whether or not patients were matched for duration of second stage or when twins were excluded.

CONCLUSIONS AND SUMMARY

The high frequency of pre-term delivery has consequences for perinatal mortality and morbidity. As a symptomatic therapy β-adrenergic drugs have a strong inhibitory action on uterine contractility. The mechanism by which β-adrenergic drugs reduce uterine contractility is thought to be a cellular action in which, through β-receptors, the enzyme adenylcyclase is activated in the cell membrane. Adenyl-cyclase, in turn, converts ATP into cyclic AMP through phosphorylases implicated in glycolysis. This form of energy promotes active sodium transport giving hyperpolarization of muscle relaxation.

Isoxsuprine, orciprenaline, ritodrine, fenoterol and terbutaline tested by means of intra-uterine pressure recording proved to be effective in inhibiting uterine activity in pregnant women. Pharmacokinetic data on these β-adrenergic drugs reveal adequate blood levels with intravenous administration and "chemical half-lives" of several hours. The degree of maternal tachycardia parallels blood levels. Clinical trials with β-adrenergic drugs to stop threatened early labor were judged according to the "ten commandments" necessary for good clinical trials. Using these criteria five studies support the ability of β-adrenergic drugs to lengthen the duration of pregnancy. Unwanted cardiovascular effects of β-adrenergic drugs include maternal tachycardia, raised maternal cardiac output, increase of maternal systolic and decrease of diastolic pressure and slight fetal tachycardia without influencing beat-to-beat variation. The criteria of success should be defined in terms of lengthening the duration of pregnancy in relation to gestational age at the onset of treatment and in terms of the final neonatal outcome.

The administration of bolus injections of β-adrenergic drugs during labor as a means of "treating" fetal acidosis and as a temporizing measure before instrumental delivery deserves attention. Uterine blood flow has been studied in human pregnancy, in sheep and in monkeys. The results suggest that different β-adrenergic drugs have qualitatively different effects on uteroplacental blood flow and that the effects are dose-dependent. The metabolic effects of β-adrenergic agents are elevation of the blood levels of glucose, insulin, lactate, triglycerides, glycerol and a decrease of potassium. In the clinical application of β-adrenergic drugs the tocolytic index is helpful in predicting the success of stopping labor.

Relative contra-indications to administration of β-adrenergic drugs are described as relative in cases of thyrotoxicosis, the use of other drugs, severe infections with fever, dystrophia myotonia, severe pre-eclampsia, diabetes, heart disease, severe blood loss, fetal growth retardation and fetal distress. The use of β-adrenergic drugs does not influence the amount of post partum blood loss.

The prerequisites for using β-adrenergic drugs in obstetric practice include a critical assessment of the hazards of keeping the fetus *in utero*, and knowledge of the mode of action of β-adrenergic substances with their indications, relative contra-indications, and side effects for both mother and fetus.

REFERENCES

1. Fuchs F and Stakemann G: Treatment of threatened premature labor with large doses of progesterone. *Am J Obstet Gynecol* 79, 172-176 (1960).
2. Johnson JWC, Austin KL, Jones GS, Davis GH and King ThM: Efficacy of 17- alpha-hydroxyprogesterone caproate in the prevention of premature labor. *N Engl J Med* 293, 675-680 (1975).
3. Fuchs F, Fuchs AR, Poblete VF and Risk A: Effect of alcohol on threatened premature labor. *Am J Obstet Gynecol* 99, 627-637 (1967).
4. Wiqvist N, Lundström N and Gréen K: Premature labour and indomethacin. *Prostaglandins* 10, 515-526 (1975).
5. Steer CM and Petrie RH: A comparison of magnesium sulfate and alcohol for the prevention of premature labor. *Am J Obstet Gynecol* 129, 1-4 (1977).
6. Landesman R, Adeodato de Souza J, Coutinho EM, Wilson, KH and Bomfin de Sousa M: The inhibitory effect of diazoxide in normal term labor. *Am J Obstet Gynecol* 103, 430-433 (1969).
7. Coutinho EM, Bomfim de Sousa M, Wilson KH and Landesman R: Inhibitory action of new sympathomimetic amine (DU 21220) on the gravid uterus. *Am J Obstet Gynecol* 104, 1053-1056 (1969).
8. Ahlquist RP: A study of the adrenotropic receptors. *Am J Physiol* 153, 586-600 (1948).
9. Lands AM, Arnold A, McAuliff JP, Luduena FP and Brown TG: Differentiation of receptor systems activated by sympathomimetic amines. *Nature* 214, 597-598 (1967).
10. Weidinger H and Wiest W: Modellvorstellung zur Wirkung betasympatikomimetischer Substanzen. *Z Geburtshilfe Perinatol* 177, 223-232 (1973a).
11. Grüber CM: The autonomic innervation of the genito-urinary system. *Physiol Rev* 13, 497-512 (1933).
12. Van Driel C, Houthoff HJ and Baljet B: The innervation of the myometrium. Some histochemical observations in man and rat. *Eur J Obstet Gynecol Reprod Biol* 3, 11-17 (1973).
13. Pose SV, Cibils LA and Zuspan FP: Effect of l′ epinephrine infusion on uterine contractility and cardiovascular system. *Am J Obstet Gynecol* 84, 297-306 (1962).
14. Buchelt L and Rominger KL: Pharmacokinetik und Metabolismus von Th 1165a beim Menschen. *Int J Clin Pharmacol* 4, 37-41 (1972).
15. Martin LE, Rees J and Tanner RJN: Quantitative determination of salbutamol in plasma, as either its trimethylsilyl or t-butyldimethylsilyl ether, using a stable isotope multiple ion recording technique. *Biomed Mass Spectrom* 3, 184-190 (1976).
16. Post LC: Pharmakinetics of beta-adrenergic agonists. In: *Pre-term labour*, Anderson A, Beard R, Brudenell JM and Dunn PM (eds), London, Royal College of Obstetricians and Gynecologists, 1977, p 134-148.
17. Leferink JG, Wagemaker-Engels I, Maas RAA, Lamont H, Pauwels R and van der Straeten M: Quantitative analysis of terbutaline in serum and urine at therapeutic levels using gaschromatography - mass spectrometry. *J Chromatography* 143, 299-305 (1977).
18. Gamissans P, Canas E, Cararach V, Ribas J, Puerto B and Edo A: A double-blind study with indomethacin in threatened preterm labour. *Eur J Obstet Gynecol Reprod Biol* 8, 123-128 (1978).
19. Richter R: Evaluation of success in treatment of threatening premature labor by betamimetic drugs. *Am J Obstet Gynecol* 127, 482-486 (1977).
20. Baumgarten K and Grüber W: Tokolyse-index. In: *Perinatale Medizin*, Dudenhausen JW and Saling E (eds), Stuttgart, Thieme Verlag, 1974, p 58-59.
21. Essed GGM, Eskes TKAB and Jongsma HW: A randomized trial of two betamimetic drugs for the treatment of threatening early labor. *Eur J Obstet Gynecol Reprod Biol* 8, 341-348 (1978).

22. Bieniarz J, Ivankovich A and Scommenga A: Cardiac output during ritodrine treatment in premature labor. *Am J Obstet Gynecol* 118, 910-920 (1974).
23. Martin CB, Jr, Murata Y, Petrie RH and Parer JT: Respiratory movements in fetal rhesus monkeys. *Am J Obstet Gynecol* 119, 939-948 (1974).
24. Meschia G, Cotter JR, Breathnach CS and Barron DH: The hemoglobin, oxygen, carbon dioxide and hydrogen ion concentration in the umbilical bloods of sheep and goats as sampled via indwelling plastic catheters. *Quart J Exp Physiol* 50, 185-195 (1965).
25. Brennan SC, McLaughlin MK and Chez RA: Effects of prolonged infusion of beta-adrenergic agonists on uterine and umbilical bloodflow in pregnant sheep. *Am J Obstet Gynecol* 128, 709-715 (1977).
26. Brettes JP, Renaud R and Gandar R: A double-blind investigation into the effects of ritodrine on uterine bloodflow during the third trimester of pregnancy. *Am J Obstet Gynecol* 124, 164-168 (1976).
27. Lippert TH, De Grandi PB and Fridrich R: Actions of the uterine relaxant, fenoterol, on uteroplacental hemodynamics in human subjects. *Am J Obstet Gynecol* 125, 1093-1098 (1976).
28. Wallenburg HCS, Mazer J and Hutchinson DL: Effects of a beta-adrenergic agent (metaproterenol) on uteroplacental circulation. *Am J Obstet Gynecol* 117, 1067-1075 (1973).
29. Kleinhout J: Foetale hartfrequentie en autonoom zenuwstelsel. *Thesis*, Free University, Amsterdam, 1975.
30. De Haan J, Cacciavillani G, Eskes TKAB, Van der Hoek JM and Arts THM: Der Einfluss von Th 1165a auf die maternelle und fetale Zirkulation beim Rhesusaffen. In: *Perinatale Medizin*, Dudenhausen JW und Saling E (eds), Stuttgart, Thieme Verlag, 1974, p 60-61.
31. Eskes TKAB and De Haan J: The influence of betamimetic catecholamines upon the fetal circulation. *Z Geburtshilfe Perinatol* 176, 97-107 (1972).
32. Eskes TKAB and De Haan J: The fetal heart frequency during treatment with betamimetic drugs. In: *Labour inhibition – Betamimetic drugs in Obstetrics*, Weidinger H (ed), Stuttgart New York, Gustav Fischer Verlag, 1977, p 57-65.
33. Rudolph AM: Cardiac output in the mammalian fetus. In: *Reviews in Perinatal Medicine*, vol I, Scarpelli EM and Cosmi EV (eds), Baltimore, University Park Press, 1976, p 35-47.
34. Nochimson DJ, Riffel HD, Yeh SY, Kreitzer MD, Paul RH and Hon EH: The effects of ritodrine hydrochloride on uterine activity and the cardiovascular system. *Am J Obstet Gynecol* 118, 523-528 (1974).
35. Caritis SN, Morishima HD, Stark RI, Daniel SS and James LS: Effects of terbutaline on the pregnant baboon and fetus. *Obstet Gynecol* 50, 56-60 (1977).
36. Borell U, Fernström I, Ohlson L and Wiqvist N: Effect of uterine contractions on the human uteroplacental blood circulation. *Am J Obstet Gynecol* 89, 881-890 (1964).
37. Caldeyro-Barcia R, Magana JM, Castillo JB, Poseiro JJ, Mendez-Bauer C, Pose SV, Escarcena L, Casacu-Berta C, Bustos JR and Giusi G: Nuevo enfoque para el tratamiento del sufrimiento fetal agudo intraparto. *Archivos de Ginecologia y Obstetricia* 24, 3-7 (1969).
38. Schmidt J and Hirdes G: Prä-operative Tokolyse vor der Schnittentbindung. *Geburtshilfe Frauenheilkd* 34, 978-982 (1974).
39. Künzel W and Reinecke J: Der Einfluss von Th 1165-a auf die Paspartialdruck und auf Kardiovaskuläre Parameter von Mutter und Fetus. Zugleich eine quantitative Analyse der Wehentätigkeit. *Z Geburtshilfe Perinatol* 177, 81-90 (1973).
40. Humphrey M, Chang A, Gilvert M and Wood C: The effect of intravenous ritodrine on the acid-base status of the fetus during the second stage of labor. *Br J Obstet Gynaecol* 82, 234-245 (1975).
41. Kastendiek E, Künzel W und Kirchhoff J: Der Einfluss von Th 1165a auf die metabolische Azidose der Feten während der Austreibungsperiode. *Z Geburtshilfe Perinatol* 178, 439-443 (1974).

42. Gamissans O, Esteban-Altirriba J and Calaf J: The treatment of intrapartum fetal acidosis by intravenous infusion of beta adrenergic drugs to the mother. In: *Perinatal Medicine*, Huntingford PJ, Beard RW and Hytten FE (eds), Basel, Karger, 1971, p 152-160.
43. Gamissans O, Carreras M, Duran P, Cararach I, Calaf J, Avril V and Esteban-Altirriba J: The treatment of foetal acidosis with betamimetic drugs. Studies on acid-base balance, blood glucose levels and uterine motility. In: *Proceedings of the International Symposium on the treatment of fetal risks*, Baumgarten K and De Casparis AW (eds), Vienna, University of Vienna, 1973, p 145-148.
44. Lipshitz J and Baillie P: Uterine and cardiovascular effects of betamimetic selective sympathomimetic drugs administered as an intravenous infusion. *South Afr Med J* 50, 1973-1977 (1976).
45. Unbehaun V, Conradt A, Schlotter CM and Schneider V: Stoffwechselveränderungen während infusion von Th-1165a. *Z Geburtshilfe Perinatol* 178, 118-127 (1974).
46. Myers RE: Nervous system effects of cardiac arrest in monkeys. *Arch Neurol* 34, 65-75 (1977).
47. Klöck FK, Chantraine H, Etzrodt A, Liedtke H und Schulte HJ: Der Einfluss des beta-stimulators Th-1165-a auf mütterliche und fetale Stoffwechselparameter. In: *Perinatale Medizin*, Dudenhausen JW and Saling E (eds), Stuttgart, Thieme Verlag, 1972, p 384-386.
48. Weidinger H and Wiest W: Die Auswirkungen langdauern der Wehenhemmung mit Th 1165-a und Isoptin auf Herz-Kreislauf-, Organ- und Stoffwechselparameter der Mutter. *Z Geburtshilfe Perinatol* 177, 238-244 (1973).
49. Weidinger H and Mohr D: Blutglukose und Immunoreaktives Insulin unter dem Einfluss von Th 1165-a und Isoptin bei Schwangeren mit und ohne tokolytische Therapie. *Z Geburtshilfe Perinatol* 177, 244-251 (1973).
50. Bergstein NAM, Stolte LAM, Flynn MJ and Van Doorn GA: An investigation into the effects of betamimetic agents on the response to intravenous glucose loads. In: *Proceedings of the International Symposium on the treatment of fetal risks*, Baumgarten K and Casparis AW (eds), Vienna, University of Vienna, 1972, p 187-189.
51. Conradt A, Schlotter CM and Unbehaun V: Lipolysis ketonaemia, estrogen-gestagen concentrations during short time infusion therapy with betamimetics. In: *Labour inhibition - Betamimetic drugs in Obstetrics*, Weidinger H (ed), Stuttgart, Fischer Verlag, 1977, p 103-110.
52. Lang N, Bellmann O, Hinckers HJ and Schlebusch H: Carbohydrate and lipid metabolism during longtime treatment with beta-adrenergic drugs. In: *Labour Inhibition - Betamimetic drugs in Obstetrics*, Weidinger H (ed), Stuttgart, Fisher Verlag, 1977, p 111-120.
53. Kubli F: Beta-adrenergic agonists. In: *Pre-term labour*. Anderson A, Beard R, Brudenell JM and Dunn PM (eds), London, Royal College of Obstetricians and Gynecologists, 1977, p 218-220.
54. Eskes TKAB and De Leeuw JHA: Circulatory aspects of amniotic fluid embolism. In: *Amniotic fluid Research and Clinical Application*, Fairweather DVI and Eskes TKAB (eds), Amsterdam, Excerpta Medica, 1978, p 441-445.
55. Wesselius-de Casparis A, Thiery M, Yo le Sian A, Baumgarten K, Brosens I, Gamissans O, Stolk JG and Vivier W: Results of double blind multicentre study with ritodrine in premature labour. *Br Med J* 3, 144-147 (1971).
56. Sivasamboo R: Premature labor. In: *Proceedings of the International Symposium on the treatment of fetal risks*. Baumgarten K and Casparis AW (eds), Vienna, University of Vienna, p 35-37.
57. Ingemarsson J: Effect of terbutaline on premature labor. *Am J Obstet Gynecol* 125, 520-524 (1976).
58. Lauersen NH, Merkatz IR, Tejani N, Wilson K, Roberson A, Mann LI and Fuchs F: Inhibition of premature labor: A multicenter comparison of ritodrine and ethanol. *Am J Obstet Gynecol* 127, 837-845 (1977).

59. Ehrenkranz RA, Walker AM, Oakes G, McLaughlin M and Chez RA: Effect of ritodrine infusion on uterine and umbilical bloodflow in pregnant sheep. *Am J Obstet Gynecol.* 126, 343-349 (1976).
60. Ehrenkranz RA, Walker AM, Oakes GK, Hamilton LA and Chez RA: Effect of fenoterol infusion on uterine and umbilical blood flow in pregnant sheep. *Am J Obstet Gynecol* 128, 177-182 (1977).
61. Rondinelli M and Vangelista R: Effects of orciprenaline (alupent) on the uteroplacental blood flow in pregnant women. In: *Perinatal Medicine*, 4th Europ Congr of Perinatal Medicine, Prague 1974, Stembera ZK, Polacek K and Sabata V (eds), Stuttgart, Georg Thieme Verlag, 1975, p 347.
62. Janish H, Leodolter S and Reinold R: Uteroplazentäre Durchblutungsverbesserung bei EPH gestose durch langzeit Therapie mit betasympathikomimetika. *Z Geburtshilfe Perinatol* 178, 202-206 (1974).

THE USE OF INHIBITORS OF PROSTAGLANDIN SYNTHESIS IN OBSTETRICS

NILS WIQVIST

The use of prostaglandin synthetase inhibitors in the treatment of pre-term labour is still a highly controversial issue. Based on theoretical and experimental evidence there seems to be no doubt that suppression of endogenous prostaglandin levels results in a reduction of uterine contractions. However, it is known from animal studies as well as from some clinical case reports that fetal hazards may be associated with this treatment.

RATIONALE BEHIND THE USE OF PROSTAGLANDIN SYNTHETASE INHIBITORS

At the beginning of this short review one should consider the major steps in the conversion of arachidonic acid to biologically active prostaglandins (table 1). The endogenous concentrations of $PGF_{2\alpha}$ and PGE_2 are to date the only parameters that have been studied to any degree in the context of pre-term labour (Keirse, this volume). Very little is known about the biological significance of the endoperoxides PGG_2 and PGH_2 or of PGI_2 (prostacyclin) and TXA_2 (trhomboxane A_2), although these compounds possess potent organ specific activities. For instance, we have found that PGI_2 affects contractility of the human uterus in a similar way to PGE_2 (1). Prostaglandin synthetase inhibitors such as aspirin, indomethacin, fenamates, naproxen and others exert their action on the enzyme cyclo-oxygenase, which converts

Table. 1. Major metabolic pathways in the conversion of arachidonic acid

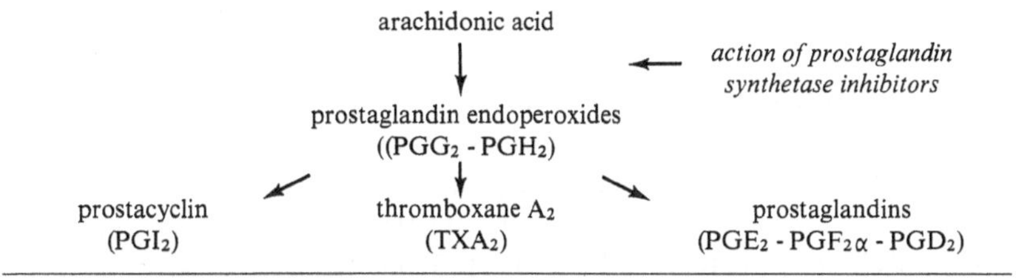

M.J.N.C. Keirse et al. (eds.), Human Parturition, 189-200.

arachidonic acid into the endoperoxides. This means that administration of prostaglandin synthetase inhibitors decreases the formation of all subsequent compounds (table 1) and that the possibility of developing organ specific inhibitors at this level is small (2).

The urinary excretion of the major metabolite of $PGF_{2\alpha}$ increases progressively during pregnancy with an acute rise in connection with normal labour (fig. 1). This is in contrast to the data of Granström and Kindahl (4) who collected daily urine samples during pregnancy and analyzed the major

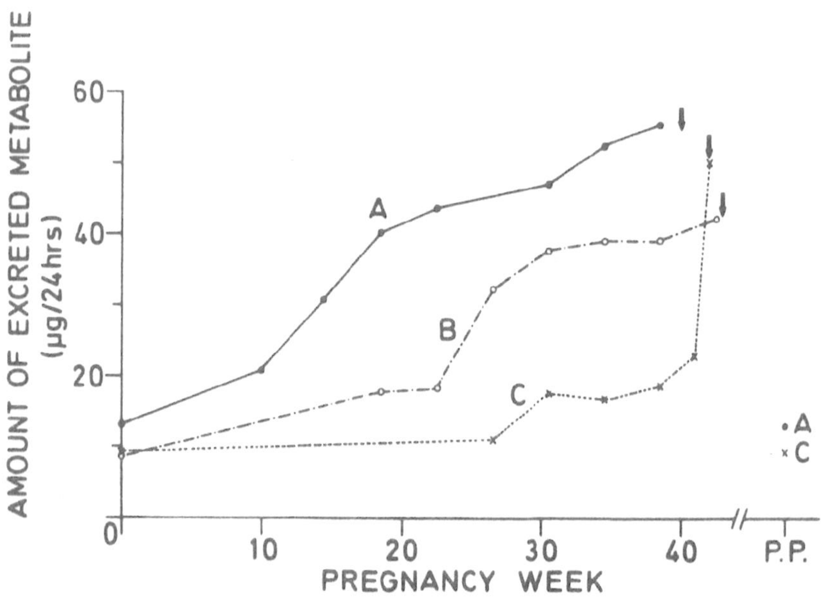

Fig. 1. Urinary excretion of the major metabolite of $PGF_{1\alpha}$ and $PGF_{2\alpha}$, 5α,7α-dihydroxy-11-keto-tetranor prosta-1,16-dioic acid (µg/24 h), in three pregnant women. Arrows indicate time of delivery. (After Hamberg, 1974 [5], with permission.)

metabolite of $PGF_{2\alpha}$. It is evident that they were unable to find any tendency towards increased levels during the last few days of pregnancy preceding normal labour (fig. 2). The involvement of prostaglandins in parturition is discussed elsewhere (Keirse, this volume).

Pre-term labour is by definition a situation in which labour-like contractions are present and one would consequently expect the $PGF_{2\alpha}$ levels to be increased. We analyzed the plasma concentration of the major serum metabolite of $PGF_{2\alpha}$, 15-keto-13, 14-dihydro $PGF_{2\alpha}$, using the GLC-mass spec-

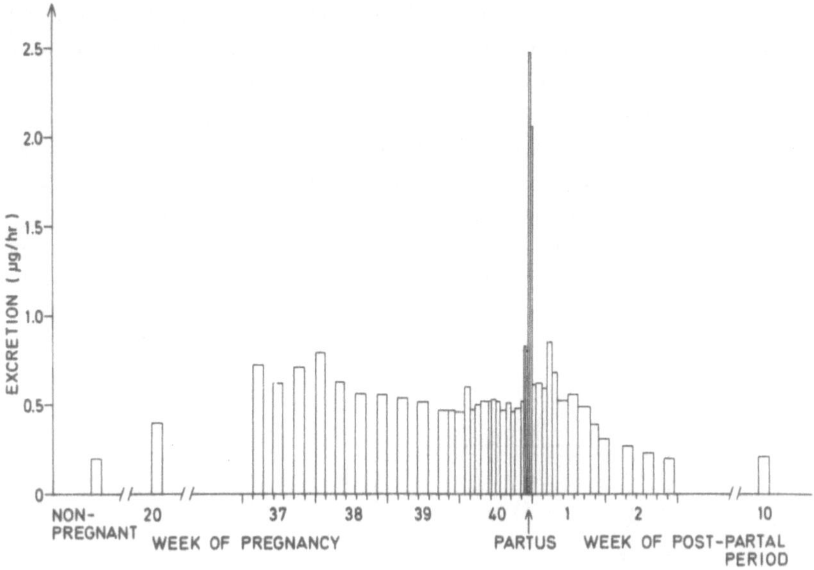

Fig. 2. Daily urinary excretion of the major metabolite of $PGF_{1}\alpha$ and $PGF_{2}\alpha$, 5α-, 7α-dihydroxy-11-keto-tetranor-prosta-1,16-dioic acid (μg/24 h) before, during and after pregnancy. (After Granström and Kindahl, 1976 [4], with permission.)

trometry method in a few cases admitted in pre-term labour. Some of these patients had levels which were consistent with normal pregnancy whereas others had values similar to those found during labour (5). Schwartz et al. have determined the same $PGF_{2}\alpha$ metabolite in plasma of 18 women in connection with pre-term labour using a radioimmunoassay (6). They found that the average level of the metabolite corresponded to 220 pg/ml. Administration of flufenamic acid resulted in a decrease in the concentration of the metabolite so that normal values were present on the day following treatment.

It seems possible that the concentration of prostaglandins is proportional to the level of uterine activity and cervical involvement and that normal or low values are present in cases of false or early pre-term labour, whereas the levels are high in patients in advanced pre-term labour.

TOCOLYTIC EFFECTS

One of the difficulties in an objective evaluation of the effect of tocolytic agents in pre-term labour is related to the criteria of selecting patients. A significant proportion of women admitted with symptoms of pre-term labour are patients with so-called 'false labour'. In other women there is a rapid spontaneous decrease in uterine contractility immediately following hospitalisation. It is therefore questionable whether a reduction in uterine contractility should be attributed to the effect of the tocolytic drug or to bed rest.

We have tried to obtain some objective information on the contractility reducing effect of prostaglandin synthetase inhibitors by external and standardized monitoring of the frequency of contractions before, during and after therapy. Figure 3 illustrates a fall in the frequency of contractions within the

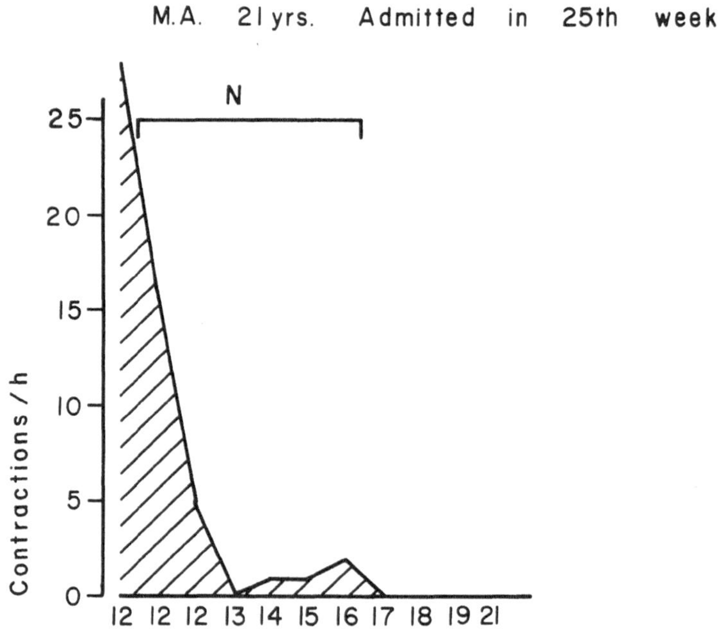

Fig. 3. Frequency of uterine contractions per hour recorded by external tocometry before and during naproxen (N) therapy.

few hours following administration of naproxen, whereas figure 4 shows a similar but significantly slower decrease in uterine contractility. It is of course difficult to judge to what extent these effects represent drug-induced tocolysis. However, intense, frequent and spastic uterine contractions are typical in many instances of severe dysmenorrhoea. This contractility pattern remains constant for many hours and significant alterations are easy to identify. Figure 5 represents a tracing from such a case. Rectal administration of 100

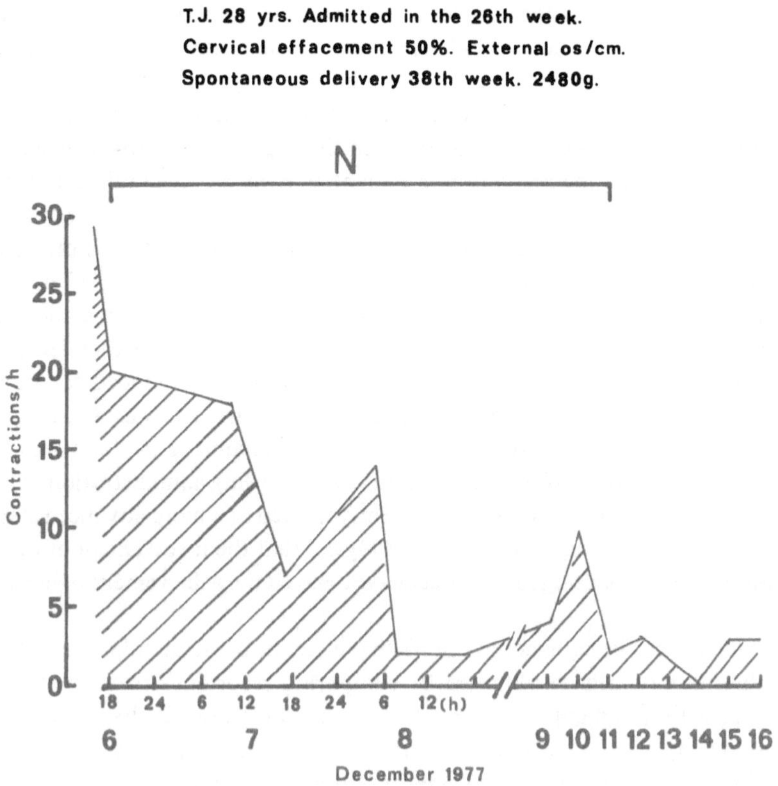

Fig. 4. See figure 3.

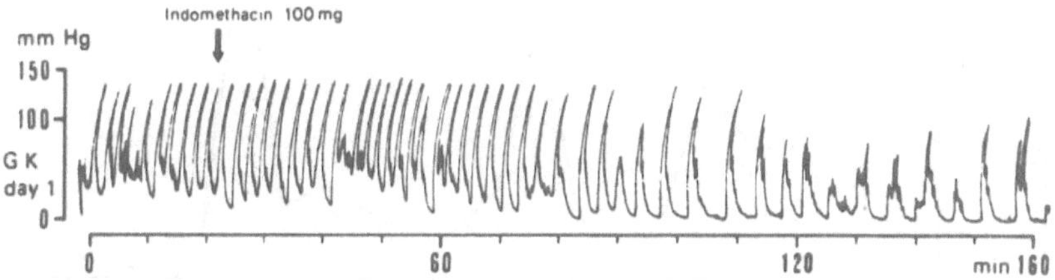

Fig. 5. The effect of rectal administration of 100 mg indomethacin on uterine contractility during menstruation (day 1) in a dysmenorrhoeic patient. (After Lundström et al., 1976 [7].)

mg indomethacin resulted in a definite decrease in amplitude and frequency of contractions (7). The pathophysiological mechanisms of dysmenorrhoea are of course completely different from those in pre-term labour. However, this tracing, among many others, illustrates that commonly used doses of prostaglandin synthetase inhibitors reach the uterus in effective concentrations and that uterine relaxation is evident as early as 60-90 min following administration of the drug.

Ten patients monitored in our department were admitted with pre-term uterine contractions corresponding to an average frequency of 17/h. The frequency decreased to 9 contractions within the hour following the oral administration of 550 mg of naproxen. After 2 h there was a further decrease of contractions to 5/h. At 24 h the contractions were reduced to 4 and remained subsequently at 2/h over the next few days. In a study by Schwartz et al. (6) on women in pre-term labour given flufenamic acid there was no significant reduction in contractility until 24 h following administration of the drug. However, their cases were apparently treated at a more advanced stage of pre-term labour than ours. It seems logical that the involvement of other contractility stimulating factors may have delayed the achievement of uterine quiescence.

Evidence on the contractility inhibiting effect of prostaglandin synthetase inhibitors may also be obtained by comparing recordings from treatment periods with treatment free intervals. Figure 6 illustrates results in a patient admitted to hospital in the 27th week of gestation. The frequency of the uterine contractions was monitored by external tocometry for at least one

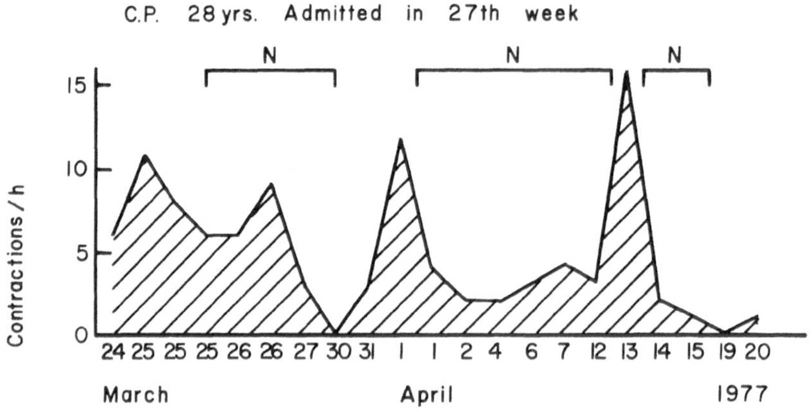

Fig. 6. See figure 3. Note the tendency towards recurrent uterine contractions in the treatment free intervals.

hour more or less daily during one month. Naproxen was administered during three periods. The decrease in frequency during the treatment was obvious as was the recurrence of uterine contractions in between the treatment periods. Following the last treatment course the uterus remained in a relaxed state and pregnancy continued uneventfully until term. Figure 7 illustrates a similar course of events in another patient.

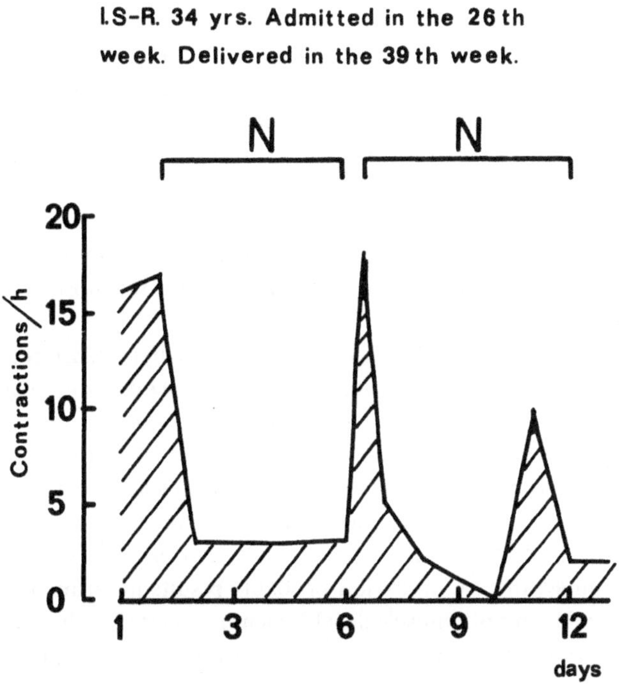

Fig. 7. See figures 3 and 6.

POTENTIAL FETAL HAZARDS

If we now turn to the problem of potential fetal hazards there are a number of items to be considered (table 2). Disregarding for a moment the consequences related to the cardio-pulmonary circulation I would like to comment on the possibility that fetal renal function may be impaired. Novy (8) has observed that pregnant rhesus monkeys developed oligohydramnios following treatment with indomethacin. This drug is known to exert a renal vasoconstrictor and antidiuretic effect associated with decreased renal PGE_2 synthesis. It is

Table 2. Potential fetal hazards of prostaglandin synthetase inhibitors

Inluence on cardio-pulmonary circulation
Reduction of cerebral blood circulation
Longer bleeding time
Hyperbilirubinemia
Impairment of renal function

believed that the decrease in amniotic fluid volume is related to an impairment of fetal urine excretion. However, the duration of therapy was considerable in these experiments and the dose of indomethacin very high. Oligohydramnios has not been observed in any of the clinical trials so far reported.

Indomethacin has been shown to reduce cerebral blood flow in the baboon (9). In the rat fetus indomethacin has been shown to increase the number of areas of neuronal micro-necrosis in the brain (10). These observations are of course of a serious nature and there is clearly a need for more animal work within this particular field.

Closure of the ductus arteriosus and pulmonary hypertension as a result of prostaglandin synthetase inhibitors is to the best of our knowledge the only complication documented in clinical case material. Basic facts do not seem to be in dispute, i.e. E prostaglandins cause relaxation of the ductus, F prostaglandins contraction and synthetase inhibitors also lead to contraction. The exact mechanisms are still incompletely known but there is evidence that PGI_2 and thromboxanes play a major role in this context (2). Chronic prostaglandin synthetase inhibition probably results in an increase in pulmonary vascular smooth muscle development associated with an increase in pulmonary arterial pressure and in some cases the paradoxical situation of postnatal patency of the ductus (11). A review of the current world literature on fetal hazards possibly connected with prostaglandin synthetase inhibitors reveals that there are a total of 9 cases exhibiting signs of ductal disorder or pulmonary hypertension (12, 13, 14, 15). Three of these neonates had signs of patent ductus arteriosus.

Our own study includes 18 cases admitted in pre-term labour in the 25th-32nd week of gestation. Eight women were given indomethacin (25 mg $\times$ 4) and 10 naproxen (275 mg $\times$ 2-6) orally over periods of generally 5 days. There was a significant decrease or inhibition of uterine contractions in 16 women and 15 of these went to term. One pre-term infant (2,700 g) developed respiratory distress with signs of patent ductus arteriosus. The neonate needed digitalisation and assisted ventilation for 8 days but recovered and has had a normal development subsequently. The association between ductal patency in this neonate and the administration of a prostaglandin synthetase inhibitor 5 weeks earlier seems doubtful but the incident merits careful attention. Except for the case of respiratory distress post-natal adaptation was normal as judged from blood gas analyses, arterial blood pressure, ECG and vector-cardiography. The different coagulation tests did not show any deviation from normal. Three neonates had bilirubin values exceeding 260 μM/1, one requiring phototherapy. All children appeared normal at follow-up examination.

In this context we may refer to a study by Gamissans et al. (16). Their study was a double blind trial with indomethacin and placebo in one group of patients and indomethacin and ritodrine in the other (table 3). The two groups were matched with regard to gestational age, parity and examination findings at admission (tocolytic index). The indomethacin-ritodrine group had significantly better results with regard to gain in days before delivery, number of patients delivered at term, weight of newborns and number of recurrences. There were no significant differences in neonatal morbidity or mortality (table 3). The study shows that treatment with indomethacin and ritodrine was slightly more effective than ritodrine and placebo in prolonging pregnancy.

Table 3. Results of a double-blind study comparing ritodrine and placebo to ritodrine and indomethacin in the treatment of pre-term labour. (Data from Gamissans et al., 1978 [16].)

	Group		Significance of the differences between groups
	Ritodrine + placebo	ritodrine + indomethacin	
Number of cases	22	22	
Recurrences (n)	15	7	$p < 0.02$
Pre-term deliveries (n)	14	7	$p < 0.05$
Mean gain in days	26	41	$p < 0.05$
Mean birthweight (g)	2367	2798	$p < 0.05$
Fetal and neonatal mortality (n)	4	2	not significant

Pros and cons as to the use of prostaglandin synthetase inhibitors in the treatment of pre-term labour remain controversial. The number of controlled studies totals less than 200 women which is far too small to allow any definite conclusions. There is on the other hand the world experience with aspirin, and we can compare the effect of aspirin on the prostaglandin synthesis to that of indomethacin. Figure 8 shows the effect of a fairly large dose of indomethacin (200 mg per day) on the plasma concentration of 15-keto-

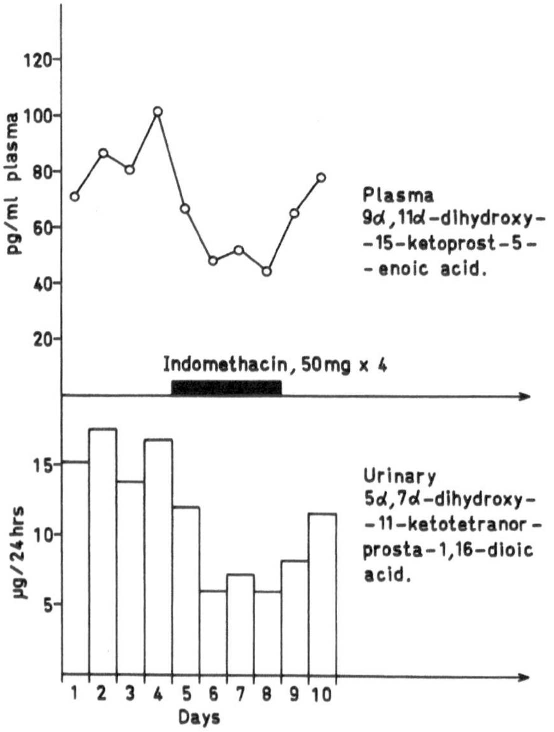

Fig. 8. $PGF_{2\alpha}$ production before, during and after administration of indomethacin measured as major metabolites in plasma (upper panel) and urine (lower panel). (After Granström and Kindahl 1976 [4], with permission.)

13,14-dihydro $PGF_{2\alpha}$. Figure 9 shows the effect of a commonly used aspirin dose (0.6 g × 4 per day). The decrease in plasma concentration of the $PGF_{2\alpha}$ metabolite was the same with indomethacin and aspirin in these experiments (4). An immediate reaction to these data is that thousands of fetuses and neonates should have been killed or born with heart failure as a consequence of the wide spread misuse of aspirin in many societies and this is obviously not the case. This is further substantiated by a recent case report (17). A mother had ingested large doses of aspirin during the last month of pregnancy and the infant appeared to have a serum salicylate level as high as 31 mg/100 ml as compared to 2.0 mg/100 ml in maternal serum. The neonate appeared to some extent malnourished and irritable but recovered rapidly following diuretics and intravenous fluids. However, there were no signs of cardio-pulmonary circulation disturbances.

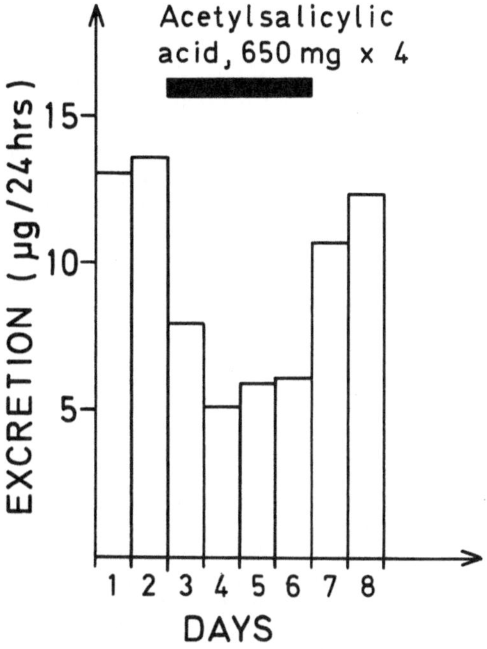

Fig. 9. Urinary excretion of 5α, 7α-dihydroxy-11-keto-tetranor-prosta-1,16-dioic acid before, during and after administration of acetylsalicylic acid.: After Granström and Kindahl, 1976 [4], with permission.)

CONCLUSIONS

Some may question whether prostaglandin synthetase inhibitors should be used at all in clinical trials until further documentation from animal studies is available. Others may be inclined to justify such trials provided that their use is limited to carefully controlled studies in a few centres with special resources. In the latter event there are a number of problems that have to be considered. Firstly, these drugs should be avoided early in pregnancy and perhaps also after the 32nd week of pregnancy. Secondly, from the literature, there is evidence that prolonged exposure to these drugs may be hazardous and therefore the treatment periods should be comparatively short. Thirdly, prostaglandin synthetase inhibitors should not be given in advanced pre-term labour were delivery is imminent as the drugs are likely to be ineffective.

REFERENCES

1. Lindblom B, Wilhelmsson L and Wiqvist N: Influence of PGI_2 (Prostacyclin) on the smooth muscle activity of the human oviduct. Congress abstract. *Vth European Congress on Sterility and Fertility*. Venice, October 2nd/6th 1978.
2. Vane JR: Inhibitors of prostaglandin, prostacyclin and thromboxane synthesis. In: *Advances in Prostaglandin and Thromboxane Research*, Vol. 4, New York, Raven Press, 1978, p 27-44.
3. Hamberg M: Quantitative studies on prostaglandin synthesis in man. 3. Excretion of the major urinary metabolite of prostaglandins $F_{1\alpha}$ and $F_{2\alpha}$ during pregnancy. *Life Sci* 14, 247-252 (1974).
4. Granström E and Kindahl H: Radioimmunoassay for urinary metabolites of prostaglandin F_2. *Prostaglandins* 12, 759-783 (1976).
5. Wiqvist N, Lundström V and Gréen K: Premature labor and indomethacin. *Prostaglandins* 10, 515-526 (1975).
6. Schwartz A, Brook I, Zor U, Kohen F, Insler V and Lindner HR: Discussion contribution (H.R. Lindner). In: *Pre-term labour. Proceedings of the Fifth Study Group of the Royal College of Obstetricians and Gynaecologists* 1977, London, 1977, The Royal College of Obstetricians and Gynaecologists, 27 Sussex Place, Regent's Park, London NW1 4RG, p 249-252.
7. Lundström V, Gréen K and Wiqvist N: Prostaglandins, indomethacin and dysmenorrhoea. *Prostaglandins* 11, 893-904 (1976).
8. Novy MJ: Effects of indomethacin on labor, fetal oxygenation and fetal development in Rhesus monkeys. In: *Advances in Prostaglandin and Thromboxane Research vol. 4, Prostaglandins and Perinatal Medicine*, New York, Raven Press, 1978 p 285-300.
9. Pickard JD and Mackenzie ET: Inhibition of prostaglandin synthesis and the response of baboon cerebral circulation to carbon dioxide. *Nature (New Biol)* 245, 187-188 (1973).
10. Sharpe GL, Krous H and Altshuler G: Perinatal use of indomethacin, *Lancet* 2, 87, 1977.
11. Rudolph AM: Effects of prostaglandins and synthetase inhibitors on the fetal circulation. In: *Pre-term Labour. Proceedings of the Fifth Study Group of the Royal College of Obstetricians and Gyneacologist*, London 1977, Royal College of Obstetricians and Gynaecologists, 27 Sussex Place, Regent's Park, London NW1 4RG, p 231-242.
12. Arcilla RA, Thilenius OG and Ranniger K: Congestive heart failure from suspected ductal closure in utero. *J Pediatr* 75, 74-78 (1969).
13. Bowes W: Discussion contribution. In: *Pre-term Labour, Proceedings of the Fifth Study Group of the Royal College of Obstetricians and Gynaecologists*, London 1977, Royal College of Obstetricians and Gynaecologists, 27 Sussex Place, Regent's Park, London NW1 4RG, p 257.
14. Levin DL, Fixler, DE, Morriss FC and Tyson J: Morphologic analysis of the pulmonary vascular bed in infants exposed in utero to prostaglandin synthetase inhibitors. *J Pediatr* 92, 478-483 (1978).
15. Manchester D, Margolis HS and Sheldon RS: Possible association between maternal indomethacin therapy and primary pulmonary hypertension of the newborn. *Am J Obstet Gynecol* 126, 467-469 (1975).
16. Gamissans O, Canas E, Cararach V, Ribas J. Puerto B and Edo A: A study of indomethacin combined with ritodrine in threatened preterm labor. *Eur J Obstet Gynecol Reprod Biol* 1, 123-128 (1978).
17. Lynd PA, Andreasen AC and Wyatt RJ: Intrauterine salicylate intoxication in a newborn. *Clin Pediatr* 15, 912-913 (1976).

THE MANAGEMENT OF THE UNRIPE CERVIX

ANDREW A. CALDER

Amid the intense interest that has recently been focussed on the control of human parturition, the importance of the uterine cervix may have been underestimated. The contractility of the myometrium of the upper uterine segment has been the subject of extensive study and important advances have been made towards defining the factors which control it. It may be as important, however, to study the behaviour of the cervix.

The pattern of rapid change in the cervix during normal labour is well known and knowledge of this pattern is fundamental to good clinical care, but while the cervix may be thought of as the uterine sphincter, closed throughout pregnancy and opening during labour, such a notion may be a misleading oversimplification. It is now well recognised that important changes occur in the structure and function of the cervix as pregnancy progresses and before labour begins. These changes have become known as "cervical ripening" and study of this phenomenon may shed valuable light on the physiological transition from pregnancy to parturition.

Failure of cervical ripening is a complication commonly seen by the clinician especially in the primigravida. This article discusses the reasons for this and the clinical problems which may result, and considers a number of therapeutic options in the management of such cases.

MEASUREMENT OF CERVICAL RIPENESS

Meaningful study and discussion of this subject must depend on definition of what is meant by cervical ripening and on our ability to measure it. Ripening consists of a change in the shape and consistency of the cervix: it becomes shorter (effaces) and begins to dilate while the tissue itself softens and becomes more compliant. This is usually accompanied by some descent in the pelvis of the fetal presenting part.

Assessment of these features depends on clinical vaginal examination and is of necessity very subjective. To try to overcome this difficulty a number of authors (1, 2, 3) have devised scoring systems which quantify cervical

M.J.N.C. Keirse et al. (eds.), Human Parturition, 201-217.

ripeness, the most widely used of which is the "pelvic score" described by Bishop in 1964 (1), which also takes into account the position of the cervix (table 1). The range of possible scores is 0 to 13 as the degree of ripeness increases. Because of some difficulties in assessing the "pelvic score" we have employed a minor modification (table 2) of Bishop's system (4). This "cervical score" has a range of 0 to 12. Such systems of measuring cervical ripeness are essential if meaningful data are to be obtained, but they suffer from a large observer error. Their value is therefore enhanced if the number of observers can be minimised.

Table 1. Pelvic scoring system devised by Bishop, 1964 (1).

	0	1	2	3
Dilatation (cm)	0	1-2	3-4	5-6
Effacement (percent)	0-30	40-50	60-70	80
Consistency	firm	average	soft	—
Position	posterior	mid	anterior	—
Level	0-3	0-2	0-1;0	+

Table 2. Modification of the Bishop system used to assess cervical ripeness (Calder et al. 1974 [4].)

	0	1	2	3
Dilatation (cm)	less than 1	1-2	2-4	more than 4
Length (cm)	more than 4	2-4	1-2	less than 1
Consistency	firm	average	soft	—
Position	posterior	mid-anterior	—	—
Level	0-3	0-2	0-1;0	+

PHYSIOLOGY OF CERVICAL RIPENING

The nature of the process of cervical ripening and the factors which may control it will now be considered. The central features of current knowledge and theory are illustrated in figure 1.

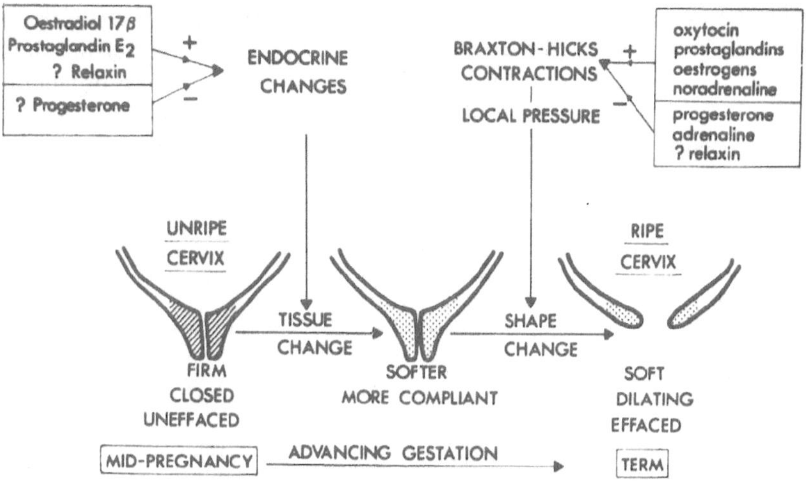

Fig. 1. Schematic representation of the factors which may control cervical ripening. (It should be noted that the tissue change and the shape change probably occur concurrently.)

Shape change

The most obvious aspect of ripening is the change in shape of the cervix. In the primigravida at mid-pregnancy it is long and closed while at term it is usually partially effaced and able to admit at least one finger. Anderson and Turnbull

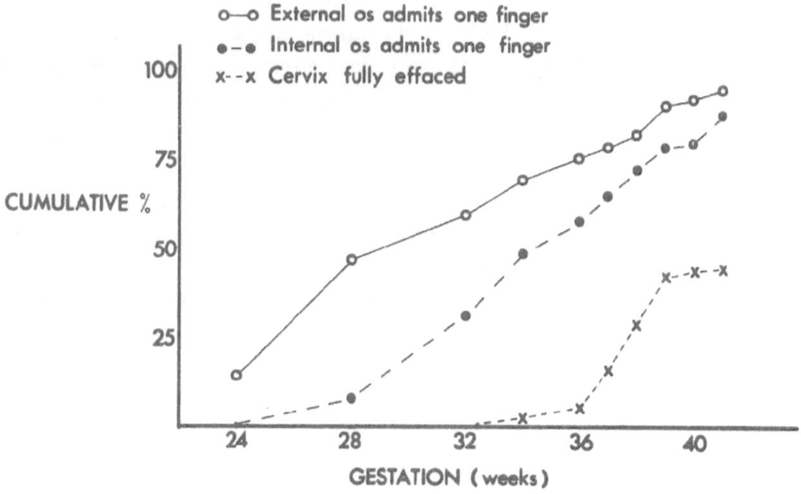

Fig. 2. Pattern of change in shape of the cervix in 90 primigravidae during the latter half of pregnancy. (Drawn from data of Anderson and Turnbull, 1969 [5].)

(5) have shown that this is a gradual process occurring mainly during the third trimester of pregnancy (fig. 2); they also demonstrated a close relationship between the development of these changes and the time of onset of labour (table 3) and found that in about 5 percent of primigravidae this shape change had not occurred by term. Similar findings were reported by Hendricks et al. (6).

Table 3. Cervical findings in primigravidae at 32 weeks gestation in relation to the time of onset of spontaneous labour (From Anderson and Turnbull, 1969 [5].)

Onset of labour	External os admits 1 finger	Internal os admits 1 finger
Before 38 weeks	100%	100%
38-39 weeks	70%	55%
40-41 weeks	55%	20%
41 weeks or later	40%	10%

Changes in the physical properties of cervical tissue

The cervix of the non-pregnant subject is firm and rigid; instrumental dilatation requires force and may result in injury. In pregnancy, especially the latter half of pregnancy, the cervix usually becomes increasingly soft and compliant.

This altered physical condition of the cervix is essential for a normal pattern of dilatation during labour. The shape change during ripening is thus simply a prelude to that which occurs during active labour and probably results from a combination of the gradual increase in uterine contractility (Braxton-Hicks contractions) during the pre-labour phase in the last few weeks of pregnancy and the direct pressure stimulus from the fetal presenting part.

It is now well established (7, 8, 9) that the increased compliance of the cervix in late pregnancy is mainly a result of changes in the nature of the collagen which is the predominant tissue component of the cervix. Detailed animal and human studies point to alterations in the binding arrangements between collagen fibres due to changes in the glycosaminoglycans and glycoproteins in the ground substance; there may also be some absolute breakdown of collagen under the influence of collagenase. These changes reduce the tensile strength of the tissue.

Endocrine changes

The build-up in uterine contractility during pre-labour (10) in the last few weeks of pregnancy may be partly responsible for cervical ripening but this is also a time in which there are changes in the endocrine activity within the uterus. These hormonal changes are very complex and not yet fully defined. It seems likely, however, that as well as influencing uterine contractility, the changing hormonal patterns may have direct effects on the collagen of the cervix and on collagenase activity.

The hormonal control of uterine contractility is discussed elsewhere in this book and will not be considered in great detail here. The evidence for direct hormonal effects on the cervix is fragmentary but in addition to the clinical effects of hormone treatment described later, a number of important observations have been reported.

Oestradiol 17β rises steadily in the peripheral circulation during the last six weeks of pregnancy (11) when cervical ripening is normally occurring. In contrast the very low levels of oestrogens found in pregnancies complicated by placental sulphatase deficiency may be associated with prolongation of pregnancy and failure of the cervix to ripen (12). Oestradiol 17β is known to modify the collagen of skin (13) and Leppi and Kinnison (14) using histochemical and electron microscopic techniques have demonstrated loosening and scattering of the collagen fibrils in the cervix of mice treated with oestradiol. In women, infusion of large doses of oestradiol 17β in late pregnancy has been claimed to produce clinical evidence of cervical softening (15).

Prostaglandins may also have a direct effect on the cervix. Conrad and Euland (16) studied the stretch modulus of human cervical tissue *in vitro* and showed that this could be reduced by addition of PGE_2 to the bathing solution. Fitzpatrick (17) has described softening and dilatation of the pregnant sheep cervix in response to direct intra-arterial infusion of $PGF_{2}\alpha$. We have measured both E and F prostaglandin levels in amniotic fluid obtained at the time of amniotomy from patients with varying cervical scores and found significantly higher levels in association with a ripe cervix (fig. 3).

The importance of seminal prostaglandins is uncertain although Anderson and Turnbull (5) found no association between the pattern of cervical ripening and the reported frequency of coitus during pregnancy. PG inhibiting analgesic agents are known to prolong human pregnancy and labour (18). They may interfere with normal cervical ripening, and habitual ingestion of, for example, salicylates during pregnancy (19) may perhaps explain some cases of unripe cervix at term.

The role of relaxin in human pregnancy remains obscure. It has long been

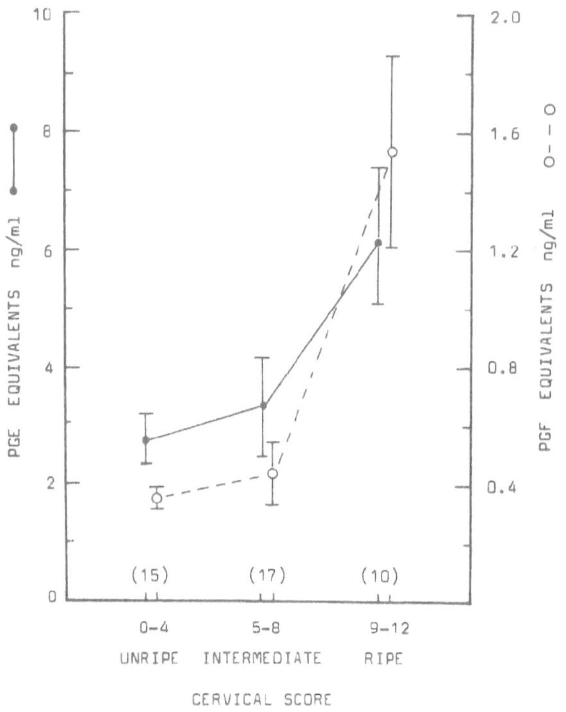

Fig. 3. Concentrations of E and F prostaglandins measured by specific radioimmunoassays in amniotic fluid obtained at the time of amniotomy in 42 primigravidae undergoing induction of labour at term and related to the ripeness of the cervix (Calder, Hillier, Anderson and Dilley, unpublished observations, 1975).

thought responsible for the increased mobility in pregnancy of joints such as the sacro-iliac joints and the pubic symphysis, perhaps by an effect on the connective tissue. Leppi and Kinnison (14) in addition to their observations with oestradiol in the mouse cervix, found a similar loosening and scattering effect on cervical collagen fibrils in response to administration of relaxin.

Progesterone has been shown in tissue culture (20) to inhibit collagenase activity in the uterus and a similar observation has recently been made in a culture of human cervical tissue (21). The uncertain role of progesterone in late human pregnancy, however, makes these observations difficult to interpret.

Relationship of cervical ripening to the onset of labour

Mention has already been made of the association shown by Anderson and

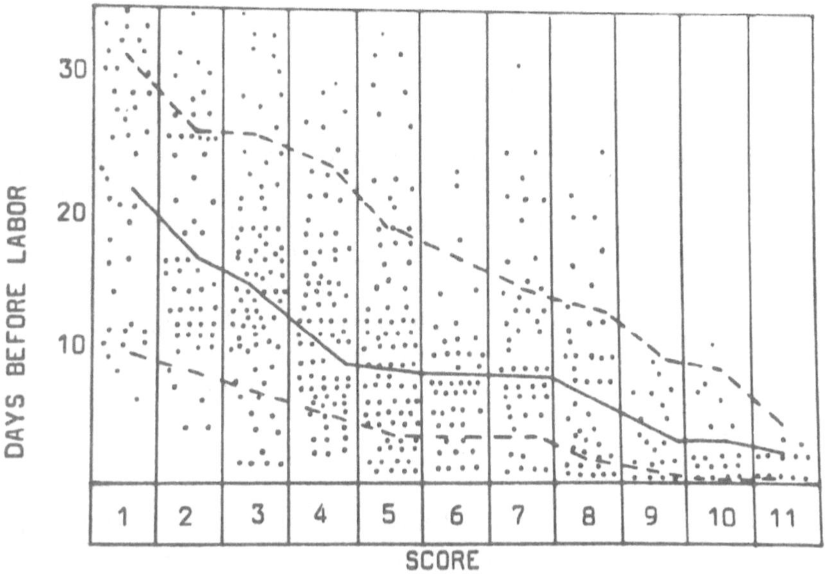

Fig. 4. Relation of the degree of cervical ripeness as measured by the pelvic score and the interval to spontaneous onset of labour. The solid line represents the mean and the dotted lines 80 percent confidence limits. (From Bishop, 1964 [1].)

Turnbull between the cervical shape change and the time of onset of labour (table 3). A similar relationship between all the elements of cervical ripening and the start of labour is seen in Bishop's original study (1) illustrated in figure 4. Pelvic scores assessed in late pregnancy are plotted against the interval until the spontaneous onset of labour and it can be seen that if the score was high (the cervix ripe) labour was imminent whereas the opposite was generally found if the score was low.

A normal pattern of cervical ripening, then, would seem to depend on a basic change in the compliance of the cervix being exploited by efficient Braxton-Hicks contractions, and this may be fairly assumed to be an integral part of the transition from pregnancy to labour. Indeed, the gradual nature of the process accords with the gradual evolution of uterine contractility which culminates in clinical labour (22). In physiological terms there is no definable moment for the onset of labour because the uterus is never entirely dormant. The patient with an unripe cervix at term represents an important departure from normality because of defects in the function of the uterus or the cervix or both. She requires to be identified and specially managed if she is to escape important perinatal complications.

CLINICAL PROBLEMS OF THE UNRIPE CERVIX

If the cervix is found to be unripe in late pregnancy it may be assumed that labour is not imminent (1, 5). The obstetrician's first response to this should be to re-examine the evidence of gestational age since the patient may simply have incorrect dates and be at an earlier point in a normal ripening pattern. This is rare in our experience and it should be remembered that the ripening process occupies most of the last trimester so that by 36 weeks the cervix is usually fairly ripe.

However, an unripe cervix cannot be regarded as indicating prematurity any more than a ripe one is definite evidence of maturity, and where there is doubt the maturity should be assessed by radiology or amniotic fluid analysis.

Response to induction of labour

The observation which has focussed most attention on the unripe cervix has been the poor results of conventional methods of labour induction. In former years when the methods available were less efficient, the likely outcome was complete failure (23, 24, 25). So long as the method did not include amniotomy no great harm resulted other than disappointment for the patient and loss of face by her attendants. If the membranes were ruptured, however, the Rubicon had been crossed and unless delivery was achieved within a very few days the dangers of intrauterine sepsis called for delivery by Caesarean section (26, 27).

The combination of amniotomy with a more rational use of oxytocin (Turnbull, this volume) has in recent years brought far greater reliability to induction of labour and is now the routine method in most clinical departments; but the problem of the unripe cervix has not been overcome.

We have studied prospectively 125 consecutive inductions by this method in term primigravidae covering the spectrum of cervical ripeness (28). In table 4 the results of those 31 patients with a cervical score of 3 or less (*i.e.* an unripe cervix) are compared with those 94 whose score was 4 or greater. As might be expected labour was significantly prolonged if the cervix was unripe, but the most striking finding was the high rate of complications in this group. The rates of maternal pyrexia and caesarean section were at least ten times greater and the incidence of birth asphyxia five times greater in this group. Of the ten patients who required caesarean section in the unripe group, seven followed a very similar pattern: in spite of seemingly adequate uterine contractility the cervix never became properly effaced and failed to dilate beyond 4 cms. Caesarean section was performed in these cases after 18 to 28 hours for what

Table 4. Influence of cervical score on the outcome of labour induced by amniotomy and intravenous oxytocin infusion.

	cervical score	
	0-3	4-11
Number of patients	31	94
Induction – delivery interval in hours (mean ± S.D.)	14.9 ± 5.5	8.2 ± 2.9
Caesarean section (%)	10 (32 %)	3 (3.2 %)
Maternal pyrexia* (%)	10 (32 %)	2 (2.1 %)
Birth asphyxia* (%)	7 (23 %)	4 (4.3 %)

* maternal pyrexia is defined as a temperature greater than 38 °C occurring during labour, and birth asphyxia as a 1 minute Apgar score of 4 or less.

was described as "failure to progress in labour". By this time most of the mothers were pyrexial and there was commonly a fetal tachycardia.

This study demonstrated that amniotomy and intravenous oxytocin therapy is associated with an unacceptable level of complications in primigravidae with an unripe cervix. A simple guideline would seem to be: if amniotomy is physically difficult to perform because of the state of the cervix it may be better to reconsider performing it.

Alternative lines of management

If conventional methods of labour induction are unsuitable what clinical options are available? Many clinicians consider that the appropriate management is to defer delivery until cervical ripening occurs. Clearly this would seem sensible if the indications for delivery are not unduly pressing but in practice we have found such an approach disappointing. Firstly, from Bishop's original data (fig. 4) it appears that a wait of several weeks may be required, introducing the dangers of prolonged pregnancy. We have seen cases of typical postmature stillbirths occurring with the cervix still unripe at 42 weeks' gestation or later. In any case it may be wrong to expect that the cervix *will* eventually ripen normally. As has been suggested earlier in this chapter the unripe cervix may be the result of a basic biological abnormality in the behaviour of the uterus and waiting may not cure it. This view is supported by the observation (29, 30) that abnormal uterine action is commoner in pregnancies which continue beyond term. The same defect may be responsible for failure of ripening, prolongation of pregnancy and unsatisfactory labour.

In the light of the poor results of induced labour some might favour delivery by elective Caesarean section. Clearly this would be wise if placental function appeared to be impaired but if the fetus is healthy and well grown, delivery by elective Caesarean section because of an unripe cervix is unduly radical.

In our study the unripe cervix group contained a very large part of the total morbidity of induced labour but an unripe cervix was not an invariable index of a poor outcome. More than half such patients responded well to the method with good labours and normal delivery of healthy babies. Caesarean section is not yet so safe that it may be employed without good reason.

Other methods of labour induction

Amniotomy and intravenous oxytocin infusion works well if the cervix is ripe. It seems likely that the endocrine conditions which are associated with ripening of the cervix also make the uterus sensitive to oxytocin. As indicated

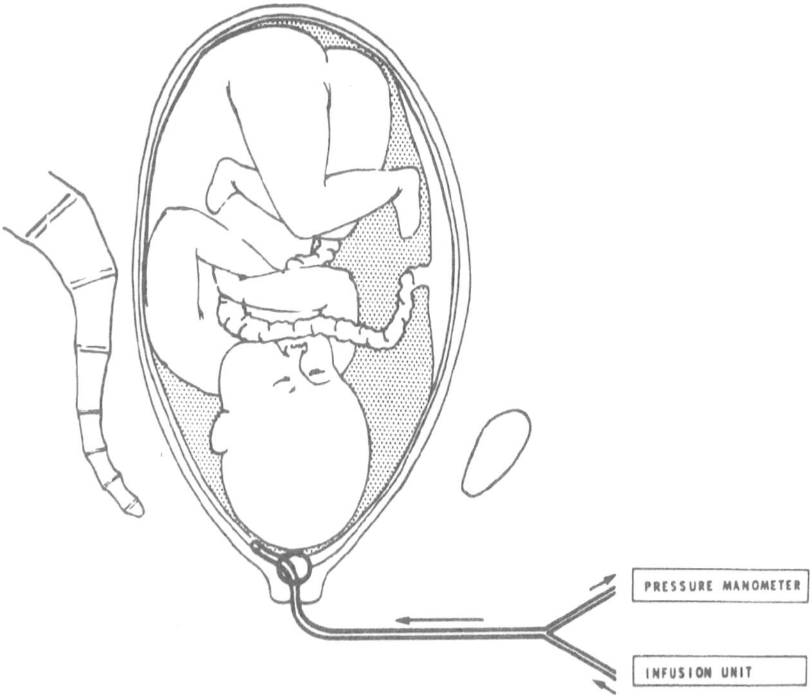

Fig. 5. Drug administration into the extra amniotic space by means of a transcervical Foley catheter.

earlier (fig. 3) prostaglandins may be deficient where the cervix is unripe and their use may be logical for such cases. Unfortunately, if systemic routes (oral, intravenous) of prostaglandin administration are employed, much may be metabolised before reaching the target organ. The higher doses required to induce labour where the cervix is unripe, especially without amniotomy, cause such troublesome side effects as to preclude their use for this purpose (31). In association with amniotomy, oral prostaglandins are really only suitable if the cervix is ripe (32) and intravenous prostaglandins show little advantage over intravenous oxytocin (33).

The route of choice for prostaglandin administration to induce labour if the cervix is unripe is by continuous infusion of a dilute solution into the extra-amniotic space (34) via a Foley or a plain catheter (fig. 5). A dose rate of 0.5 μg to 3.0 μg per minute PGE_2 of a solution containing 5 or 10 μg/ml has been found to be safe and a number of studies have confirmed the efficacy of this technique (4, 35, 36). Although this method gives much better results than amniotomy and intravenous oxytocin, it has been superseded in our practice by techniques of ripening the cervix before induction and will not be discussed further here.

THERAPY TO RIPEN THE CERVIX BEFORE INDUCTION OF LABOUR

Because the results of induction of labour are so good if the cervix is ripe at the outset, the objective where the cervix is found to be unripe should be to make it ripe in the hope that induction of labour may be successful. In the past a number of techniques have been tried.

It has long been the practice in many units to give a prolonged intravenous infusion of oxytocin, sometimes over several days, to ripen the cervix. This is endocrinologically unsound and is of little value in practice (37). The uterus with an unripe cervix behaves like a preterm uterus and is relatively insensitive to oxytocin; in any event, simply making the uterus contract is unlikely to ripen the cervix.

Oral prostaglandins have been tried to the same end but the results have been disappointing (38, 39). The rate of metabolic breakdown in the circulation appears to be too great to allow systemically administered prostaglandins to be effective but in the coming years more specific PG analogues which resist degradation may be found to be valuable for this purpose.

Another approach has been to introduce a Foley catheter through the cervix and inflate the balloon to lie just at the internal cervical os. Although it might take as long as several days, Embrey (40) found this an effective method of cervical ripening. It is still employed routinely in some departments.

Local prostaglandin gel therapy

During experience with extra-amniotic infusion of prostaglandin solution for induction of labour, it was noticed that when a Foley catheter was employed, uterine contractions began soon after the start of infusion and continued until the catheter was expelled from the cervix which was then at least 3 cm dilated. If amniotomy was performed soon after this labour generally progressed, but if not, the contractions tended to abate.

As a result of this experience a technique was developed (41) which is now our established clinical practice in the management of the unripe cervix. Prostaglandin therapy is given to ripen the cervix on the day before induction of labour. A single dose of 400 μg PGE_2 ("Prostin E_2"; Upjohn) is suspended in 5 ml 5 percent methyl hydroxyethyl cellulose ("Tylose" MH 300; Hoechst) and delivered via a trascervical Foley catheter (20 ml balloon) into the extra-amniotic space (fig. 5). The patients generally experience mild uterine contractions or backache for 3 to 6 h after which the catheter is extruded via the cervix which is now 3-4 cm dilated and beginning to efface. Thereafter the contractions generally wear off although in a proportion of patients they continue into established labour; the majority are able to enjoy a good night's sleep before coming fresh to induction of labour the following morning with a ripe cervix.

Our initial study concerned 106 primigravidae with cervical scores of 3 or less (mean 2.3). Their selection criteria were otherwise identical to the primigravidae in the study of induction of labour by amniotomy and intravenous oxytocin described in table 4 i.e. they were all greater than 152 cm in height with a cephalic presenting fetus at 38 to 42 weeks' gestation.

The morning after treatment 21 patients had either already delivered or become well established in labour. The mean cervical score of the remainder had improved to 6.3, an increase of 4.0. These patients then had labour induced by amniotomy and intravenous oxytocin therapy. The results are shown in table 5 and compared with those of the 31 comparable patients in the earlier study where no ripening therapy was given. As might be expected the labours were shorter but the most striking feature was the reduction in the rates of Caesarean section, maternal pyrexia and birth asphyxia. All patients in both studies had full continuous electronic monotoring of labour and fetal wellbeing throughout.

The technique has proved to be safe, highly effective and well accepted by the patients. In a large experience in several centres (42-45) there have been no reports of serious maternal or fetal complications. Some clinicians have expressed reluctance to apply the technique because of worries about in-

Table 5. Results of cervical ripening with PGE_2 in viscous gel prior to induction of labour by amniotomy and intravenous oxytocin infusion.

	Pre-treatment with PGE_2 in viscous gel	Control patients (no pre-treatment)
Number of patients	106	31
Induction – delivery interval in hours (mean ± S.D.)	11.1 ± 4.8	14.9 ± 5.5
Caesarean section rate	9 %	32 %
Maternal pyrexia rate (< 38 °C)	4 %	32 %
Birth asphyxia rate (1 minute Apgar score 4 or less)	6 %	23 %

troducing infection to the uterus but this has not been seen in practice. The one important contraindication to PG gel therapy is the rare occurrence of bleeding at the time of catheter insertion. Experience with PG induced abortions in the second trimester has shown that when this occurs PG administration may be followed by uterine hyperstimulation probably because of rapid absorption of PG into the circulation. It is therefore considered unwise to give bolus PG therapy in the event of bleeding at catheter insertion in term pregnant subjects.

Recently MacKenzie and Embrey (46) have described a greatly simplified technique of PG gel therapy for cervical ripening. Using a very much larger dose of PGE_2 (2.0 mg or 5.0 mg) in a different gel (2 or 4 percent sodium carboxymethyl cellulose) simply given high into the posterior vaginal fornix 16 to 18 h before induction of labour, they achieved results in 168 primigravidae which were largely similar to those obtained with the intrauterine (extra-amniotic) route. The mean length of induced labour was 10.5 h and the rates of Caesarean section and birth asphyxia were 12.4 percent and 8.9 percent respectively. They reported no serious fetal or maternal complications or side effects.

This represents a considerable improvement over the extra-amniotic technique especially because of its simplicity for both the patient and the obstetrician. The absorption of prostaglandins from the vagina has generally been thought to be systemic with no local vascular route to the uterus, and in the past, vaginal therapy has appeared to have no obvious benefit over and similar side effects to other systemic routes (31). The impressive results in this series may then be the result of direct PG absorption by the cervix or of the nature and speed of vaginal absorption from the gel formulation used. Without the need for an intrauterine catheter the potential problems of bleeding, infection and accidental membrane rupture are also avoided.

Local oestradiol gel therapy

As an alternative to prostaglandin gel therapy the use of oestradiol in gel has been investigated and shown to have benefit for cervical ripening (47). In a small series of 25 primigravidae extra-amniotic administration with a Foley catheter of a large dose (150 mg) of oestradiol valerate in 6 ml 5 percent Tylose was compared with a matched control group of 25 primigravidae who had identical treatment but for omission of oestradiol from the gel. Both groups showed cervical changes but these were more marked in the treatment group and the morbidity following induction of labour was reduced in this group (table 6). There were no side effects of the treatment. Only one patient in each group went into labour before induction and the lack of uterine contractility was the only obvious difference from PG gel therapy. This has potential advantages in the management of very high risk cases or in the event of bleeding at catheter insertion. It might also be suitable for outpatient treatment.

Table 6. Results of cervical ripening with oestradiol prior to induction of labour: comparison between treatment and control groups.

	Pre-treatment with oestradiol in viscous gel	Pre-treatment with viscous gel alone
Number of patients	25	25
Mean improvement in cervical score (± S.D.)	3.2 ± 0.9	1.1 ± 0.6
Induction – delivery interval in hours (mean ± S.D.)	10.5 ± 3.6	14.3 ± 3.9
Caesarean section rate	12 %	28 %
Maternal pyrexia rate (> 37.5 °C)	0 %	20 %
Birth asphyxia rate (1 minute Apgar score of 4 or less)	0 %	12 %

CONCLUSIONS

Our understanding of the normal process of cervical ripening is far from complete. Much more basic research is required both in women and in laboratory animals to elucidate the factors controlling cervical function. The cellular biochemistry of the cervix and the behaviour of collagen must be studied in depth if we are to understand the role of the cervix in normal and abnormal pregnancy and labour. The different roles of prostaglandins and steroids and their inter-relationships need to be defined; the importance of relaxin in the human remains largely unexplored; the action of one agent may be mediated by other agents or they may have independent but complementary roles.

For the meantime an unripe cervix must be recognised to be biologically abnormal. The associated obstetric risk must be appreciated and steps taken to minimise them. The techniques at present available for cervical ripening are not capable of restoring complete biological normality but they do improve the prospects of a normal outcome to induction of labour.

It is to be hoped that they will soon seem rather crude as more effective prostaglandins or other compounds and more sophisticated delivery and releasing systems are developed. The existing methods entail effort and inconvenience for both the patient and the clinician but to ignore the unripe cervix is to invite unnecessary fetal and maternal morbidity.

Our ultimate objective must be a full understanding of the physiology of parturition including the process of cervical ripening. Without this and without the ability to reproduce it clinically if required, we must expect to fall short of optimal care for mother and child.

REFERENCES

1. Bishop EH: Pelvic scoring for elective induction. *Obstet Gynecol* 24, 266-268 (1964).
2. Embrey MP: The effects of intravenous oxytocin on uterine contractility. *J Obstet Gynaecol Br Commonw* 69, 910-917 (1962).
3. Friedman EA, Niswander KR, Bayonet-Rivera NP and Sachtleben MR: Relation of prelabor evaluation to inducibility and the course of labour. *Obstet Gynecol* 28, 495-501 (1966).
4. Calder AA, Embrey MP and Hillier K: Extra-amniotic prostaglandin E_2 for the induction of labour at term. *J Obstet Gynaecol Br Commonw* 81, 39-46 (1974).
5. Anderson ABM and Turnbull AC: Relationship between length of gestation and cervical dilatation, uterine contractility and other factors during pregnancy. *Am J Obstet Gynecol* 105, 1207-1214 (1969).
6. Hendricks CH, Bremner WE and Kraus G: Normal cervical dilatation pattern in late pregnancy and labor. *Am J Obstet Gynecol* 106, 1065.82 (1970).
7. Bryant WM, Greenwell JE and Weeks PM: Alterations in collagen organisation during dilatation of the cervix-uteri. *Surg Gynecol Obstet* 126, 27-39 (1968).
8. Danforth DN, Veis A, Breen M, Weinstein HG, Buckingham J and Manalo P: The effect of pregnancy and labor on the human cervix: changes in collagen, glycoproteins and glycosaminoglycans. *Am J Obstet Gynecol* 120, 641-651 (1974).
9. Kleissl HP, Vander Rest M, Naftolin F, Glorieux FH, Deleon A: Collagen changes in the human uterine cervix at parturition. *Am J Obstet Gynecol* 130, 748-753 (1978).
10. Caldeyro-Barcia R: Uterine contractility in obstetrics. *Proceedings of the Second International Congress of Gynecology and Obstetrics*, vol 1, Montreal, 1958, p 65.
11. Turnbull AC, Patten PT, Flint APF, Keirse MJNC, Jeremy JY and Anderson ABM: Significant fall in progesterone and rise in oestradiol levels in human peripheral plasma before onset of labour. *Lancet* 1, 101-104 (1974).

12. France JT, Seddon RJ and Liggins GC: A study of a pregnancy with low oestrogen production due to placental sulphatase deficiency. *J Clin Endocrinol Metab* 36, 1-9 (1973).
13. Henneman DH: Effects of estrogen and growth hormone on collagen. In: *Endocrinology*, New York, Elsevier, 1973, p 1109.
14. Leppi JT and Kinnison PA: The connective tissue ground substance in the mouse uterine cervix. *Anat Rec* 170, 97-117 (1971).
15. Pinto RM, Fisch L, Schwarz RL and Montuori E: Action of estradiol 17β upon contractility and the milk-ejecting effect in the pregnant woman. *Am J Obstet Gynecol* 90, 99-107 (1964).
16. Conrad JT and Euland K: Reduction of the stretch modulus of human cervical tissue by prostaglandin E_2. *Am J Obstet Gynecol* 126, 218-223 (1976).
17. Fitzpatrick RJ: Effects of prostaglandin $F_{2\alpha}$ on the cervix of the pregnant sheep. In: *The Fetus and Birth*, Ciba Foundation Symposium no. 47, Amsterdam, Elsevier/Excerpta Medica/North-Holland, 1977, p 33-39.
18. Lewis RB and Schulman JD: Influence of acetylsalicylic acid an inhibitor of prostaglandin synthesis on duration of human gestation and labour. *Lancet* 2, 1159-1161 (1973).
19. Collins E and Turner G: Maternal effects of regular salicylate ingestion in pregnancy. *Lancet* 2, 335-338 (1975).
20. Jeffrey JJ, Coffey RJ and Eizen AZ: Studies of uterine collagenase in tissue culture II: Effect of steroid hormones on enzyme production. *Biochim Biophys Acta* 252, 143-149 (1971).
21. Hillier K: Biochemical changes in the cervix in parturition. Presented to the Blair Bell Research Society, Southampton, September 1977.
22. Wood C: Myometrial and tubal physiology. In: *Human Reproductive Physiology*, Oxford, Blackwell, 1972, p 350.
23. Garrett WJ: Prognostic signs in surgical induction of labour. *Med J Aust* 1, 929-931 (1960).
24. Embrey MP: Induction of labour. In: *The Management of Labour*, London, Royal College of Obstetricians and Gynaecologists, 1975, p 62.
25. Turnbull AC and Anderson ABM: Induction of labour. Part I: Amniotomy. *J Obstet Gynaecol Br Commonw* 74, 849-854 (1967).
26. MaCallum MF and Govan ADT: The bacteriology of surgical induction of labour. *J Obstet Gynaecol Br Commonw* 70, 244-250 (1963).
27. MacVicar J: Failed induction of labour. *J. Obstet Gynaecol Br Commonw* 78, 1007-1009 (1971).
28. Calder AA: The Unripe Cervix. *57th William Blair Bell Memorial Lecture*. Royal College of Obstetricians and Gynaecologists, London. June 1977.
29. Clayton SG: Foetal mortality in postmaturity. *J Obstet Gynaecol Br Emp* 48, 450-460 (1941).
30. Stewart DB and Bernard RM: A clinical classification of difficult labour and some examples of its use. *J Obstet Gynaecol Br Emp* 61, 318-328 (1954).
31. Embrey MP: *The Prostaglandins in Human Reproduction*, Edinburgh, Churchill-Livingstone, 1975, p 48.
32. Leading Article: Prostaglandins and the uterus. *Lancet* 2, 829-830 (1973).
33. Calder AA and Embrey MP: Comparison of intravenous oxytocin and prostaglandin E_2 for induction of labour using automatic and non-automatic techniques. *Br J Obstet Gynaecol* 82, 728-733 (1975).
34. Calder AA and Embrey MP: Prostaglandins and the unfavourable cervix. *Lancet* 2, 1322-1323 (1973).
35. Miller AWF and Mack DS: Induction of labour by extra-amniotic prostaglandins. *J Obstet Gynaecol Br Commonw* 81, 706-708 (1974).
36. Neuberg R: The uninducible cervix. Induction of labour using extra-amniotic prostaglandin E_2. *Int J Gynaecol Obstet* 13, 171-173 (1975).
37. Lillienthal CM and Ward JP: Medical induction of labour. *J Obstet Gynaecol Br Commonw* 78, 317-321 (1971).
38. Friedman EA and Sachtleben MR: Preinduction priming with oral prostaglandin E_2. *Am J Obstet Gynecol* 121, 521-523 (1975).

39. Weiss RR, Tejani N, Israeli I, Evans MI, Bhakthavathsalan A and Mann LI: Priming of the uterine cervix with oral prostaglandin E_2 in the term multigravida. *Obstet Gynecol* 46, 181-184 (1975).
40. Embrey MP and Mollison BG: The unfavourable cervix and induction of labour using a cervical balloon. *J Obstet Gynaecol Br Commonw* 74 44-48 (1967).
41. Calder AA, Hillier K and Embrey MP: Prostaglandin therapy for cervical ripening prior to induction of labour. In: *Advances in Prostaglandin and Thromboxane Research*, Vol. 2, New York, Raven Press, 1076, p 993.
42. Calder AA, Embrey MP and Tait T: Ripening of the cervix with extra-amniotic prostaglandin E_2 in viscous gel before induction of labour. *Br J Obstet Gynaecol* 84, 264-268 (1977).
43. Shepherd J, Sims C and Craft I: Extra-amniotic prostaglandin E_2 and the unfavourable cervix. *Lancet* 2, 709-710 (1976).
44. Thiery M, Defoort P, Benijts G, Van Eyck J, Hennay T, Van Kets H and Martens G: Effectiveness of extra-ovular injection of prostaglandin E_2 in Tylose gel to ripen the cervix prior to elective induction of labour at term. *Prostaglandins* 14, 381-388 (1977).
45. Thiery M, Defoort P, Benijts G, Derom R, Martens G, Amy JJ, Van Kets H and De Schrijver D: Fetal effects of cervical ripening with extra-amniotic prostaglandin E_2 in gel. *Prostaglandins* 15, 175-186 (1978).
46. MacKenzie IZ and Embrey MP: Cervical ripening with intravaginal PGE_2 gel. *Br Med J* 2, 1381-1384 (1977).
47. Gordon AJ and Calder AA: Oestradiol applied locally to ripen the unfavourable cervix. *Lancet* 2, 1319-1321 (1977).

EPIDEMIOLOGY OF PRE-TERM LABOUR

MARC J.N.C. KEIRSE

For some, interest in the onset of labour stems from a genuine desire to unravel this physiological enigma. For most, it stems from a constant awareness that delivery too early in pregnancy is the most frequently occurring factor in infant death and morbidity. As such this has become the largest single problem in contemporary obstetrics and paediatrics and one of the major public health problems of the present time. Therefore, it is an excellent field for epidemiologists to leap into; epidemiology being concerned mainly with the patterns of disease and their social and environmental ramifications in human populations. Yet, there is a considerable lack of information about the epidemiological aspects of pre-term labour. This is not due to a lack of interest on the part of professional epidemiologists or others, and is in sharp contrast with the number of studies which have or appear to have been devoted to it. Most of these however include apples and oranges – pre-term infants and low-weight babies – all in one single category. It is difficult to assess to what extent they are applicable to the epidemiology of pre-term labour, pre-term birth, intrauterine growth retardation or combinations of those and other factors.

In this paper we shall deal less with epidemiological data as such than with their shortcomings, the reasons for these and their relevance to both public health and clinical practice. Epidemiology is more than an esoteric academic exercise completely divorced from the practical problem at hand. Therefore we shall try to analyze the problems which bedevil this particular field and hopefully indicate some ways in which they may at least to some extent be solved.

DEFINING THE PROBLEM

One of the first requirements to solve a problem is to clearly define it or at least to attempt to do so. Judging by this characteristic pre-term labour appears to be an overwhelming problem for neither pre-term nor labour can be fully defined at present.

M.J.N.C. Keirse et al. (eds.), Human Parturition, 219-234.

Pre-term

Firstly there has been world-wide confusion in terminology. In 1950 the World Health Organization (WHO) recommended the term prematurity to denote infants born with a birthweight of 2500 g or less (1). This recommendation was based upon the constructive thought that birthweight, being relatively easy to measure, could be made readily available for every baby born. However, it ignored the fact that 40 percent of these infants are not born too early but too small (2,3). It also gave official backing to those who persuaded mothers, who gave birth to an unexpectedly small infant, at least to their own satisfaction, that she was wrong about her "dates" thereby invalidating any later analysis of gestational ages. By 1961 it was recognized how much trouble was caused by the earlier recommendation and the definitions were altered to denote infants born before 37 completed weeks from the first day of the last menstrual period as premature and infants with a birthweight of 2500 g or less as of low birthweight (4). It is hardly surprising that a new source of confusion arose with prematurity being defined by some workers in terms of birthweight and by others in terms of gestational age. Its impact is illustrated in a recent book entitled *The Epidemiology of Prematurity* the preface of which starts with 'Prematurity is a term used to describe various combinations of being born too early, or too small, or both" (5). The remainder of the book or at least most of it lives up to that expectation, thereby invalidating much of the useful information which it contains. It may be difficult to aggravate a Babylonic confusion initiated at a world-wide level. Authors who do not feel compelled to disclose what their working definition of prematurity is based upon certainly succeed in doing so.

To avoid that confusion wide agreement has been reached that the term prematurity should no longer be used in relation to either birthweight or gestational age (6-8). The current WHO recommendations (6) are that infants delivered before 37 completed weeks (less than 259 completed days) from the first day of the last menstrual period should be classified as pre-term (table 1)

Table 1. Current definitions recommended by WHO and FIGO.

pre-term	less than 37 completed weeks (less than 259 completed days)
term	from 37 completed weeks to less than 42 completed weeks (259 to 293 days)
post-term	42 completed weeks or more (294 days or more)

and infants weighing less than 2500 g as of low birthweight. Although these definitions have also been accepted by the Fédération Internationale de Gynécologie et d'Obstétrique, FIGO (9, 10), there is still little reason for enthusiasm.

Hopes that all confusion has now ended may be thoroughly dashed by a cursory look at the literature. There are at least two reasons for the apparent lack of enthusiasm in applying the new definition. Firstly, although it is now clear how late in pregnancy a baby may be considered pre-term, it remains arbitrary how early in pregnancy a baby may be born to be considered pre-term. Neither WHO nor FIGO have recommended a lower limit of gestation. Individuals are therefore left to choose between the cut-off points used to define perinatal period and birth, both of which are different and based upon weight rather than gestational age (9, 10). If the efforts made by WHO to reach agreement on perinatal definitions (11) prove successful in that national statistics will include all fetuses and infants delivered weighing at least 500 g (or, when birthweight is unavailable the corresponding gestational age (22 weeks) or body length (25 cm crown-heel)) a major advance will have been made. This is still a long way, however, from what was achieved in Norway with the Medical Registration of Births which provides information on all births with a gestational age of 16 weeks or more (12). Secondly although FIGO and WHO define pre-term as less than 37 weeks, at the same time it is recommended that countries provide statistics by gestational age in the following manner: 32 weeks to less than 36 completed weeks, 36 weeks to less than 38 completed weeks, etc. (9, 10). Certainly this must be a tremendous tribute to the guessing power of epidemiologists, who are left to imagine how many of the infants born in the period from 36 weeks to less than 38 completed weeks should be labeled as pre-term.

The deplorable lack of clarity in and support for world-wide definitions raises a further drawback which is often ignored by those who have never, when moving from one country to another or otherwise, been compelled to adopt other working definitions. This drawback is both a nationalist and a linguistic problem. Firstly, several countries including the Netherlands have their own definitions for delivery too early in pregnancy. Secondly, the English language, being particularly suited for international scientific communication is also singularly suited to translate the content but not the meaning of words used in other languages. The best-known example may be that of the American Academy of Fetus and Newborn which recommended that pre-term be delivery at less than 38 completed weeks (less than 266 days). Until recently this cut-off point also applied to the definition of *partus praematurus* in the Netherlands, which adds another 4 to 5 percent of all births to the incidence of so-called prematurity (13). National differences may be far more difficult to discern as illustrated by the study of Vanderslikke and Treffers (14). These Dutch authors studied the influence of induced and spontaneous abortions upon gestational length in subsequent pregnancies. Their conclusion that spontaneous abortions do not influence the length of gestation in subsequent pregnancies (14) appears to be at variance with several other studies (15-18) which demonstrated that spontaneous abortions carry an increased risk of early delivery in subsequent pregnancies. This finding remains unexplained until it is realized that spontaneous abortion is not spontaneous abortion but the translation of what Dutch definitions recognize as being spontaneous abortion. When it is realized that in the Netherlands spontaneous abortions invariably occur under 16 weeks' gestation, pregnancies which end after 16 weeks (112-196 days) being labeled as *partus immaturus* (13), the discrepancy between the Dutch and other data largely disappears. In fact these data then conform to those of a study conducted in the United Kingdom (18) which demonstrated that mainly second trimester (14-27 weeks) abortions but not first trimester (< 14 weeks) abortions increased the likelihood of pre-term delivery in subsequent pregnancies.

Length of gestation

Apart from the confusion in terminology, some reluctance to the use of pre-term is based upon the general unreliability of gestational age. Defining pre-term naturally depends upon the accuracy of determining the length of gestation. From a clinical point of view the use of ultrasound and scoring of gestational age at birth (19, 20) have helped much to solve this problem. On the other hand the widespread use of oral contraception, the largely unconfirmed belief (21) that pre-term deliveries occur more often in women who have received only perfunctory antenatal care, and the finding that some of these women consider antenatal care as largely superfluous (22) again aggravate it. In most women the date of conception is unknown and in a proportion of them also the onset of the last menstrual period is an absolute enigma.

That much of this depends upon the ethnic and cultural background of the population under study is well-known (Kloosterman, this volume). In Western societies however it must be possible to define the length of gestation either prospectively or retrospectively with a high degree of accuracy in at least 80 percent of pregnancies. If 10 to 15 percent of pregnancies have unreliable dates this can be accounted for in any scientific analysis as well as an inter-assay variability of 15 percent can be accounted for in biochemical studies. Furthermore if there is a 2-week error in determining the length of gestation this may be quite serious but it still accounts for a mere 5 percent of the length of gestation at term and 10 percent at 20 weeks. Any biochemist would be happy with an assay which shows an inter-assay variability of just above 5 percent; he certainly would not dream of discarding it. There is error in any scientific study and we should accept this fact rather than to refrain from scientific evaluation. If there are factors, epidemiological or other, which are really involved in pre-term labour they will, as Milton Terris pointed out (23), show up despite the errors.

Labour

If defining pre-term may be difficult, defining labour is an even greater problem. The records of any obstetric department can exemplify this with the incidence of so-called false labour on the one hand and with the number of women who despite adequate antenatal care and attention unexpectedly reach full dilatation and delivery on the other hand.

Since neither the onset of labour nor the mechanism which is responsible for it can be accurately determined, the definition of labour is of necessity more of a practical than of a scientific nature. At term it is usually defined as the development of regular, frequent and strong uterine contractions which lead to progressive dilatation of the cervix and delivery of the baby. When applying the same definition to labour pre-term, the most powerful criteria of progressive cervical dilatation and delivery, become at once the very facts which we try to prevent. Therapeutic measures to achieve this effect jeopardize by their very nature the accuracy of our diagnosis. The difficulties in establishing the effectiveness of these measures as compared to placebo or non-specific forms of treatment (Eskes and Essed, this volume) clearly exemplify it. Some studies have shown that up to 40 percent of women admitted in pre-term labour will, despite the classical signs of the onset of labour, continue their pregnancy for a considerable length of time without any special treatment (Anderson, this volume). Usually the diagnosis of labour is initially a diagnosis made by the patient which is then either accepted or with some difficulty refuted by her attendants. According to O'Driscoll (24), for labour at term there is a 10 percent error in patient diagnosis, whereas the error in diagnosis for pre-term labour lies in the region of 80 percent (24). Although this estimate is likely to be too generous in order to be applicable to all centres it clearly emphasizes the inadequacies of diagnosing pre-term labour.

This may well be the main reason why epidemiological data on pre-term, if at all available, relate to pre-term delivery more than to pre-term labour. From the data discussed above this may appear to be an advantage.

Stillbirth and lethal malformation

When epidemiology is not to be divorced from public health and clinical medicine there are other factors which should be considered. Firstly, fetal death *in utero* will inevitably lead to delivery whether labour occurs spontaneously or is induced (25). In the 1958 British Perinatal Mortality Survey, when the total perinatal mortality was 33 per 1000, less than half of these occurred under 37 weeks (26). With the general decline in perinatal mortality – in the Netherlands from 32.3 per 1000 in 1952 to 13.9 per 1000 in 1975 (27) – and the current more active management of intrauterine death (25) far more than half of the stillbirths now occur under 37 weeks (28-30). Rush et al. (28, 29) demonstrated in two totally different populations that for stillborn infants pre-term delivery is the consequence rather than the cause of fetal death. Hence these cases should be considered separately in epidemiological studies for they relate to the epidemiology of intrauterine death and not to the epidemiology of pre-term labour and delivery. Secondly, infants with lethal congenital deformities should be excluded from or considered separately in such studies for two reasons in particular. The first reason is that delivery as soon as possible can be considered as the most successful outcome of preg-

Table 2. Contribution of stillborn infants and infants with lethal malformations to the incidence and perinatal mortality of pre-term birth. (Data from Rush et al. on Oxford [28] and Cape Town [29] births.)

Type of pre-term birth	Oxford births		Cape Town Births	
	No. of births	No. of deaths	No. of births	No. of deaths
Stillbirth with lethal deformity	14	14	3	3
Stillbirth without lethal deformity	36	36	338	338
Live birth with lethal deformity	7	7	9	9
Live birth without lethal deformity	429	34	1979	187
Total	486	91	2329	537
Number of stillbirths and/or lethal deformities as a percent of the total births	11.7	62.6	15.–	65.2

nancy in these cases and that is what public health or clinical medicine is or should be most concerned about. A second reason can be found in the fact that some of these malformations may lead to pre-term delivery. At least two of these are well-known: anencephaly (Swaab and Boer, this volume) and Potter's syndrome or bilateral renal agenesis (31, 32), though the mechanism by which they lead to early delivery is unknown. Both categories, stillbirths and lethal deformities, now account for more than 10 percent of pre-term deliveries and for more than 60 percent of the perinatal mortality associated with it (table 2).

Live births

Even when only the remainder of pre-term deliveries, i.e. those which result in a live birth without lethal malformations, are studied it is obvious that they do not form a single well-defined category. The data from two studies (28, 29) which have used identical methods in two greatly different populations illustrate this (tables 3 and 4). The tables show the numbers of pregnancies, births and early neonatal deaths related to the reason for pre-term delivery in a predominantly Caucasian population in Oxford (table 3) and in a Coloured population in Cape Town (table 4). The incidence of pre-term delivery in infants born alive without lethal deformity was 4.2 percent in Oxford (28) and 9.5 percent in Cape Town (29). Although the difference in

Table 3. Infants born alive without lethal malformations: Number of births and early neonatal deaths related to type of pre-term delivery. (From Rush et al. [28], data from Oxford.)

Type of pre-term delivery	Pregnancies		No. of live births	First-week deaths		Early neonatal mortality rate (per 1000 live births)
	No.	Percent		No.	Percent	
Spontaneous labour of unknown aetiology	148	38	148	12	35	81.1
Spontaneous labour with maternal and/or fetal pathology	96	24	96	10	29	104.2
Multiple pregnancy	40	10	76	9	27	118.4
Elective delivery (57 caesarean sections and 52 induced labours)	109	28	109	3	9	27.5
Total	393	100	429	34	100	79.3

Table 4. Infants born alive without lethal malformations: number of births and early neonatal deaths related to type of pre-term delivery. (From Rush et al. [29], data from Cape Town.)

Type of pre-term delivery	Pregnancies		No. of live births	First-week deaths		Early neonatal mortality rate (per 1000 live births)
	No.	Percent		No.	Percent	
Spontaneous labour of unknown aetiology	883	47	883	97	52	109.8
Spontaneous labour with maternal and/or fetal pathology	522	28	522	52	28	99.6
Multiple pregnancy	93	5	185	16	8	86.4
Elective delivery (149 caesarean sections and 240 induced labours)	389	20	389	22	12	56.5
Total	1887	100	1979	187	100	94.5

incidence of pre-term delivery testifies to the difference between the two populations studied the conclusions which can be reached are remarkably similar.

Firstly, any epidemiological study on pre-term delivery may for 20 percent or more consist of pregnancies which ended too early because of deliberate intervention by the obstetrician (tables 3 and 4). Any associations found will naturally relate more to other pathology and the reasons for this intervention than to pre-term delivery as such. It is again obvious that pre-term labour is by no means identical to pre-term delivery. If the former does not necessarily lead to delivery, the latter is not necessarily the consequence of pre-term labour.

Secondly both tables show that, even for the simple purpose of studying early neonatal mortality rates of pre-term infants, it is necessary to separate elective deliveries from those which follow the spontaneous onset of labour. In both studies the mortality rate of single infants was significantly lower when pre-term delivery was the result of obstetric intervention. There are several reasons for this difference not in the least the fact that the whole purpose of obstetric intervention is usually aimed at decreasing perinatal mortality. Elective pre-term delivery therefore tends to occur later in pregnancy than spontaneous pre-term labour. Combining these groups may introduce a considerable bias.

That twin pregnancies are at increased risk of pre-term delivery is well-known. In the Oxford study (28) the incidence of pre-term delivery in twin pregnancies was 47.1 percent. In the Cape Town study (29) it was 37 percent and in our department it is 42 percent. Although most epidemiological studies distinguish single pregnancies from multiple pregnancies, even then more than 50 percent of the pregnancies have other maternal or fetal pathology most frequently antepartum haemorrhage, fetal growth retardation and hypertension (28, 29). To the best of our knowledge there are no epidemiological data which pertain especially to the group of spontaneous pre-term labour and delivery without other fetal or maternal pathology, less than half of all pre-term deliveries. This point may not be too serious for it is conceivable that spontaneous pre-term labour associated with e.g. fetal growth retardation or hypertension is distinctly different from term labour with the same pathology. There may however be another bias which cannot be discerned in these (28, 29) or other studies. When pre-term births are used as a starting-point for the study, those of unknown aetiology will more frequently have resulted from failure to arrest pre-term labour than those associated with maternal and/or fetal pathology. In the latter group labour is often a welcome event which will be promoted rather than inhibited. At present one can only speculate to what extent this may influence data currently available.

It would appear however that many studies have to be done over again in order to determine which factors belong to which entity.

NEONATAL MORTALITY AND MORBIDITY

That pre-term delivery is the single most important factor in early neonatal mortality has been recognized for a long time. Virtually all studies show that although pre-term deliveries range from about 5 to just over 8 percent in Western Europe (13, 28, 33-36) and probably remain below 10 percent in most parts of the world (29, 37), they account for well over 50 percent of early neonatal mortality. For instance, at Leiden University Medical Centre all of the 1976 perinatal mortality of 21 per 1000 was accounted for by pre-term deliveries and congenital malformations (30).

Apart from elective delivery, the reason for pre-term delivery appears to have but a limited influence on the early neonatal mortality rate of pre-term infants (tables 3 and 4). Early neonatal death rates however are closely linked to both gestational age and birth weight (tables 5 and 6).

Neonatal morbidity is exceedingly high in pre-term infants who provide reason for the very existence of neonatal care units. The important question however is how much of that morbidity is carried on into later life and whether this differs according to the cause of pre-term birth. Very limited information is available to answer this question, since attention has been

Table 5. Early neonatal (1st week) mortality rate of liveborn pre-term infants without lethal deformity in relation to gestational age. (Data from Rush et al. on Oxford [28] and Cape Town [29] births.)

Gestational age in weeks	Oxford births		Cape Town births	
	No. of births	Mortality rate per 1,000	No. of births	Mortality rate per 1,000
23 - 25	4	1000	9	1000
26 - 27	12	750	35	914
28 - 29	26	346	71	690
30 - 31	23	217	103	388
32 - 33	55	54.5	318	101
34 - 35	139	21.6	621	27.4
36	170	5.9	822	9.7
Total	429	79.3	1979	94.5

Table 6. Early neonatal (1st week) mortality rate of liveborn pre-term infants without lethal deformity in relation to birthweight (Data from Rush et al. on Oxford [28] and Cape Town [29] births).

Birthweight in grams	Oxford births		Cape Town births	
	No. of births	Mortality rate per 1,000	No. of births	Mortality rate per 1,000
<750	7	857	17	1000
750 - 999	8	625	43	814
1000 - 1249	22	364	107	421
1250 - 1499	34	235	154	227
1500 - 1749	29	69	243	78
1750 - 1999	53	57	296	57
2000 - 2249	74	27	305	39
2250 - 2499	84	0	389	10
⩾2500	118	0	425	7
Total	429	79.3	1979	94.5

devoted more to birthweight than to gestational age, although the outcome of infants who are born too soon appears to be slightly better than those who are born too small (38). Several studies have attested to the falling incidences of major handicap to about 10 percent along with falling mortality rates in infants with very low birthweight, most of whom will be pre-term (39-41).

Stewart (41) showed that of 589 infants weighing less than 1500 g at birth and all but six born pre-term (from 24 weeks onwards) 40 percent died within the first 28 days of life. Another 6 percent died before the age of 2 years and 8.5 percent of the remainder were significantly handicapped at their last follow-up assessment after 18 months of age. The latter percentage amounted to 8 and 13 percent for infants weighing respectively 1001-1500 g and 500-1000 g at birth. Of infants with a birthweight over 1000 g who were mechanically ventilated for hyaline membrane disease, a typical hazard of the pre-term infants, and survived between 1970 and 1975, only 7 percent had major handicaps at the age of 18 months or more (41).

EPIDEMIOLOGICAL FACTORS IN SPONTANEOUS PRE-TERM BIRTH

Sociobiological and environmental

Epidemiological studies have indicated that low birthweight and/or pre-term delivery are associated with a variety of sociobiological and environmental variables (42, 43). Most of these studies suffer from the drawback that it is difficult to determine to what extent they relate to pre-term birth, not to mention spontaneous pre-term labour and delivery as compared to obstetric intervention pre-term. Fedrick and Anderson (43) specifically examined several of these factors in a group of women who went into spontaneous labour and were delivered before 37 weeks of an infant which weighed less than 2500 g and showed neither maceration nor major congenital malformations. The risk of spontaneous pre-term birth in that study was shown to be related to low maternal age, low maternal weight rather than height, low social class, illegitimacy and maternal smoking. These data however are based upon the 1958 British Perinatal Mortality Survey and one may wonder whether and to what extent this still applies in 1978, despite the fact that the percentage of deliveries with certain gestational age which occur between 28 and 37 weeks has hardly changed in Britain from 5.3 percent in 1958 to 5.2 percent in 1970 (44). There is little doubt that some of these factors, smoking in particular (45), relate to a shorter length of gestation but the quantitative importance and the nature of such relationships remain to be determined.

Reproductive history

In multigravidae spontaneous pre-term birth was shown to be related to various aspects of their previous obstetric history. High incidences of spontaneous pre-term birth have been found in women with a previous history of perinatal loss, antepartum haemorrhage, spontaneous abortion, induced abortion, low birthweight livebirths and pre-term birth (12, 17, 18, 43).

For some of these factors, particularly induced abortion, the associations are not as clear as they appear to be. Whereas some authors found a positive correlation between induced abortion and subsequent "second trimester spontaneous abortion" and/or spontaneous pre-term delivery (17, 46-48), others have found no such associations in carefully controlled studies (14, 49). The mechanism by which induced abortions would lead to pre-term birth in subsequent pregnancies is open to question, but cervical damage and subsequent cervical incompetence through forceful dilatation are currently the most favoured explanations. Methods and techniques used for terminating pregnancy as well as experience, duration of pregnancy and several other factors may well influence the effect upon gestational length in subsequent pregnancies. At least in the Netherlands there are presently no indications that induced abortions in the first trimester of pregnancy significantly increase the likelihood of spontaneous pre-term labour and delivery in subsequent pregnancies (14).

A history of previous livebirths weighing less than 2500 g increases the likelihood of spontaneous pre-term birth in subsequent pregnancies from 2 to 7-fold depending upon the number of previous <2500 g infants (43). The birth of infants weighing more than 4000 g on the other hand lowered the incidence of pre-term births in subsequent pregnancies (43). Bakketeig (12) showed however that the incidence of pre-term delivery in a second single pregnancy correlates far better with gestational age than with birthweight of the first single birth. Although these data do no separate various causes of pre-term delivery they are based on the analysis of records from 76,938 women for whom birthweight and gestational age were known for both first and second births from 16 weeks of gestation onwards (12). The over-all risk of pre-term delivery in the second pregnancies was 4.9 percent, but this increased to over 20 percent if the birthweight of the first birth was 2500 g or less and the gestational age less than 34 weeks. The relative risk of a subsequent pre-term delivery was 4 times higher for mothers who had previously delivered pre-term compared to those who had not.

In a retrospective analysis of more than 8000 single live births, from which infants with lethal deformities and pre-term deliveries due to obstetric intervention were excluded, pre-term delivery following the spontaneous onset of labour accounted for 3 percent of these births (18). The incidence of pre-term delivery was significantly higher in patients who were gravidae three or more (4 percent) than in the rest of the population (2.6 percent), but in gravidae three or more without a history of early delivery the incidence of pre-term delivery was only 2.3 percent. The incidence of spontaneous pre-term delivery was related to whether they had a history of two or more pregnancies ending spontaneously in the first trimester(< 14 weeks), the second trimester (14-27) or from 28 to less than 37 completed weeks. Table 7 shows that the incidence of spontaneous pre-term delivery, whether or not associated with maternal and/or fetal pathology, is influenced by both the number and the gestational age of previous pregnancies which ended too early. The risk of spontaneous pre-term delivery was highest in patients with previous deliveries between 28 and 37 weeks and lowest in those with only first trimester abortions.

Table 7. Incidence of pre-term delivery in patients with at least two previous pregnancies which ended spontaneously before 37 weeks. (From Keirse et al. [18].)

Previous pregnancies which ended spontaneously before 37 weeks*	No. of patients	Pre-term delivery in present pregnancy	
		No.	Percent
Abortions only, no pre-term births			
2 abortions	244	14	5.7
2 or more abortions	330	27	8.2
3 or more abortions	86	13	15.1
2 or more abortions but			
0 in second trimester	216	8	3.7
1 in second trimester	95	14	14.7
2 or more in second trimester	19	5	26.3
3 or more abortions but			
0 in second trimester	60	4	6.7
1 in second trimester	18	5	27.8
2 or more in second trimester	8	4	50.0
Pre-term births			
1 pre-term birth			
plus 1 or more abortions	30	11	36.7
2 pre-term births	8	5	62.5
2 or more pre-term births	10	7	70.0
All patients	370	45	12.2

* For this study these previous pregnancies were subdivided into spontaneous first trimester abortions (< 14 weeks), second trimester abortions (14-27 weeks) and pre-term births (28-36 weeks).

CONCLUSIONS AND SUMMARY

Spontaneous pre-term labour and delivery tends to be a repetitive process in successive pregnancies. It is associated with a high neonatal mortality and a high neonatal morbidity some of which is carried on into later life. It has a distinct though poorly understood link with sociobiological and environmental variables. Clearly, all of these are major reasons for epidemiological concern. Even at a purely descriptive level this is bedevilled by semantic problems. Pre-term may be difficult to define, pre-term labour and pre-term delivery are by no means identical to each other and both may induce several biases. In conclusion, many of the current studies will have to be done over again in order to obtain valid data on the epidemiology of spontaneous pre-term labour and delivery. There is a need to use clearly defined and preferentially widely accepted terminology, and to consider pre-term infants in terms of both weight and gestational age, presence of lethal deformities and life at birth and/or at the onset of labour. The considerable improvement in prognosis for infants born with very low birthweight and gestational age will probably lead to a further increase in elective delivery of pre-term infants. There is likely to be agreement that these pregnancies and infants will need to be studied separately. Over the next few years it may remain difficult to answer the question whether pre-term delivery as a consequence of spontaneous labour, needs to be studied separately according to the presence or absence and the type of associated pathology. It may well prove to be useful however to study separately pre-term labours which do and those which do not lead to pre-term delivery. Such studies may perhaps help to gain an insight, which is still lacking at the present time, into the mechanism of the onset of spontaneous labour.

ACKNOWLEDGEMENT

I am grateful to Miss H. Wittenberg for typing the manuscript.

REFERENCES

1. Expert group on prematurity final report, World Health Organization, Technical report series no 27, 1950.
2. Alberman E: Factors influencing perinatal wastage. *Clin Obstet Gynaecol* 1, 1-15 (1974).
3. Usher R, McLean F and Scott KE: Judgment of fetal age. II. Clinical significance of gestational age and an objective method for its assessment. *Pediatr Clin North Am* 13, 835-848 (1966).

4. Public Health aspects of low birthweight. World Health Organization, Technical report series no 217, 1961.
5. Reed DM and Stanley FJ: Preface. In: *The epidemiology of prematurity*, Reed DM and Standly FJ (eds), Baltimore, Urban & Schwarzenberg, 1977.
6. Prevention of perinatal morbidity and mortality, World Health Organization, Public Health Papers no 42, 1969.
7. Working party to discuss nomenclature based on gestational age and birthweight. *Arch Dis Child* 45, 730 (1970).
8. Committee on fetus and newborn: Nomenclature for duration of gestation, birthweight and intrauterine growth. *Pediatrics* 39, 935-939 (1967).
9. FIGO news: Lists of gynecologic and obstetrical terms and definitions. *Int J Gynaecol Obstet* 14, 570-576 (1976).
10. WHO: Recommended definitions, terminology and format for statistical tables related to the perinatal period and use of a new certificate for cause of perinatal deaths. *Acta obstet gynaecol Scand* 56, 247-253 (1977).
11. Dunn PM: Definition of perinatal mortality, *Lancet* 1, 1357-1358 (1977).
12. Bakketeig LS: The risk of repeated pre-term or low birth weight delivery. In: *The epidemiology of prematurity*, Reed DM and Stanley FJ (eds), Baltimore, Urban & Schwarzenberg, 1977, p 231-241.
13. Kloosterman GJ: Abnormale duur van de zwangerschap. In: *De voortplanting van de mens*, Kloosterman GJ (ed), Haarlem, Centen, 1977, p 332-342.
14. Van der Slikke JW and Treffers PE: Influence of induced abortion on gestational duration in subsequent pregnancies. *Br med J* 1, 270-272 (1978).
15. MacNaughton MC: Pregnancy following abortion. *J Obstet Gynaecol Br Commonw* 68, 789-792 (1961).
16. Speert H: Pregnancy prognosis following repeated abortion, *Am J Obstet Gynecol* 68, 665-673 (1966).
17. Papaevangelou G, Vrettos AS, Papadatos C and Alexiou D: The effect of spontaneous and induced abortion on prematurity and birthweight, *J Obstet Gynaecol Br Commonw* 80, 418-422 (1973).
18. Keirse MJNC, Rush RW, Anderson ABM and Turnbull AC: Risk of pre-term delivery in patients with previous pre-term delivery and/or abortion. *Br J Obstet Gynaecol* 85, 81-85 (1978).
19. Farr V, Mitchell RG, Neligan GA and Parkin JM: The definition of some external characteristics in the assessment of gestational age in the newborn infant, *Dev Med Child Neurol* 8, 507-511 (1966).
20. Dubowitz LMS, Dubowitz V and Goldberg CG: Clinical assessment of gestational age in the newborn infant, *J Pediatr* 77, 1-10 (1970).
21. Terris M and Gold EM: An epidemiologic study of prematurity. II. Relation to prenatal care, birth interval, residential history, and outcome of previous pregnancies, *Am J Obstet Gynecol* 103, 371-379 (1969).
22. Vaughan DH: Some social factors in perinatal morbidity, *Br J Prev Soc Med* 22, 138-145 (1969).
23. Terris M: Descriptive and analytic studies of etiology. In: *The epidemiology of prematurity*, Reed DM and Stanley FJ (eds), Baltimore, Urban & Schwarzenberg, 1977, p 335-338.
24. O'Driscoll M: Discussion remark. In: *Pre-term labour*, Anderson ABM, Beard RW, Brudenell JM and Dunn PM (eds), London, Royal College of Obstetricians and Gynaecologists, 1977, p 369.
25. Keirse MJC and Bennebroek Gravenhorst J: Het inleiden van de baring bij intra uteriene vruchtdood, *Ned Tijdschr Geneesk* 123, 1195-1199 (1979).
26. Gruenwald P: Stillbirth and early neonatal death. In: *Perinatal problems*, Butler NR and Alberman ED (eds), Edinburgh-London, Livingstone, 1969, p 163-183.

27. Hoogendoorn D: De relatie tussen de hoogte van de perinatale sterfte en de plaats van bevalling: thuis, dan wel in het ziekenhuis, *Ned Tijdschr Geneesk* 122, 1171-1178 (1978).
28. Rush RW, Keirse MJNC, Howat P, Baum JD, Anderson ABM and Turnbull AC: Contribution of pre-term delivery to perinatal mortality. *Br med J* 2, 965-968 (1976).
29. Rush RW, Davey DA and Segall ML: The effect of preterm delivery on perinatal mortality, *Br J Obstet Gynaecol* 85, 806-811 (1978).
30. Fetal and neonatal mortality at Leiden University Medical Centre, unpublished.
31. Ratten GJ, Beischer NA and Fortune DW: Obstetric complications when the fetus has Potter's syndrome, *Am J Obstet Gynecol* 115, 890-896 (1973).
32. Keirse MJNC, Anderson ABM and Laurence KM: *unpublished observations.*
33. Butler NR and Alberman ED (eds), *Perinatal problems.* Edinburgh-London, Livingstone, 1969, p 49.
34. Saling E: Prämaturitäts und Dysmaturitäts Präventions-Programm (PDP Programm), *Z Geburtsh Perinatol* 176, 70-81 (1972).
35. Kucera H, Pavelka R, Rudelsdorfer B and Reinold E: Einfluss Sozialer Faktoren auf die Ergebnisse eines gezielten Frühgeburten Präventions Programmes, *Wien Klin Wochenschr* 89, 307-311 (1977).
36. Papiernik-Berkhauer E: Discussion. In: *Pre-term labour.* Anderson ABM, Beard RW, Brudenell JM and Dunn PM (eds), London, Royal College of Obstetricians and Gynaecologists, 1977, p 29-39.
37. Boldman R and Reed DM: Worldwide variations in low birth weight. In: *The epidemiology of prematurity*, Reed DM and Stanley FJ (eds), Baltimore, Urban & Schwarzenberg, 1977, p 39-51.
38. Neligan GA, Kolvin I, Scott DM and Garside RF (eds), *Born too soon or born too small*, Clinics in Developmental Medicine no 61, London, Heinemann, 1976.
39. Davies PA and Tizard JPM: Very low birth weight and subsequent neurological defect, *Dev Med Child Neurol* 17, 3-17 (1975).
40. Versluys C: Loont 'neonatale intensive care' de moeite? *Tijdschr Kindergeneesk* 45, 149-163 (1977).
41. Stewart A: Follow-up of pre-term infants. In: *Pre-term labour*, Anderson ABM, Beard RW, Brudenell JM and Dunn PM (eds), London, Royal College of Obstetricians and Gynaecologists, 1977, p 372-384.
42. Reed DM and Stanley FJ (eds), *The epidemiology of prematurity*, Baltimore, Urban & Schwarzenberg, 1977.
43. Fedrick J and Anderson ABM: Factors associated with spontaneous pre-term birth. *Br J Obstet Gynaecol* 83, 342-350 (1976).
44. Alberman E: Sociobiologic factors and birth weight in Great Britain. In: *The epidemiology of prematurity*, Reed DM and Stanley FJ (eds), Baltimore, Urban & Schwarzenberg, 1977, p 145-156.
45. Pirani BBK: Smoking during pregnancy, *Obstet Gynecol Survey* 33, 1-12 (1978).
46. Lembrych S: Schwangerschafts-, Geburts- und Wochenbettverlauf nach künstlicher Unterbrechung der ersten Gravidität, *Zentralbl Gynäkol* 94, 164-168 (1972).
47. Liu DTY, Melville HAH and Martin T: Subsequent gestational morbidity after various types of abortion, *Lancet* 2, 431 (1972).
48. Wright CSW, Campbell S and Beazley J: Second-trimester abortion after vaginal termination of pregnancy, *Lancet* 1, 1278-1279 (1972).
49. Daling JR and Emanuel I; Induced abortion and subsequent outcome of pregnancy. A matched cohort study, *Lancet* 2, 170-173 (1975).

PREVENTION OF PRE-TERM LABOUR

ANNE B.M. ANDERSON

The ultimate achievement of preventing pre-term labour and delivery will depend both on understanding the aetiological factors involved in the spontaneous onset of uterine contractions too early in gestation and on the availability of methods to predict and prevent the problems. These ideals are not likely to be realised in the foreseeable future, unfortunately, since the prevention of pre-term labour appears to depend on finding a solution to almost all the major problems in obstetrics. A study of all pre-term births in Oxford in 1973 and 1974 (1) showed that delivery occurred following the spontaneous onset of labour before 37 completed weeks of pregnancy in 62 percent of cases where the infant was born alive and without deformity which proved lethal; the other 38 percent of pre-term births occurred in association with multiple pregnancy (10 percent) or were delivered electively by the obstetrician (28 percent). But where pre-term labour started spontaneously it did so in 40 percent of cases in asssociation with a pathology in either the mother or fetus or in both. These pathologies included haemorrhage, severe retardation of fetal growth, uterine abnormality, pre-eclampsia or severe hypertension, infection, and congenital abnormality of the fetus. It is not known if the pathologies are causally related to the premature onset of labour but it may well be that in these cases the fetus is wisely triggering its own birth in the presence of a hostile intrauterine environment. In most of these cases it would clearly be neither safe for the mother or fetus or of benefit to the fetus to attempt to prevent pre-term labour and delivery.

Prevention of pre-term birth in an individual can only be worthwhile where the fetus is alive without lethal deformity, does not have severe growth retardation, is not jeopardised *in utero* and the mother has no serious complication of pregnancy such as haemorrhage or pre-eclampsia. Thus, even with the perfect prediction systems and very effective and safe means of preventing pre-term labour only a part of the problem of pre-term birth (about 40 percent in Oxford) would be solved. On the other hand, this goal would at first sight be worth achieving since perinatal mortality is high in this group. For example, in our Oxford study (1) after exclusion of infants born with lethal deformity 35 percent of the early neonatal deaths (i.e. death in the

M.J.N.C. Keirse et al. (eds.), Human Parturition, 235-245.

first week of life irrespective of gestational age) in pre-term infants were in the group where spontaneous labour started pre-term for no obvious reason and with a singleton fetus; the early neonatal mortality rate in this group was high at 81 per 1000 live births. This, in contrast to an overall early neonatal death rate for the hospital of 4.2 per 1000 in the same years, again excluding lethal deformities which accounted for about one-third of all perinatal deaths. It can be calculated, however, that even if all the early neonatal deaths had been prevented in the group where pre-term labour and delivery occurred unexpectedly whether with a single or multiple pregnancy, the overall perinatal death rate in the hospital for 1973-74 would have fallen from 15.5 per 1000 to 13.3 per 1000 (from 10.4 to 8.2 per 1000 if all lethal abnormalities are excluded). Although many pre-term infants are stillborn our analysis (1) showed that 28 percent of stillborn infants had a lethal deformity and only two deaths occurred in the group with spontaneous labour, both before admission to hospital in labour. Thus very little further reduction in perinatal mortality would be achieved by prevention of stillbirths in association with unexplained pre-term labour.

A critical analysis of all pre-term births in Oxford therefore forces the conclusion that prevention of unexpected pre-term labour in the absence of fetal or maternal pathology would not decrease overall perinatal mortality to any large extent in our community although some reduction would be achieved and we have not measured morbidity which would undoubtedly be reduced. It is important to realise that "unexplained" pre-term labour leading to delivery is only the tip of the iceberg as far as the total problem of pre-term birth is concerned and that given the best pharmacological agents to inhibit uterine contractility only a fraction of the problem would be solved and very little impact made on overall perinatal mortality rates.

Despite the introduction in recent years of a plethora of drugs aimed at preventing pre-term delivery by suppressing uterine activity, it is disappointing that so little appears to have been achieved. National figures available for England and Wales (2) show that over the past 25 years there has been no change in the incidence ($\sim$6.5 percent) of babies weighing less than 2500 g at birth although a reduction in the percentage of infants delivered pre-term could be concealed within these data and factors such as increasing numbers of termination of pregnancy may, if cervical damage is caused, mitigate against any demonstrable improvement. National trends reporting separately infants delivered pre-term (at less than 37 completed weeks of pregnancy) from infants of low birthweight (weighing less than 2500 g at birth) are not available in Britain so that the plethora of treatment at present being used for the "prevention" of pre-term birth cannot be assessed at a national level. From West Germany Kubli reported (3) that there was no change in the incidence of liveborn infants weighing 500 to 2500 g over the years 1972 to 1975, the incidence varying between 5.5 percent and 5.8 percent in these years. This, during a period of time in West Germany when according to Kubli (3) the beta-mimetic drug, fenoterol was introduced to that country (on the open market in 1974) and is now used at the estimated yearly rate of 1 million 0.5 mg ampoules plus about 6 million 5 mg tablets. These data of Professor Kubli are in sharp contrast to the German results as presented by Wynn and Wynn (4) who claim that many series written mainly in the German language, show that "the new drugs" (referring to beta-mimetics) are "highly effective in delaying birth". The same authors (4) also state that "the right use of these drugs is of the greatest importance to women, to their children, and to society".

It may be considered timely to challenge some of the wellestablished concepts relating to the prevention of pre-term birth and to attempt to review critically current knowledge concerning the prediction and prevention of such an important cause of human morbidity and mortality.

PREDICTION OF PRE-TERM LABOUR

The early antenatal identification of women "at risk" of pre-term labour could be useful in clinical practice if only to make the obstetrician more aware of the possibility of such an event although, as will be discussed later, "preventive" measures may not be helpful and require reappraisal. Several approaches have been tried to allow the obstetrician to identify warning signs for pre-term birth by taking account of socio-biological variables, previous reproductive performance, hormonal factors, the physical characteristics of the cervix on palpation, or the contractility of the uterine musculature. The predictive value of each of these will be discussed.

Scoring systems

Several scoring systems have been devised (e.g. 5, 6, 7, 8, 9) and are in use in several countries throughout the world. In Britain, the only attempt to produce an accurate scoring system for spontaneous pre-term labour was made by Fedrick in Oxford (8) based on data from the British Perinatal Mortality Survey in 1958. In addition to socio-economic variables such as social class, age, parity, height, weight, smoking habits, Fedrick also took into account bleeding during the present or in a previous pregnancy, previous obstetric history particularly previous spontaneous abortion, previous low birthweight babies or perinatal deaths. The survey did not unfortunately provide information on previous termination of pregnancy nor did it identify previous pre-term births as opposed to previous low birthweight infants. Scores were awarded for the various parameters based on calculation of relative risks; they were then multiplied to give a composite score for each woman – the higher the score, the greater the risk of spontaneous pre-term labour and delivery. The score was a much better predictor of pre-term delivery in multiparous than in nulliparous women. For multiparous women a previous obstetric history of perinatal death, low birthweight or bleeding in pregnancy, increased the probability of pre-term delivery; for primigravidae with no past reproductive behaviour as a guide, socio-economic factors were not powerful enough predictors of pre-term delivery to be helpful.

In terms of effectiveness of such a scoring system one must examine the total number of women who would have to be screened in order to select out the patients who will actually deliver pre-term. Fedrick (8) found that although a high score was given to almost 30 percent of primiparae who went into pre-term labour, they represented only 9 percent of the total number of patients in the population who would be given a high score. For multiparae the results were more encouraging, a high score identifying 25 percent of the total population who would go into pre-term labour. Such a scoring system is therefore of very limited practical use, being effective at predicting only a relatively small proportion of patients likely to go unexpectedly into pre-term labour. Rather better results were shown by Papiernik using his scoring system (5, 6) which when tested on a control population, could predict 75 percent of pre-term births in 35 percent of the population. Although these figures appear impressive they mean that in a population of 5000, (approximately the total number of yearly births in Oxford) and given a 5 percent pre-term birth rate (250 births/year), we would predict $\sim$190 of these pre-term births but in a total of 1750 pregnant women in our community. But, for 1560 of these pregnant patients we would have made a false prediction of pre-term delivery which would not only be a constant worry to a vast number of women but might tempt the obstetrician to intervene with "preventive therapy" – bed rest, cervical suture or drugs which might suppress uterine activity – in cases where there was never any risk of pre-term birth. Since these preventive measures may in themselves have dangers and adversely affect the physical and mental health of the mother and the well-being of the fetus, we should be cautious in advocating the application of complex scoring systems in clinical practice. In the future perhaps the inclusion of new variables will be helpful but only if the final scoring system is such a powerful discriminant that a large proportion of women at risk of pre-term delivery can be identified in a very small number of the total population of pregnant women. It seems unlikely that this Utopia will arrive in the near future.

On the other hand, identification of risk factors can contribute a great deal to a better understanding of the physiological factors likely to be involved in initiating pre-term labour and hence point out the direction in which the development of preventive measures might go. Lesinski (10) points out that if the aim of identifying risk factors is to try and give women the best outcome for their pregnancy by means of an improvement in certain aspects of antenatal care, then many of the variables used in the scoring systems might be questioned. For example, socio-economic status, age or parity cannot be altered therapeutically and would have to be altered long before conception if the risk of pre-term birth due to these variables was to be reduced. But some variables such as smoking, poor working conditions or long daily commuting time (6), could be altered and this might have some effect in reducing the incidence of pre-term birth.

Contractility of the uterus and dilatation of the cervix

Another approach to the prediction of pre-term labour has been to measure the contractions of the uterus combined with an assessment at intervals of the dilatation and effacement of the cervix. Results are conflicting. Wood et al. (11), found that pre-term labour could be predicted if the cervix was dilated and effaced by the 34th week and the patient also had an unduly active uterus. On the other hand Anderson and Turnbull (12) did not confirm these findings and showed that in one-third of primigravidae the cervical canal was dilated to allow the index finger to be passed through the internal os by the 32nd week. Although the four patients who subsequently delivered pre-term (in the total of 77 patients studied) were in the group with an open cervical canal by 32 weeks, most of the women delivered near term. The study of Anderson and Turnbull (12) appears to be the only published work in English describing serially the clinically detectable changes in dilatation of the cervical canal in human pregnancy. Their results apply to primigravidae only and it is likely that in multiparae cervical dilatation may occur earlier in pregnancy. Thus, although early detection of shortening or dilatation of the cervix is said to be an important predictive observation for pre-term labour (13) there is no proof that this is so and a prospective study of cervical changes is required in a large enough group of women who are at risk of pre-term birth. There is so little information on the physiological changes in the cervix in pregnancy that there is a great danger of misinterpreting these physiological changes as pathological. Hence, we should be sure we have defined the normal cervical changes for our population before instituting preventive measures such as cervical sutures.

We have recently shown that both vaginal examination in pregnancy (14) and cervical encerclage (15) will raise prostaglandin levels in the maternal circulation within minutes of these procedures and if we advocate repeated vaginal examination throughout pregnancy or cervical sutures we may be creating a hormonal environment in which the uterus finds it easy to contract – the very situation we are aiming to prevent. Trying to prevent all prematurity by putting a suture around the cervix is in any case an excessively mechanistic approach.

Undoubtedly there are patients who have had previous cervical damage and there may be rare cases of congenital cervical incompetence but the diagnosis of "cervical incompetence" is often made on the basis of a past history of abortions or pre-term birth, situations in which there is no evidence that the physiology of the cervix has been disturbed in any way. Although a past history of spontaneous second trimester abortion or spontaneous pre-term labour and delivery is associated with an increased risk of pre-term birth (16, 17) there is no evidence that cervical encerclage would help to prevent the repetitive tendency to deliver pre-term.

Endocrine parameters

Another approach to the prediction of spontaneous pre-term labour we have used, is to examine the hypothesis that there may be changes in steroid hormones in the maternal circulation before the onset of unexplained pre-term labour. Over the past few years in Oxford an attempt has been made to test the hypothesis that plasma levels of 17β-oestradiol might rise and levels of progesterone might fall before the onset of spontaneous pre-term labour of unknown aetiology since we had found that such endocrine changes precede the onset of spontaneous labour at term (18). This approach has proved disappointing in the final analysis. In about 15 patients with a singleton pregnancy and where adequate numbers of samples have been obtained throughout pregnancy before spontaneous pre-term labour and delivery with no fetal or maternal pathology, circulating levels of oestradiol and progesterone in the week or weeks preceding pre-term labour were on average no different to levels found in patients at a similar stage of gestation but who progressed to deliver at term.

We have also recently measured circulating levels of prostaglandins, particularly 13,14-dihydro-15-keto-PGF (PGFM), in patients in pre-term labour

(19). Surprisingly the levels of PGFM are not raised in early pre-term labour when the cervix is less than 4 cm dilated although levels do rise later in pre-term labour. In early pre-term labour the levels of PGFM are low compared with levels in early labour at term. These data suggest that the mechanism of spontaneous pre-term labour may be different to that of term labour. The factors initiating pre-term labour have not yet been elucidated, and although it is possible that we are missing some vital endocrine link which may improve the prediction of pre-term delivery, with this lack of knowledge our ability to predict it will remain restricted. At present therefore attempts to predict pre-term labour by examining changes in circulating levels of steroid hormones or of prostaglandins seems unlikely to be fruitful.

PREVENTION OF PRE-TERM LABOUR

If we could predict pre-term labour with confidence, what measures can we usefully take to prevent its occurrence?

In general the risk of pre-term labour can be assessed at the first antenatal visit taking into account a previous history of pre-term birth or second trimester abortion in particular, as well as features suggesting the possibility of cervical incompetence. Moreover the patients general health and physique, social circumstances, diet, smoking habits and drug history may all point to an increased hazard of pre-term birth. More intensive antenatal care than average may thus be indicated in such patients and as pregnancy advances, complications such as threatened abortion or antepartum haemorrhage may indicate a risk that labour may start too early in gestation.

Multiple pregnancy or polyhydramnios may also be detected as added hazards and cervical dilatation and effacement before the 24th week probably carry an added risk of pre-term birth particularly if the membranes begin to bulge through the cervix.

Preventive management may therefore include appropriate general advice, dietetic counselling, stopping smoking and getting adequate rest and sleep. Ultrasound assessment to confirm gestational age and to detect multiple pregnancy at an early stage is valuable. Cervical encerclage may be considered necessary if early signs of pathological effacement and dilatation of the cervix are detected. But unfortunately, although attention to these particular features may alert the obstetrician to the possibility of pre-term labour being a hazard, there is no proof that any measure taken including bed rest, cervical encerclage or drug therapy will lower the incidence of pre-term delivery.

Cervical encerclage

Objective evidence of the value of this procedure in the prevention of pre-term birth is difficult to find. A retrospective study in Oxford (16) examined the influence of cervical suture in the present pregnancy in 59 of 370 patients with a history of two or more pregnancies ending in spontaneous abortion and/or pre-term delivery. There was no statistical difference in the incidence of pre-term delivery whether or not a cervical suture had been inserted on the basis of a past history of spontaneous first trimester abortions, at least one second trimester abortion, two or more second trimester abortions or previous pre-term delivery.

Another retrospective study from England on twin pregnancy (20) compared 60 twin pregnancies treated by bed rest in hospital, 37 treated by cervical suture and 36 who were given no treatment. The incidence of spontaneous onset of labour before 36 weeks' gestation, mean gestational age at delivery, mean birthweights of the first and second twins and the incidence of fetal growth retardation was similar in the three groups. Thus, although it may be helpful and clinically important in some respects to detect multiple pregnancy early in gestation, there is no evidence at present that we can prevent spontaneous pre-term labour in twins by intervention in the form of cervical sutures or bed rest. The effect on the mother and the family of separation, and economic considerations should make us wary of advocating prolonged hospitalisation in these circumstances until the efficacy of such treatment has been proven. There is an urgent need for prospective randomised controlled trials to examine the efficacy of cervical sutures in the prevention of pre-term birth.

Drug therapy

The prevention of pre-term labour by the oral administration of β-sympathomimetic drugs in the antenatal period has not been found helpful either in twin pregnancy using fenoterol (21) or using ritodrine in primigravidae where the internal cervical os admitted one or more fingers at 28 to 32 weeks of pregnancy (22). A recent review of the benefits of drugs used (hormones, ethanol, β-sympathomimetics) to prevent premature birth (23) concluded that in eight methodologically adequate trials where drugs were given prophylactically, in only one (24) did the drug favourably affect the outcome for the infant. The drug used by Johnson et al (24) was 17α-hydroxyprogesterone caproate but that trial could be criticized since subjects and controls were not matched for variables such as previous abortions, incidence of cervical sutures, race and incidence of twin pregnancies, so that there may have been unintentional bias in this study.

Prophylaxis using drugs aimed at preventing premature uterine contractility does not therefore seem a hopeful approach and despite the inadequacies of some of the trials it seems unlikely that different conclusions would be reached from further controlled trials.

PREVENTION OF PRE-TERM BIRTH: TREATMENT OF PRE-TERM LABOUR

Even when pre-term labour is diagnosed, the prediction of outcome i.e. delivery, is difficult despite classical signs of the onset of labour. This is best illustrated by reference to publications which testify to the apparent effectiveness of non-specific forms of treatment for pre-term labour, with a high percentage of success due to placebo effect. Thus, in three trials (25, 26, 27) of betamimetics for the treatment of pre-term labour where results are given after 7 days of therapy, approximately 40 percent (25 of 65) of patients with unruptured membranes and given placebo therapy only had not been delivered one week after a diagnosis of pre-term labour was made by the obstetrician. If all women in pre-term labour are treated with betamimetics then about 40% will be needlessly given drugs which in themselves are not without danger. Trials examining the efficacy of β-sympathomimetic drugs or prostaglandin synthetase inhibitors in the suppression of pre-term labour may show the ability of these drugs to prolong gestation but do not appear to have examined in detail the long term outcome for the baby (23). We still await good follow-up studies on pre-term infants when these drugs have been used in an attempt to postpone their birth.

The pros and cons of therapy aimed at delaying pre-term birth as opposed to conservatism in allowing pre-term labour to proceed to pre-term delivery is difficult to assess especially in hospitals with expert neonatal paediatric units.

For the patient at risk of pre-term delivery, "treatment" could mean hospitalisation, separation from her family, and intervention which may involve a general anaesthetic for insertion of a cervical suture or drugs which may have side effects affecting herself or the fetus. We have to be certain that such treatment is safe and has a high chance of being successful if we advocate that pregnant women should be given it. In addition, even if we have effective treatment we must know who to treat otherwise women not at risk could find themselves the recipients of therapy.

In summary, I think our ability to predict pre-term birth is still very limited, that intervention may not be without hazard and has not been shown in prospective randomised controlled trials to offer improvement in the quality of survival for the baby. So many factors are involved in the aetiology of pre-term birth that a single approach to the problem will not be successful and some of the aetiological factors such as fetal abnormality or haemorrhage cannot be predicted or prevented by any known means. Improvement in standards of neonatal paediatric care may be the best investment for the future development of the pre-term infant.

ACKNOWLEDGEMENTS

Studies in Cardiff and Oxford have been supported by the Medical Research Council (UK) through a Programme Grant to Professor AC Turnbull. I am grateful to Mrs Pat Moon for typing the manuscript.

REFERENCES

1. Rush RW, Keirse MJNC, Howat P, Baum JD, Anderson ABM and Turnbull AC: Contribution of pre-term delivery to perinatal mortality. *Br Med J* 2, 1-12 (1976).
2. Department of Health and Social Security. In: *Annual Reports of the Chief Medical Officer "On the State of Health of the Nation"*, London, Her Majesty's Stationery Office, 1952-1977.
3. Kubli F: Discussion remark In: *Pre-term Labour*, Anderson ABM, Beard R, Brudenell JM and Dunn PM (eds), London, Royal College of Obstetricians and Gynaecologists, 1977, p 218.
4. Wynn M and Wynn A (eds): *The Prevention of Pre-term Birth*, London, Foundation for Education and Research in Child-Bearing, 1977, p 10-21.
5. Papiernik-Berkhauer E: Coefficient de risque d'accouchement prématuré. *Presse Med* 77, 793-794 (1969).
6. Papiernik E and Kaminski M: Multifactorial study of the risk of prematurity at 32 weeks of gestation. I. A study of the frequency of 30 predictive characteristics. *J Perinat Med* 2, 30-36 (1974).
7. Kaminski M, Goujard J and Rumeau-Rouquette C: Prediction of low birthweight and prematurity by a multiple regression analysis with maternal characteristics known since the beginning of pregnancy. *Int J Epidemiol* 2, 195-204 (1973).
8. Fedrick J: Antenatal identification of women at high risk of spontaneous pre-term birth. *Br J Obstet Gynaecol* 83, 351-354 (1976).
9. Hobel CJ: ABC's of perinatal medicine. In: *Major Mental Handicap: Methods and Costs of Prevention*, Ciba Foundation Symposium no 59, Amsterdam, Elsevier/Excerpta Medica/North-Holland, 1978, p 53-72.
10. Lesinski J; High-risk pregnancy. Unresolved problems of screening, management and prognosis. *Obstet Gynecol* 46, 599-603 (1975).
11. Wood C, Bannerman RHO, Booth RT and Pinkerton JHM: The prediction of premature labor by observations of the cervix and external tocography. *Am J Obstet Gynecol* 91, 396-402 (1965).
12. Anderson ABM and Turnbull AC: Relationship between length of gestation and cervical dilatation, uterine contractility, and other factors during pregnancy. *Am J Obstet Gynecol* 105, 1207-1214 (1969).

13. Papiernik-Berkhauer E. In: *Pre-term Labour*. Anderson ABM, Beard R, Brudenell JM and Dunn PM (eds), London, Royal College of Obstetricians and Gynaecologists, 1977, p 29-41.
14. Mitchell MD, Flint APF, Bibby J, Brunt J, Arnold JM, Anderson ABM and Turnbull AC: Rapid increases in plasma prostaglandin concentrations after vaginal examination and amniotomy. *Br Med J* 2, 1183-1185 (1977).
15. Bibby JG, Brunt J, Mitchell MD, Anderson ABM and Turnbull AC: The effect of cervical encerclage on plasma prostaglandin concentrations during early human pregnancy. *Br J Obstet Gynaecol* 86, 19-22 (1979).
16. Keirse MJNC, Rush RW, Anderson ABM and Turnbull AC: Risk of pre-term delivery in patients with previous pre-term delivery and/or abortion. *Br J Obstet Gynaecol* 85, 81-85 (1978).
17. Bakketeig LS: The risk of repeated pre-term or low birth weight delivery. In: *The Epidemiology of Prematurity*. Reed BM and Stanley FJ (eds), Baltimore-Munich, Urban and Schwarzenberg, 1977, p 231-241.
18. Turnbull AC, Patten PT, Flint APF, Keirse, MJNC, Jeremy JY and Anderson ABM: Significant fall in progesterone and rise in oestradiol levels in human peripheral plasma before the onset of labour. *Lancet* 1, 101-104 (1974).
19. Mitchell MD, Flint APF, Bibby J, Brunt J, Arnold JM, Anderson ABM and Turnbull AC: Plasma concentrations of prostaglandins during late human pregnancy; influence of normal and pre-term labor *J Clin Endocrinol Metab* 46, 947-951 (1978).
20. Weekes ARL, Menzies DN and de Boer CH: The relative efficacy of bed rest, cervical suture and no treatment in the management of twin pregnancy. *Br J Obstet Gynaecol* 84, 161-164 (1977).
21. Marivate M, De Villiers KQ and Fairbrother P: Effect of prophylactic outpatient administration of fenoterol on the time of onset of spontaneous labor and fetal growth rate in twin pregnancy *Am J Obstet Gynecol* 128, 707-708 (1977).
22. Walters WAW and Wood C: A trial of oral ritodrine for the prevention of premature labour. *Br J Obstet Gynaecol* 84, 26-30 (1977).
23. Hemminki E and Starfield B: Prevention and treatment of premature labour by drugs: review of controlled clinical trials. *Br J Obstet Gynaecol* 85, 411-417 (1978).
24. Johnson JWC, Austin KL, Jones GS, Davis GH and King TM: Efficacy of 17α-hydroxyprogesterone caproate in the prevention of premature labor. *N Engl J Med* 293, 675-680 (1975).
25. Wesselius- de Casparis A, Thiery M, Yo Le Sian A, Baumgarten K, Brosens I, Gamissans O, Stolk JG and Vivier W: Results of double-blind, multicentre study with ritodrine in premature labour. *Br Med J* 2, 144-147 (1971).
26. Thiery M, Baumgarten K, Brosens I, Esteban-Altirriba J, Gamissans O, Yo Le Sian A, Flynn M and Van Strik R: A multicentre trial with ritodrine in the treatment of premature labour in patients with intact membranes. In: *Yutopar, ritodrine*, Philips-Duphar, 1976.
27. Ingemarsson I: Effect of terbutaline on premature labor. *Am J Obstet Gynecol* 125, 520-524 (1976).

EPIDEMIOLOGY OF POSTMATURITY

GERRIT JAN KLOOSTERMAN

There are two ways to define postmaturity: a statistical one and a clinical one.

STATISTICAL POSTMATURITY

According to the statistical approach a pregnancy is postmature when there is a considerable prolongation of pregnancy beyond its mean duration. There has been some dispute about the amount of prolongation (10 days, 2 weeks, 3 weeks) which is required. However WHO and FIGO have accepted as a world wide definition of postmaturity a pregnancy that goes beyond an amenorrhoea of 294 completed days (beyond 42 completed weeks, i.e. more than 14 days beyond the calculated date of delivery). In addition they have recommended that these pregnancies be labeled as post-term rather than postmature.

This definition stands or falls with the accuracy of the data on the first day of the last period and the regularity of the menstrual cycle. If these data are unreliable, it becomes impossible to give a calculated date of delivery and consequently of postmaturity.

In our department the percentage of women with uncertain or unknown duration of pregnancy decreased from 1952 till 1963, but has risen considerably thereafter (table 1) and is now much higher than it was 25 years ago. The initial improvement in all probability is due to an earlier start of

Table 1. Percentage of single pregnancies with uncertain dates at Wilhelmina Gasthuis, University of Amsterdam, from 1952 to 1976 (total no. of single pregnancies = 44 504).

Period	Primiparae	Multiparae
1952-'56	205 of 4921 = 4.2%	358 of 5830 = 6.1%
1957-'63	184 of 6905 = 2.7%	286 of 7796 = 3.7%
1964-'68	335 of 4826 = 6.9%	353 of 4471 = 7.9%
1969-'73	331 of 3769 = 8.8%	383 of 3517 = 10.9%
1974-'76	254 of 1984 = 12.8%	247 of 1835 = 13.5%

M.J.N.C. Keirse et al. (eds.), Human Parturition, 247-261.

prenatal care and a greater awareness of the signficance of reliable "dates" on the part of the public. The negative change in the second half of the sixties is due to the introduction of oral contraception in The Netherlands in 1963. With 46 percent of the female population between 15-44 years using oral contraception, this country was in 1976 on the top of the world list of per capita use of oral contraception (1). In later years the influx of a considerable number of women from other countries has become a second factor (table 2). In the years 1974 to 1976 they formed 28 percent of the women who delivered in our department. In 1977 their number had risen to almost 40 percent. The surprisingly great number of uncertain durations of pregnancy among women from neighbouring countries is due to the fact that the University Clinic is rather popular in "hippy" circles.

Table 2. Number of pregnancies with unreliable dates in various ethnic groups delivered at the Wilhelmina Gasthuis, University of Amsterdam in 1974-1976.

Cultural and/or ethnic group	No. of pregnancies	No. with uncertain duration of pregnancy	No. caused by inexpert use of oral contraception
Foreigners	1054	239 (22.7%)	49 (21%)
Turkey, Morocco Lebanon, Egypt	210	77 (36.7%)	5 (6%)
Creoles from Suriname	313	77 (24.6%)	21 (27%)
China, Japan, India, Indonesia, Hindustani from Suriname	189	33 (17.5%)	3 (9%)
Spain, Portugal, Italy, Yugoslavia, Greece	130	13 (10 %)	10 (77%)
Germany, Britain, France, Belgium, Scandinavia	109	27 (24.8%)	6 (22%)
Dutch women married to a foreigner	103	12 (11.7%)	4 (33%)
Dutch	2765	262 (9.5%)	64 (24.4%)
Total	3819	501 (13.1%)	113 (22 %)

Nevertheless, if we leave out all pregnancies with unreliable "dates" and only consider the other ones, the true length of gestation appears to be by no means constant. In 1954 I studied this problem for the first time by examining 4000 single pregnancies with reliable data (2, 3). In 1978, we repeated this investigation, studying nearly 58000 single pregnancies (fig. 1 and 2). The difference is slight. In our first study we found that 29 percent of pregnancies ended between 277 and 283 days' amenorrhoea. In the second study this

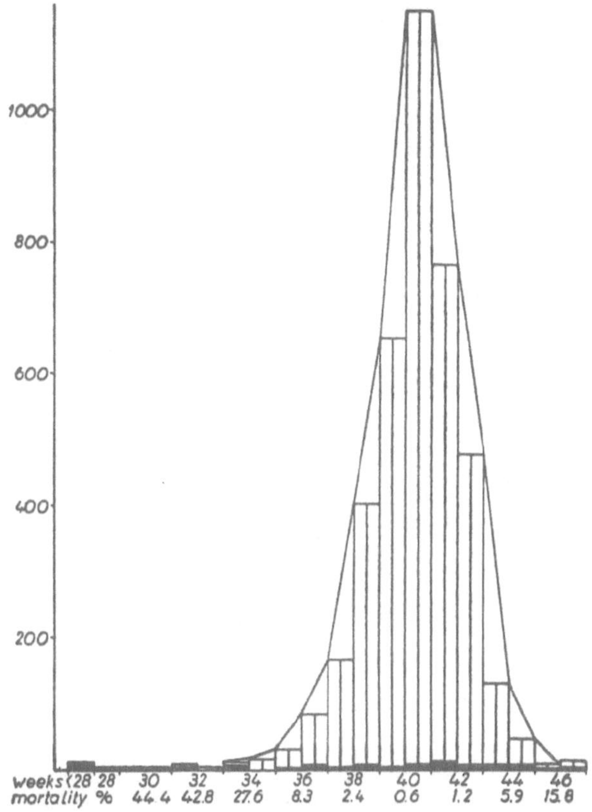

Fig. 1 Duration of pregnancy in 4 000 single pregnancies of at least 20 weeks' amenorrhoea. The data show the number of women delivered after completed weeks of pregnancy ± 3 days (e.g. 40 weeks = 277-283 days). The deliveries took place in the hospital of the School for Midwives in Amsterdam between 1947 and 1952.

proportion was 25 percent. The difference can be explained by the fact that the first study was conducted in the hospital attached to the School for Midwives in Amsterdam and the second in the Department of Obstetrics of the University of Amsterdam. In the latter institution the number of high-risk and pathological pregnancies is considerably higher. In both curves the number of pregnancies that went beyond 294 days was almost 10 percent. Pregnancies with less than 266 days' amenorrhoea also reached almost 10 percent of all pregnancies in the School for Midwives but 15.3 percent in the University Hospital.

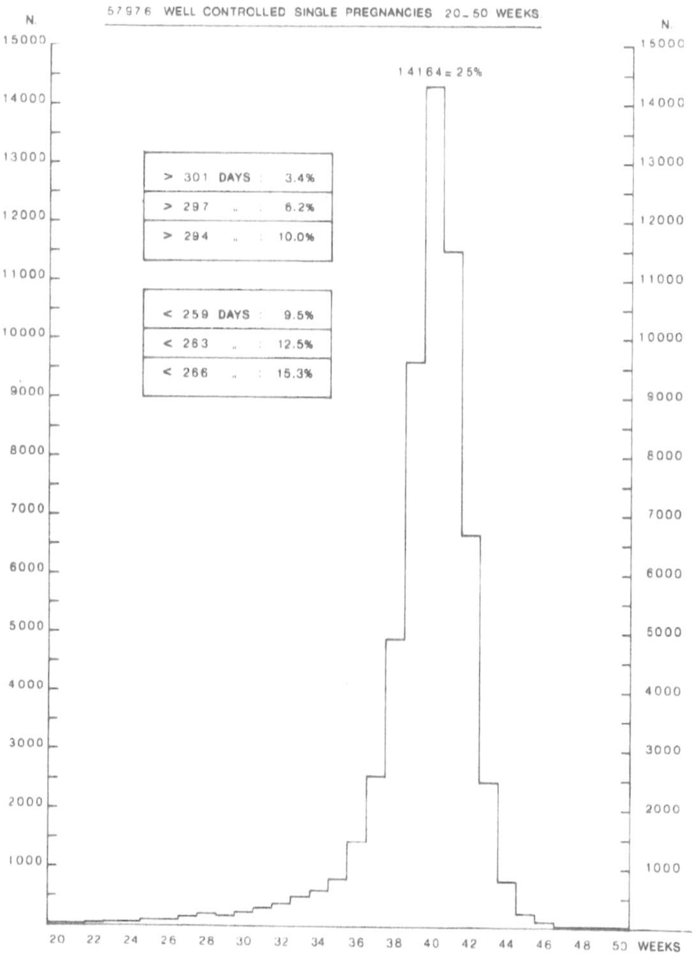

Fig. 2. Distribution of 57 976 single pregnancies of at least 20 weeks according to the duration of pregnancy at delivery (in groups of one week defined as for figure 1; e.g. 40 weeks = 277-283 days). These deliveries took place in the Obstetric Department of the University of Amsterdam (1952-1977) and in the School for Midwives (1947-1957).

From a statistical point of view this appears to answer the question on the incidence of postmaturity. Gestational length in the human (like in monkeys) is not very constant; certainly much less so than in other mammals as rabbit, sheep and rat. If we define postmaturity as a pregnancy that goes more than 14 days beyond the calculated date, then ± 10 percent of all pregnancies will become postmature. If another 3 days are added, then 6 percent go beyond

297 days and if we accept 43 weeks (more than 301 days) then 3.4 percent will be called postmature.

Yet, what is the clinical significance of such a definition? Even after a duration of pregnancy of 46 weeks a healthy baby can be born and although the Dutch law recognized this as a maximum, it is highly probable that healthy children can be born after an even longer period of gestation. In our series of 57 976 well-controlled single pregnancies there was one anencephalic child, live-born after an amenorrhoea of 50 weeks (this child died 8 days later) and one normal child after 49 weeks of amenorrhoea.

On the other hand it is now generally accepted that postmaturity carries an increased risk of intrauterine fetal death. The old adage that every child is born at the point of time that is most appropriate for it, is no longer accepted. Ballantyne (4) already had his doubts about the wisdom of this statement. Wijsenbeek (5) drew attention to the fact that infants, stillborn after a markedly prolonged pregnancy, were more often boys than girls. Runge (6) described the syndrome of postmaturity in the newborn child; but in the early fifties many clinical investigations appeared, which demonstrated beyond any doubt the danger of postmaturity (2, 3, 7, 8, 9). All investigators reached the conclusion that perinatal mortality was lowest in pregnancies which lasted 40 weeks and rose almost symmetrically, if the duration of pregnancy was shorter or longer. There was also agreement that postmaturity was a particular hazard to the first born and especially so to the child of a mother of advanced age. The increased mortality in postmature children was only to a minor extent due to higher neonatal mortality and arose mainly from an increase in intra-uterine deaths.

We (23) could also show that fetal death in postmaturity occurred almost 4 times more often in boys than in girls and that especially pregnancies with a low placental weight (below 500 g), a low placental index (ratio between placental weight and birthweight below 0.12) or a placenta with a high degree of infarction, were endangered.

However if we reach the conclusion that fetal or neonatal death by postmaturity is a rather rare occurrence (even after a pregnancy of 43 completed weeks more than 80 percent of all children are born in a normal and healthy condition) and that the course of disaster has to be sought in placental insufficiency, then we arrive at a clinical definition of postmaturity.

CLINICAL POSTMATURITY

The clinical definition of postmaturity is quite different from the statistical one. It could be phrased as follows:

> "postmature is every fetus that dies before or during labour or shows signs of severe fetal distress during a normal labour, whereas its development and degree of maturity would have guaranteed survival as a healthy individual if it had been brought into the outer world at a slightly earlier date".

Placental insufficiency, shortcomings of the fetal supply line, death by unknown causes are the diagnoses under which these cases appear in statistical records. If we consider the problem of postmaturity in this way, "statistical postmaturity" is no more than a warning sign that the possibility of "postmaturity in the clinical sense" is enhanced. However the possibility of "postmaturity in the clinical sense" is then also present in the period of gestation named mature or at term, and even in the period named pre-term. To study this problem we plotted the number of fetuses stillborn by "unknown" causes, in the obstetric department of the University of Amsterdam during the 19 years from 1958 to 1976. In 29 985 single pregnancies (all booked cases with a certain duration of pregnancy and a living fetus at the moment that a gestation of 193 completed days' amenorrhoea was reached), this occurred 208 times (6.9 per 1000). Causes of fetal mortality which were excluded were: eclampsia, severe toxaemia (diastolic blood pressure above 100 mmHg) abruptio placentae, placenta praevia, maternal diabetes, true knot in the umbilical cord, haematoma or aneurysms in the umbilical cord, tumor of the placenta, massive feto-maternal transfusion, intra-uterine infarctions (syphilis, herpes simplex, listeria, vaccania, rubella, cytomegaly), ascending infections after rupture of the membranes, vase praevia, birth trauma (fractures of skull, epi- and subdural haematoma, tentorial tear) and severe congenital malformations incompatible with life after birth. Fetal mortality of unknown cause was virtually synonymous with placental insufficiency. The only "clinical" diagnoses which we included were: growth retardation without signs of toxaemia, previous fetal death of unknown cause and prolongation of pregnancy after the expected date of delivery. That the cause of fetal death in these cases should be sought in the direction of placental insufficiency (or shortcomings in the fetal supply line as Gruenwald (10) prefers to call it) is supported by the fact that a great number of these children had a very low birthweight (table 3). In fact, of the whole group 85 percent were below the 50th centile, 65 percent below the 10th centile and 42 percent below the 2.3rd centile. As to placental weight (table 4) these figures were 88 percent, 63 percent and 34 percent respectively. The centiles of birth weight and placental weight in our community are based on the data of Kloosterman and Huidekoper (11, 12). Another important fact pointing in

Table 3. Stillbirth of unknown cause at various gestational ages in single pregnancies: total number of stillborn infants and number with birthweights below the 50th, 10th and 2.3rd centile (2 cases with unknown birthweight are excluded; birthweight was compared to the growth curve of Kloosterman [11] based upon nearly 80 000 single pregnancies in Amsterdam from 1930 to 1968).

Duration of pregnancy in weeks	28 - 32	33 - 36	37 - 41	>41	Total
Number (percent) of stillbirths with a birthweight					
<2.3rd centile	13 (35)	33 (60)	38 (42)	3 (13)	87 (42)
<10th centile	23 (62)	44 (80)	54 (59)	12 (52)	133 (65)
<50th centile	35 (95)	50 (91)	75 (82)	14 (61)	174 (85)
Total number (percent) of stillbirths	37 (100)	55 (100)	91 (100)	23 (100)	206 (100)

Table 4. Stillbirth of unknown cause at various gestational ages in single pregnancies: total number of stillborn infants and number with placental weights below the 50th, 10th and 2.3rd centile (2 cases with unknown birthweight and 2 with unknown placental weight are excluded; placental weight was compared to the data on placental weight compiled from nearly 40 000 placentae examined at the School for Midwives and the University Hospital, Amsterdam from 1948 to 1970).

Duration of pregnancy in weeks	28 - 32	33 - 36	37 - 41	>41	Total
Number (percent) of stillbirths with a placental weight					
<2.3rd centile	8 (22)	25 (45)	34 (37)	2 (10)	69 (34)
<10th centile	24 (65)	43 (78)	53 (58)	8 (38)	128 (63)
<50th centile	35 (95)	52 (95)	76 (84)	17 (81)	180 (88)
Total number (percent) of stillbirths	37 (100)	55 (100)	91 (100)	21 (100)	204 (100)

the direction of placental insufficiency is that 97 of these 204 placentae (48 percent) showed a marked degree of infarction, whereas the same degree of infarction was found in only 9 percent of the remaining 29 000 placentae.

If we now consider the population of 15 207 women who expected their first child, had a single pregnancy with a living fetus at the time that the duration of pregnancy reached 193 completed days (table 5) the risk of stillbirth of unknown cause in the period from 28 to 32 weeks was 6 in 15 207 (0.4 per 1000). This is far less than the survival rate of liveborn children in that same period. If one would try to avoid unexpected intrauterine death by induction

Table 5. Number of pregnancies, number of births and number of stillbirths in relation to gestational age in nulliparous and multiparous women. (Weeks of gestation in this and other tables refer to completed weeks ± 3 days; e.g. 40 weeks = 277-283 days.)

Weeks of gestation	Nulliparous women				Multiparous women			
	No. of pregnancies	No. of births	Stillbirths of "unknown" cause		No. of pregnancies	No. of births	Stillbirths of "unknown" cause	
			No.	per 1000			No.	per 1000
28	15207	27	0	0	14778	31	1	0.07
29	15180	22	1	0.07	14713	34	2	0.14
30	15158	24	1	0.07	14747	52	5	0.34
31	15134	38	4	0.26	14661	62	8	0.55
32	15096	52	8	0.50	14599	59	8	0.55
33	15044	60	5	0.33	14540	81	3	0.21
34	14984	95	8	0.53	14459	145	6	0.42
35	14889	165	8	0.54	14314	171	8	0.56
36	14724	317	9	0.61	14143	326	8	0.57
37	14407	599	11	0.76	13817	632	6	0.43
38	13808	1259	16	1.16	13185	1280	8	0.61
39	12549	2532	10	0.80	11905	2590	6	0.50
40	10017	3793	8	0.80	9315	3733	14	1.50
41	6224	3200	8	1.29	5582	2970	4	0.72
42	3024	1943	8	2.66	2612	1587	3	1.15
43	1081	778	2	1.85	1025	628	4	3.90
44	303	217	0		397	243	3	
45	86	55	0		154	99	1	
46	31	19	0		55	46	2	
47	12	8	0	3.30	9	7	0	15.11
48	4	2	1		2	1	0	
49	2	1	0		1	1	0	
50	1	1	0					

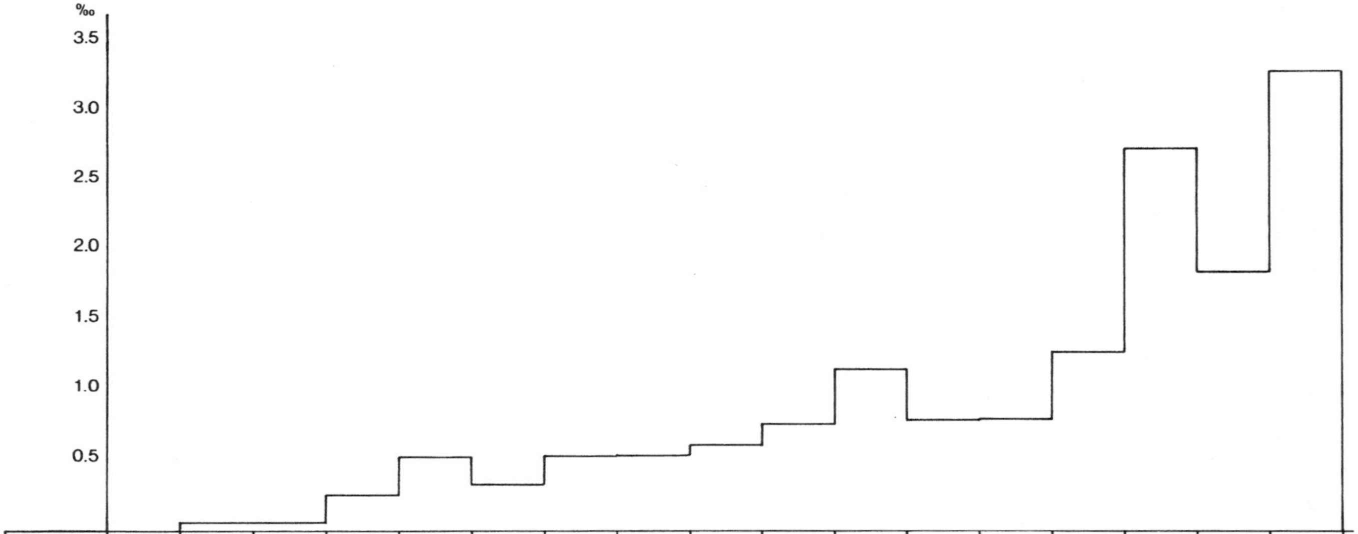

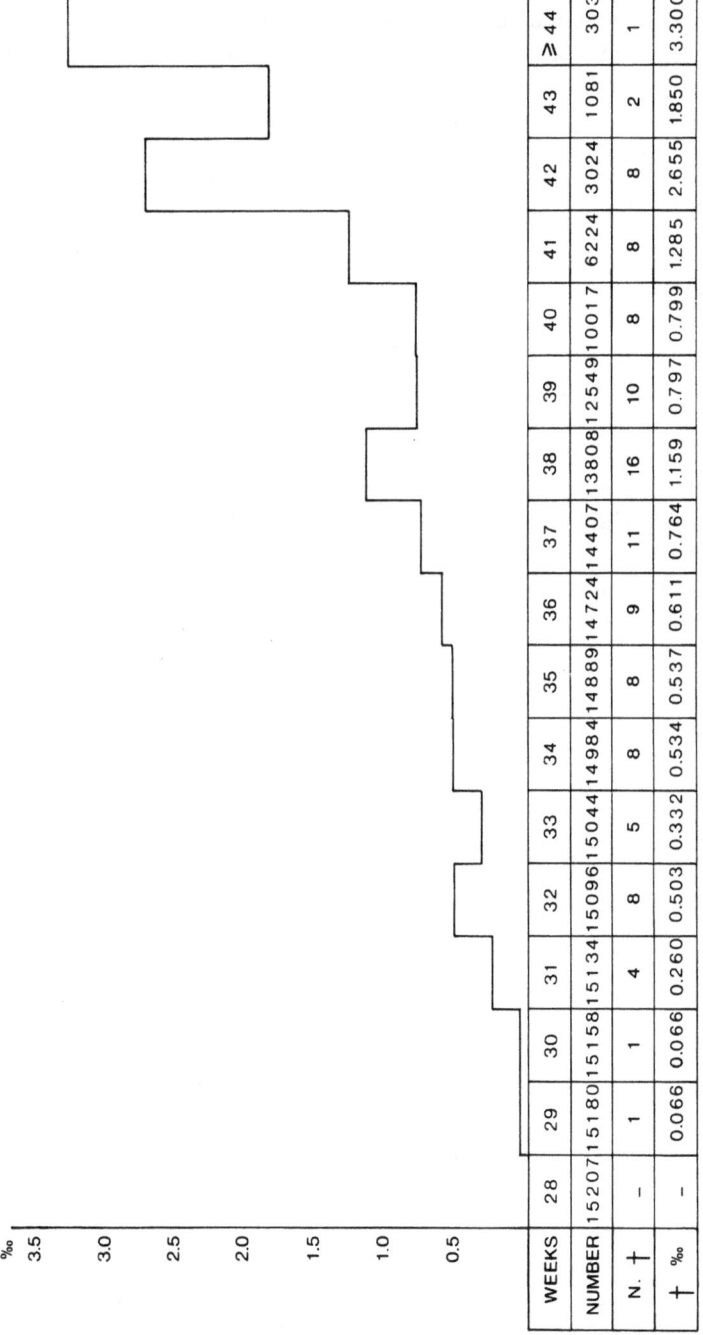

WEEKS	28	29	30	31	32	33	34	35	36	37	38	39	40	41	42	43	≥ 44
NUMBER	15207	15180	15158	15134	15096	15044	14984	14889	14724	14407	13808	12549	10017	6224	3024	1081	303
N. †	–	1	1	4	8	5	8	8	9	11	16	10	8	8	8	2	1
† ‰	–	0.066	0.066	0.260	0.503	0.332	0.534	0.537	0.611	0.764	1.159	0.797	0.799	1.285	2.655	1.850	3.300

Fig. 3. Incidence of stillbirth of 'unknown'' cause in relation to gestational age in 15 207 nulliparous women with single pregnancies. The stillbirth rate is based upon the number of stillbirths per 1000 pregnancies, whereas the number of pregnancies refers to pregnancies which proceed up to or beyond that particular week of gestation.

of labour in that period of gestation, one would have to interrupt 2500 pregnancies to save one child and loose several hundreds of children by "prematurity". In the period 32 to 35 weeks the stillbirth rate was 29 of 15 096 (1.9 per 1000). In the period 36 to 37 weeks the rate of unexpected intrauterine death was 20 of 14 724 (1.3 per 1000), in the period 38 to 39 weeks 26 of 13 808 (1.9 per 1000), at 40 to 41 weeks 16 of 10 017 (1.6 per 1000) and at 42 weeks or beyond 11 of 3 024 (3.6 per 1000). In figure 3 these data are shown in a histogram. From the histogram it is clear that the tendency towards intra-uterine death became higher with increasing duration of pregnancy. In reality this tendency has been even stronger than is shown in the histogram since after 42 completed weeks (>297 days of amenorrhoea) almost all primiparae have been hospitalized for treatment with bedrest, low salt diet and close observation. In almost 50 percent of these cases medical induction of labour has been tried every three days (without rupturing the membranes). On the other hand it is also obvious that even after 43 weeks of pregnancy only a small minority of all pregnancies are in real danger. In an absolute sense it is even true that more children die unexpectedly before birth in the 37th and 38th week (between 256 and 269 days of amenorrhoea) than after 42 weeks of gestation (fig. 4). In that figure we also gave data on the week in which the

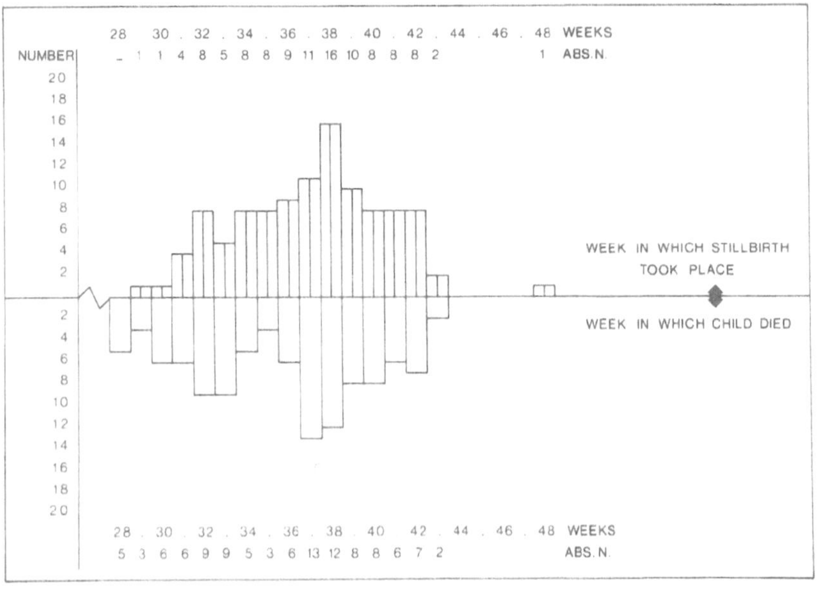

Fig. 4. Number of stillbirths of "unknown" cause at various weeks of gestation in nulliparous women (single pregnancies only; n=15,207; 1958-1976). Despite the stillbirth rate shown in figure 3 the highest number of deaths occurred at 37-38 weeks.

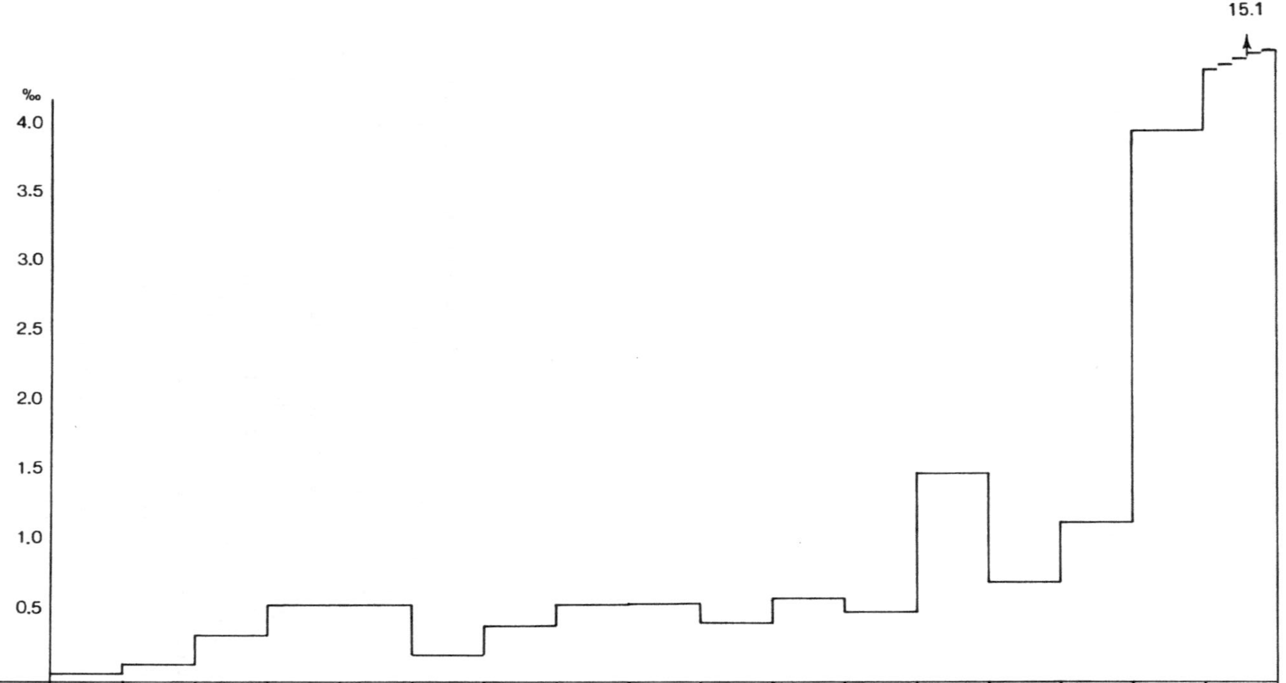

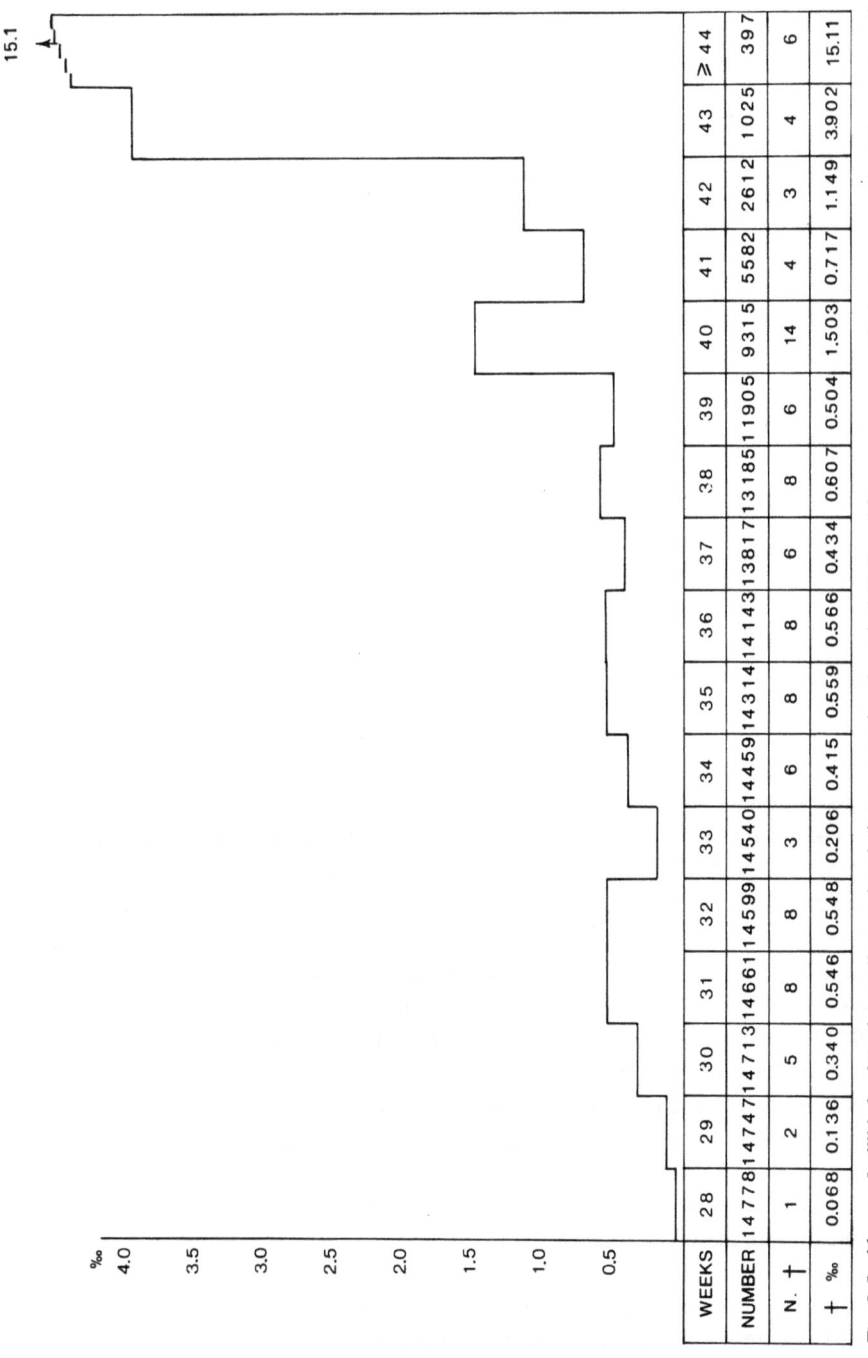

WEEKS	28	29	30	31	32	33	34	35	36	37	38	39	40	41	42	43	≥ 44
NUMBER	14778	14747	14713	14661	14599	14540	14459	14314	14143	13817	13185	11905	9315	5582	2612	1025	397
N. †	1	2	5	8	8	3	6	8	8	6	8	6	14	4	3	4	6
† ‰	0.068	0.136	0.340	0.546	0.548	0.206	0.415	0.559	0.566	0.434	0.607	0.504	1.503	0.717	1.149	3.902	15.11

Fig. 5. Incidence of stillbirth of "unknown" cause in relation to gestational age in 14 778 multiparous women with single pregnancies. The number of pregnancies refers to pregnancies which proceed up to or beyond that particular week of gestation.

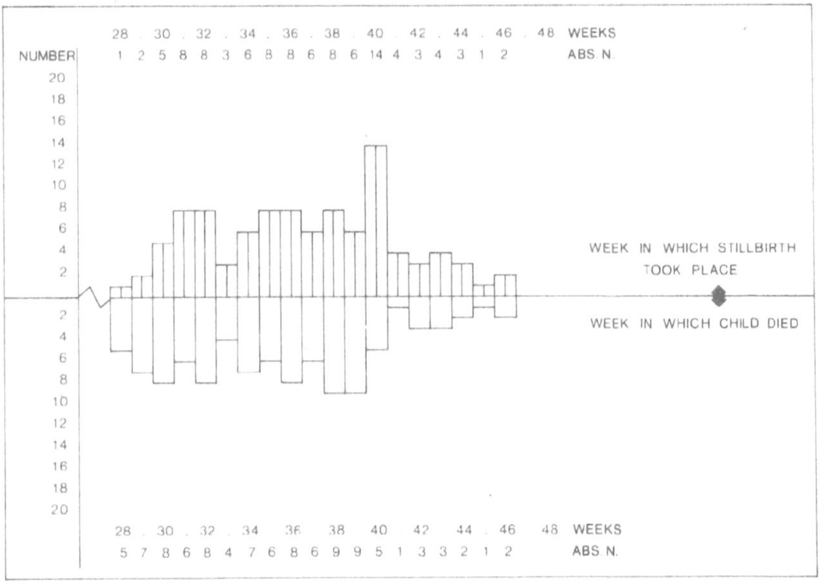

Fig. 6. Number of stillbirths of "unknown" cause at various weeks of gestation in multiparous women. As for fig. 4, the data apply to single pregnancies only (n=14,778; 1958-1976).

fetus probably died. Figure 3 and table 5 are based on the moment of birth as this is a reliable date, whereas the time of intra-uterine death sometimes was a supposition rather than an established fact.

The data on 14778 single pregnancies in multiparae, collected in the period from 1958 to 1976 in our department are given in table 5, figure 5 and figure 6. In general a study of the pregnancies in multiparous women leads to the same conclusions. Whereas the total number of fetal deaths by "cause unknown" in nulliparae was 108 out of 15 207 pregnancies (7.1 per 1000), in multiparae it was 100 out of 14 778 (6.8 per 1000). In the same way as in nulliparae the likelihood of intra-uterine death increases with the duration of pregnancy. The increase after 42 weeks in multiparae is even more obvious than in nulliparae. Here it becomes apparent however that our almost completely conservative attitude towards postmaturity in multiparae must be the explanation of this phenomenon. Our studies in 1955 and 1956 showed that postmaturity was a real danger for the fetus of a nulliparous woman. At that time the risk increased up to 112 per 1000 after 44 weeks in nulliparae (13, 14), whereas we could find no significant increase in the intra-uterine death rate and perinatal mortality in multiparae.

More intensive prenatal and natal care in the period after 1957 in nulliparae led to a striking reduction of fetal mortality after 42 weeks from 19.2 per 1000 to 2.8 per 1000. The mortality in multiparae from the same cause changed only from 11.1 per 1000 to 9.8 per 1000. So it remained virtually the same and is now higher than in primiparae. We are aware of this problem and, in the last 10 years, we are devoting more attention to multiparae who go beyond 42 weeks of amenorrhoea. Nevertheless we still think that it is superfluous to hospitalize every multipara who reached more than 294 or 297 days of amenorrhoea, whereas we do advocate this approach for nulliparous women.

If we compare figure 5 and figure 3, these histograms show that the relative risk of intra-uterine death by unknown (read: placental) cause in multiparae increases quite impressively and even more so than in nulliparae (fig. 3). The explanation for this rather unnatural phenomenon was discussed above. Without our close observations, treatment and interference, these histograms would have shown a much steeper rise in nulliparae than in multiparae. If we now compare figure 6 and figure 4, then we see that, in spite of the fact that our interference rate in postmature multiparae has been negligibly small, the majority of fetal mortality by unknown cause in both groups occurred before 40 weeks of pregnancy.

CONCLUSIONS

In concluding we should like to stress the fact that "statistical" postmaturity or rather post-term pregnancy (that is a pregnancy that goes more than 14 days beyond the expected date of delivery) is associated with a rise in fetal mortality from placental insufficiency. Knowledge of this fact must lead to an intensification of prenatal control, watchfulness and close observation.

Interruption of pregnancy in all women who go beyond a certain length of amenorrhoea is perhaps acceptable in nulliparae with reliable data about the probable moment of conception who go beyond 294 days of gestation. Even then we must realize that we do cause some harm to 4 women to benefit one at the utmost. If we extend this type of treatment to larger groups, for example to all women who go beyond the expected day of delivery, then we harm more than 300 women to benefit one. In addition, the greatest part of the problem would remain unsolved, for in our investigation the majority of intra-uterine deaths by "unknown" cause took place before 40 weeks' amenorrhoea (150 of 208, or 72 percent).

Postmaturity in the statistical sense of the word (post-term) is a warning sign of minor importance, if we compare it for example to the significance of the diastolic bloodpressure (fig. 7). It is true that the relative risk of fetal

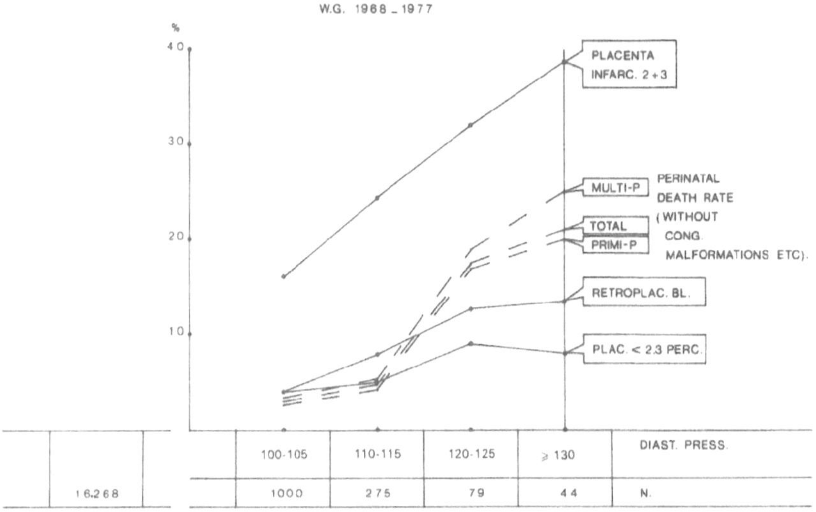

Fig. 7. Influence of diastolic blood pressure on various parameters at birth. The data are based upon 16 268 pregnancies at Wilhemina Gasthuis, University of Amsterdam from 1968 to 1977. Only these cases are illustrated in which the diastolic blood pressure, measured on at least two occasions, rose to or above 100 mm Hg (n = 1,398). The influence of diastolic blood pressure on the degree of placental infarction, perinatal mortality, the occurrence of retroplacental clots and placental weight is obvious.

death by placental insufficiency increases with the duration of pregnancy, but in a absolute sense this phenomenon (postmaturity in the clinical sense of the word) takes place more often before the pregnancy reaches 280 days of amenorrhoea than thereafter. Induction of labour only because a certain duration of pregnancy is reached is bad obstetrics. It confuses statistical postmaturity with clinical postmaturity. The solution will come from improvements in prenatal care that will enable us to diagnose impending clinical postmaturity. Then we will benefit the fetuses who are in danger without harming the healthy ones.

REFERENCES

1. Sontoul JH, Renaud M and Lecomte P: La contraception dans le monde en 1977. *Assises Nation Méd* 100, 75-95 (1978).
2. Kloosterman GJ: Overdragen zwangerschap. *Ned Tijdschr Verlosk Gynaecol* 55, 232-246 (1955).
3. Kloosterman GJ: Prolonged pregnancy. *Gynaecologia* 142, 373-388 (1956).
4. Ballantyne JW: *Manual of Antenatal Pathology and Hygiene.* Part I, The Foetus, Edinburgh, W. Green and Sons, 1902.
5. Wijsenbeek IA: Ongewoon langdurende zwangerschappen. *Geneesk Gids* 4, 709-716 (1926).
6. Runge H: Über einige besondere Merkmale der übertragenen Frucht. *Zbl Gynäkol* 66, 1202-1206 (1942).
7. Walker J: Foetal anoxia. *J Obstet Gynaecol Br Emp* 61, 162-180 (1954).
8. Clifford SH: Postmaturity – with placental dysfunction. *J Pediatr* 44, 1-13 (1954).
9. Hosemann H: Normale und abnormale Schwangerschaftsdauer, In: *Biologie und Pathologie des Weibes*, Bd VII, Berlin, Urban und Schwarzenberg, 1952 p 828-899.
10. Gruenwald P: Growth of the human fetus. *Am J Obstet Gynecol* 94, 1112-1119 (1966).
11. Kloosterman GJ: On intra-uterine growth. *Int J Gynaecol Obstet* 8, 895-912 (1970).
12. Kloosterman GJ: The Amsterdam growth curve. In: *De Voorplanting van de Mens*, Haarlem, Centen, 1977, p 81-83.
13. Kloosterman GJ: Post maturity. *Mémoires de l'Académie Royale de Médicine de Belgique*, Bruxelles, Imprimerie médicale et scientifique, 1967, p 175-190.
14. Kloosterman GJ: The obstetrician and dysmaturity. In: *Aspects of Praematurity.* Nutricia Symposium no 2, Jonxis JHP, Visser HKA and Troelstra JA (eds), Leiden, HE Stenfert Kroese, 1968, p 263-280.

INDEX OF SUBJECTS